CNS Infections

Juan Carlos García-Moncó
Editor

CNS Infections

A Clinical Approach

Springer

Editor
Juan Carlos García-Moncó, MD
Department of Neurology
Hospital de Galdakao-Usansolo
Galdakao
Vizcaya, Spain

ISBN 978-1-4471-7043-3 ISBN 978-1-4471-6401-2 (eBook)
DOI 10.1007/978-1-4471-6401-2
Springer London Heidelberg New York Dordrecht

Softcover reprint of the hardcover 1st edition 2014

Printed on acid-free paper

Springer is part of Springer Science+Business Media (www.springer.com)

To my wife Beatriz, and to my children Carlos, Pablo, and Sofia, for they all have been taken away many hours during the preparation of this book.

To Jorge Benach, once my mentor then my friend, for his continuous help and support.

To our patients, for they are a continuous source of inspiration.

Preface

This book was first envisioned in June 2012, during the annual meeting of the European Neurological Society held in Prague. Joanna Bolesworth, from Springer, kindly approached me to delve into my interest in editing a book on central nervous system (CNS) infections.

I soon became excited about the idea since neurologic infection has been the topic I have devoted the most time over the last two decades. Furthermore, it is a stimulating field with continuous advances in which specialists from Internal Medicine and Neurology often converge, a feature that makes the readership rather heterogeneous.

It was obvious, though, that we should provide an attractive material in a field where several good textbooks already exist. With this in mind, I prepared a table of contents that was primarily oriented to the practicing, busy physician who cares for patients with infections of the CNS, and who needs easily applicable management directives. Today, there are unparalleled opportunities to make substantial progress in managing infections. The genomes of all the important pathogens as well as the genome of man are known. Monitoring global gene expression or performing genome-wide mutagenesis is now routine in the study of many pathogens, and there is the real possibility that personalized medicine will be a reality. New bioinformatic tools, molecular structures, and imaging technologies are providing an unprecedented view of both pathogens and hosts in the infection process.

Although the wealth of information and new powerful technologies have transformed the management of infections, they have also presented the field with new challenges. To take full advantage of these changes, clinicians and laboratories must implement multidisciplinary approaches, which often require the incorporation of new technologies beyond the capabilities of an individual clinician. We have been mindful of this, and have asked each author to consider the latest advances that have an impact in the management of patients in each of their respective fields.

From the very beginning, a group of experts in the different areas were put together, all of them enthusiastically agreeing to participate. It is their collaboration what provides the added value to this book. In what seems almost a record of time (several months) we have been able to finish the work, which would have been impossible without the invaluable help of Michael Griffin, the project's development editor.

The book is divided into 15 chapters encompassing general aspects of CNS infection, specific etiologic agents, and particular conditions such as immunosuppression states and anatomic locations such as spinal cord infections.

The first chapter is devoted to the analysis and interpretation of the different CSF values, a crucial aspect in dealing with patients with suspected CNS infections. It is followed by an updated chapter on community-acquired bacterial meningitis, and by a difficult-to-find detailed chapter on meningitis and ventriculitis occurring after different surgical procedures and shunting devices for CSF drain.

Viral infections represent the commonest CNS infections, and are segregated into three chapters. The first of them covers the viral meningitis, a common, usually benign condition. The second chapter deals with acute viral encephalitis, focusing on the most common and severe sporadic encephalitis, herpes encephalitis; it also discusses other viruses as well as postinfectious conditions. The third chapter includes tropical viral infections, quite frequent in certain parts of the globe, and that require special consideration in a globalized world of continuous travelling.

Fungal infections involve not only immunosuppressed patients but also healthy individuals, and are detailed in a separate chapter.

Tuberculosis is a public health problem around the world, often posing a diagnostic and therapeutic challenge, particularly in the context of nervous system disease, and is separately discussed, with mention of other mycobacterial pathogens.

Likewise, parasitic CNS infections represent a clinical dilemma, mimicking other noninfectious disorders and requiring expertise to establish proper diagnosis and therapy.

Spinal cord infection is covered on a separate chapter. It involves different pathogens, but the particular anatomic location and clinical manifestations led us to reserve a specific section for this topic.

Human CNS trepanomatoses and borrelioses span the old neurosyphilis with the more recent Lyme disease and relapsing fever, and are thoroughly covered in two separate chapters.

Often neglected, drugs can result in meningitis, a condition that represents a challenge to the clinician suspecting a CNS infection, particularly if the drug involved is an antibiotic. A separate section covers this area.

Finally, the last two chapters are devoted to patients with immune suppression, be it by different medical conditions (i. e., hematological neoplasias) or by HIV infection, a condition whose prognosis and management has drastically changed over the years since the early 1980s. The vast variety of conditions that revolve around immunosuppressed patients clearly justify these two sections.

I believe that we have achieved our goals, and that we have come up with a practical material that covers most of the infectious conditions involving the CNS. Some of them are difficult to find in other sources, and I hope that this book will help clinicians manage their patients, which in the end is our real goal. If so, all the efforts will have been completely worthy.

Galdakao, Vizcaya, Spain Juan Carlos García-Moncó, MD

Contents

Contributors

Francisco Javier Carod-Artal, MD, PhD Health Sciences and Medicine Faculty, Universitat Internacional de Catalunya (UIC), Barcelona, Spain

Department of Neurology, Raigmore Hospital, Inverness, Highlands, UK

Mausumi Barthakur, MD Department of Clinical Neurophysiology, GNRC Hospitals, Guwahati, Assam, India

Adarsh Bhimraj, MD Section of Neurologic Infectious Diseases, Department of Infectious Diseases, Cleveland Clinic Foundation, Cleveland, OH, USA

Iñigo Corral, MD, PhD Department of Neurology, Ramón y Cajal Hospital, Madrid, Spain

Oscar H. Del Brutto, MD School of Medicine, Universidad Espiritu Santo – Ecuador, Guayaquil, Ecuador

Maurizio Del Poeta, MD Department of Molecular Genetics and Microbiology, Stony Brook University, Stony Brook, NY, USA

Pere Domingo, MD, PhD Infectious Diseases, Hospital de la Santa Creu I Sant Pau, Barcelona, Spain

Juan Carlos García-Moncó, MD Department of Neurology, Hospital de Galdakao-Usansolo, Galdakao, Vizcaya, Spain

Marian Gomez-Beldarrain, MD Department of Neurology, Hospital de Galdakao-Usansolo, Galdakao, Vizcaya, Spain

John J. Halperin, MD Department of Neurosciences, Overlook Medical Center, Summit, NJ, USA

Sanjeev K. Handique, MD Department of Radiology, GNRC Hospitals, Guwahati, Assam, India

José Luis Sánchez-Menoyo, MD Department of Neurology, Hospital de Galdakao-Usansolo, Galdakao, Bizkaia, Spain

Germán Morís, MD Department of Neurology, Hospital Universitario Central de Asturias, Oviedo, Asturias, Spain

Mansa Amul Munshi, MS Microbiology Department of Molecular Genetics and Microbiology, Stony Brook University, Stony Brook, NY, USA

Javier Ruiz-Ojeda, MD Department of Neurology, Hospital de Galdakao-Usansolo, Galdakao, Bizkaia, Spain

Virginia Pomar, MD Infectious Diseases Unit, Hospital de la Santa Creu I Sant Pau, Barcelona, Spain

Amy A. Pruitt, MD Department of Neurology, University of Pennsylvania, Perelman School of Medicine, Philadelphia, PA, USA

Carmen Quereda, MD, PhD Department of Infectious Diseases, Ramóny Cajal Hospital, Madrid, Spain

Antonella Rella, PhD Microbiology Department of Molecular Genetics and Microbiology, Stony Brook University, Stony Brook, NY, USA

Aida Rodriguez-Sainz, MD Department of Neurology, Hospital de Galdakao-Usansolo, Galdakao, Vizcaya, Spain

Juan C. Salazar, MD, MPH Department of Pediatrics, Connecticut Children's Medical Center, Hartford, CT, USA

Chapter 1
Lumbar Puncture and CSF Analysis and Interpretation

Marian Gomez-Beldarrain and Juan Carlos García-Moncó

Abstract Cerebrospinal fluid (CSF) analysis is essential in the diagnosis of the infectious diseases of the central nervous system. It is also helpful in the differential diagnosis of other conditions that simulate infectious disorders and in monitoring the effects of antibiotic therapy.

The CSF is formed by the choroid plexuses of the ventricles. Its volume in adults is 150 ml. Most of the CSF is reabsorbed by the arachnoid granulations, located along the superior sagittal sinus toward the venous system. The main CSF function is mechanical, protecting the brain from acute or sudden changes in pressure.

The lumbar puncture (LP) to obtain CSF is not without risks, and the complications, such as brain herniation, spinal hematoma, and iatrogenic CNS infection, which, although rare, can be serious. Nevertheless, LP remains the gold standard procedure for the diagnosis of CNS infections. The LP should be performed in aseptic conditions with the patient assuming a lateral recumbent position. Local anesthesia at the needle insertion point makes the procedure easier. Using atraumatic needle is associated with less post-puncture headache, which is the commonest complication.

The normal CSF appears sparkling clear; any change in this characteristic is pathologic. The normal total CSF leukocyte counts are $<5/mm^3$ in adults, the normal glucose level is between 45 and 80 mg/dl, and the normal total protein is between 15 and 50 mg/dl. An increased intrathecal synthesis of immunoglobulins indicates a chronic infection of the CSF. Microbiological analysis of the CSF includes stains; aerobic and anaerobic cultures for bacteria, fungi, virus, and tuberculosis; serologic testing; and viral and bacterial screen by PCR.

M. Gomez-Beldarrain
Department of Neurology, Hospital de Galdakao-Usansolo, Galdakao, Vizcaya, Spain

J.C. García-Moncó, MD (✉)
Department of Neurology, Hospital de Galdakao-Usansolo,
Barrio Labeaga S/N, Galdakao, Vizcaya 48960, Spain
e-mail: hospit05@sarenet.es

J.C. García-Moncó (ed.), *CNS Infections*,
DOI 10.1007/978-1-4471-6401-2_1,

Keywords Cerebrospinal fluid • Physiology • Composition • Function • Lumbar puncture • Indications • Contraindications • Complications • Technique • Diagnosis • CNS infections

Introduction

The analysis of the cerebrospinal fluid (CSF) is essential in the diagnosis of the infectious diseases of the central nervous system (CNS). To this end, it is necessary to become familiar with the normal composition of the CSF as well as with the different CSF profiles that may indicate not only the location of infection (encephalitis vs. meningitis) but also the organism implicated.

The analysis of the CSF is also helpful in the differential diagnosis of other conditions that simulate an infection, such as inflammatory processes, subarachnoid hemorrhage, or cancer. CSF analysis is irreplaceable in the diagnosis and monitoring of the effects of antibiotic therapy.

The term meningitis refers to an infection limited to the subarachnoid space. When the infection crosses the pial cell lining and spreads through the perivascular spaces of Virchow-Robin to the brain parenchyma, the term meningoencephalitis is used [1, 2].

Anatomy and Physiology of the CSF

The CSF occupies the ventricles and subarachnoid spaces. The subarachnoid space separates the arachnoid membrane from the pia mater, and this space also contains vessels that enter or leave the CNS. The CSF is mainly formed by the choroid plexuses of the lateral, III, and IV ventricles, at a rate of production of 0.35 mL/min or about 500 mL/day. The total volume of the CSF in adults is 150 ml and is renewed four to five times daily. Infants and children have lower amounts, ranging from 30 to 60 ml in the neonate to 100 in adolescents. The CSF also comes from the water produced by oxidative metabolism and from an ultrafiltrate through the blood-brain barrier of the cerebral capillaries [2]. At both sites, the choroid plexuses and cerebral capillaries, the Na+/K+-ATPase pump creates an osmotic gradient that pulls water from the blood. The blood-brain barrier (BBB) includes the apical surface of the choroid plexuses, the cerebral endothelial cells, and the arachnoid. At each side of the BBB, high-resistance junctions between cells restrict the transport of substances between brain and the outer space. While lipid-soluble molecules (i.e., some drugs) readily diffuse across the choroid plexuses to gain access to the CSF, ionically charged molecules require active transport systems [1].

The CSF circulates downward from the point of production in the lateral ventricles following a descending pressure gradient. It exits the ventricles through the foramina of Monro to the III ventricle and through the median foramen of Magendie and the lateral foramina of Luschka to the IV ventricle, perimedullary space, and ambiens cisterna. After exiting the foramina of the IV ventricle, the CSF enters the subarachnoid space, and from there it flows downward around the spinal cord and to the lateral and superior surface of the brain toward the superior sagittal sinus, where it is reabsorbed.

Some of the CSF is reabsorbed by the ependyma lining the lateral ventricles, but most is reabsorbed by the arachnoid granulations toward the venous system. Granulations are more common on the superior surface of the brain hemispheres, and when large are known as Pacchionian granulations, located along the superior sagittal sinus. They are also present in the basal cisterns and along the spinal roots. At the spinal level, drainage takes place at the root sleeves, where the pia and arachnoid fuse with the connective tissue of the spinal nerves. Arachnoid granulations protrude through the dura into the superior sagittal sinus and act as one-way valves. As CSF pressure increases, more fluid is absorbed. When CSF pressure falls below a threshold value, the absorption of CSF ceases so that CSF pressure remains constant [3].

Cells and CSF are transported across the arachnoid villi within vesicles, which may become obstructed by bacteria during meningitis or by red blood cells during bleeding, thus resulting in hydrocephalus.

The main CSF function is mechanical, protecting the brain from acute or sudden changes in pressure. The CSF provides a flotation layer around the brain and spinal cord that protects them from trauma. Since there is no lymphatic system in the CNS, the CSF permits the degradation of cerebral metabolism products such as CO_2, lactate, and hydrogen. The CSF aids in regulating the pH and electrolyte balance of the extracellular space of the CNS and permits the circulation of electrolytes, neurotransmitters, hormones, antibodies, etc. [4].

Other CSF functions include getting rid of metabolic by-products linked to the biological activity of the CNS. Recent work demonstrates that sleep contributes to this function, since tracer molecules injected into the CSF of mice are cleared twice as fast when the mice are sleeping or anesthetized as compared to their awakened state [5].

The mechanisms whereby microorganisms cross the blood-brain barrier to gain access to the CNS are incompletely understood but involve the attachment of specific bacterial surface components to endothelial cells.

When an organism invades the CNS, an inflammatory response is initiated in the meninges and there is a secondary release of cytokines and chemokines. Cytokines, including tumor necrosis factor-α and interkleukin-6 are elevated in the CSF of patients with bacterial meningitis and contribute to secondary tissue damage. In a similar manner, proteases and free radicals attack brain capillaries, the components of the blood-brain barrier.

In bacterial meningitis, matrix metalloproteinases (MMPs) increase considerably and contribute to the severity of the infection. Steroids and some antibiotics (e.g., doxycycline) suppress the expression of MMPs and have a beneficial effect in reducing inflammation and thus the course of the meningeal infection. Pneumococcal meningitis is associated with significantly higher CSF concentrations of IFN-γ and of MMPs 9, and is associated with a higher case fatality rate than meningitis caused by *N. meningitidis* or *H. influenzae* [6].

Cerebrospinal Fluid Examination: The Lumbar Puncture

The LP to obtain CSF is not without risks and requires knowledge of the indications and contraindications, the pertinent anatomy, and the methods to minimize the risk of complications which, although rare, can be serious [7]. LP remains the gold standard procedure for CNS infections. Other indications are detailed on Table 1.1.

Lumbar Puncture Technique

A video describing the procedure is available on reference [7].

It should be performed in aseptic conditions to avoid iatrogenic infection of the subarachnoid space from the patient's skin flora or from the operator's oropharynx flora. Wearing sterile gloves is required, and wearing a chirurgical mask is optimal.

The patient should assume a lateral recumbent position, with the head, spine, and extremities flexed, adopting a fetal position, so that the distance between the dorsal processes and lamina of adjacent vertebrae increases, making it easier to insert the needle. The recumbent position allows proper CSF opening pressure evaluation, unlike the sitting position that makes pressure measurement unreliable, although allows a better identification of the spinous processes (Fig. 1.1). The lumbar spine should be perpendicular to the table with the patient in the sitting position and parallel to the table with the patient in the lateral recumbent position.

The lower lumbar area should be cleaned with povidone-iodine, chlorhexidine, or 70 % alcohol applied in widening concentric circles, and a sterile drape should be applied. Local anesthesia with 1 % lidocaine at the insertion point facilitates the patient's relaxation and makes the procedure easier and painless.

The needle should be in the vertebral interspace between L3 and L4 or L4 and L5, because these points are below the termination of the spinal cord (usually at L2 level in adults, lower in children). As a reference, the line between the superior aspects of the iliac crests intersects the midline at the L4 spinous process.

Small caliber (20 or 22 gauge) needles are preferred, since they are associated with less post-puncture headache. For the same reason, the American Academy of Neurology endorses the use of atraumatic needles (22-G Sprotte) instead of the more commonly used cutting needle (20-G Quincke) [8].

The needle should be inserted with the bevel parallel to the long axis of the spine, thus separating the fibers of the dura without transecting them and reducing the leakage of the CSF. The needle should be directed cephalad to parallel the slant of

Table 1.1 Indications, contraindications, and complications of lumbar puncture

Indications	Contraindications	Complications
Diagnosis of CNS infection	Lumbar skin infection	Transtentorial brain herniation
Antibiotic therapy monitoring	Severe bleeding disorders	Headache and post-puncture syndrome
Subarachnoid bleeding diagnosis	Cervical cord lesions	Back pain
Diagnosis of neoplastic CNS invasion	Increased intracranial pressure other than pseudotumor cerebri	Spinal bleeding
Pseudotumor cerebri diagnosis (pressure measurement)		Cranial nerve palsies
Inflammatory or demyelinating CNS diseases (protein evaluation)		Iatrogenic infection
Intrathecal chemotherapy administration or anesthesia		

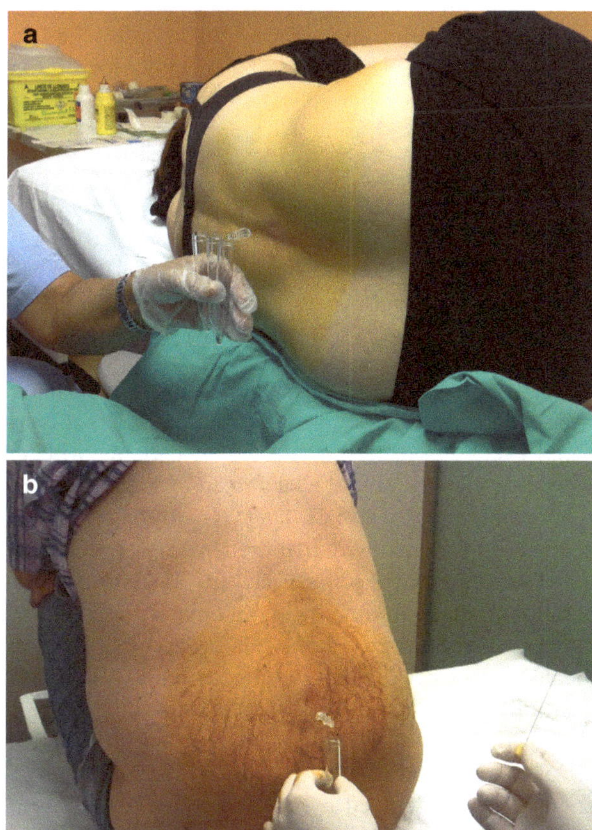

Fig. 1.1 Lateral recumbent (**a**) and sitting positioning (**b**) for lumbar puncture

the dorsal spine of the vertebrae. When the needle enters the subarachnoid space from the dura, a slight "pop" is felt. Sometimes the needle comes up against bone (usually spinous processes or lamina of the vertebrae); in that case, it should be retired and reintroduced following a nearby trajectory. To arrive into the subarachnoid space, the needle goes through the skin, subcutaneous fat, supraspinosus ligament, interspinosus ligament, yellow ligament, epidural fat, dura mater, and finally the arachnoid. Occasionally, the CSF flow stops due to (a) displacement of the tip of the needle or incomplete penetration, (b) a nerve root has fallen over the level of the needle, and (c) a blood clot is deposited in the needle lumen [9].

For diagnostic purposes, approximately 10–15 ml of CSF should be withdrawn from adults and 3–5 ml in neonates or children. For the diagnosis of a CNS infection, it is recommended to obtain three or four tubes to be sent for biochemical, microbiological, and pathologic examination.

The first obtained tube should contain at least 2 ml (40 drops) and should be sent to the biochemical laboratory. Simultaneous blood glucose levels should be measured. The second tube should be sent to the microbiological laboratory; if an uncommon infection is suspected, this tube should contain a great volume of CSF (10 ml) and often will require additional samples in different days. The last tube should go to the pathology laboratory for cellular analysis and must be processed straightaway as cells are degraded quickly after the LP.

Currently, the development of a checklist for LP to avoid unnecessary risks and make the technique safer is being validated [10].

Lumbar Puncture Contraindications (Table 1.1)

LP should be avoided in patients with evidence of brain herniation or increased intracranial pressure, with progressive headache, or with suspicion of a mass lesion of the CNS. In those cases, CSF removal may result in pressure changes that will displace downward the cerebellar amygdala with the ensuing brain herniation, coma, and death. Although brain herniation as a consequence of LP is a greatly feared event, its occurrence, even in patients with papilledema and intracranial hypertension, is quite low. The quoted incidence of herniation in patients with acute bacterial meningitis is 5 % [11]. Neuroimaging before LP is commonly recommended in patients with papilledema, suspected intracranial hypertension and depressed level of consciousness [12]. It should be remembered that antimicrobial therapy should be initiated without delay if meningitis is suspected.

Coagulopathies represent a relative contraindication for an LP and can be complicated by spinal bleeding (subarachnoid, subdural, or epidural) at the point of insertion. When platelet count is <50,000/μl, many experts recommend platelet transfusion.

Anticoagulation should be reversed before LP, and administration of anticoagulants should be delayed by at least 1 h after LP. With heparin therapy protamine should be administrated, and if the patient is on warfarin, frozen plasma and vitamin K should be injected before the LP to minimize the bleeding risk [13].

Relative contraindications are also the presence of a cervical cord lesion, where CSF removal could result in cord shifting against the lesion with quadriplegia, and skin infection of the lumbar area.

Lumbar Puncture Complications

The most frequent complications after an LP are post-LP headache and a post-LP low CSF volume syndrome, bleeding on the point of puncture, cranial nerve palsies (the commonest is the cranial nerve VI), and back and radicular pain. Other, less frequent complications are the transtentorial or transforaminal herniation of the brain and iatrogenic infection.

Post-LP Headache

It occurs in one-fourth of patients, lasts between 2 and 8 days, and is likely due to a persistent CSF leakage through the dural puncture site that exceeds the rate of CSF production and leads to CSF hypotension. This causes the brain to sink down with traction on pain-sensitive structures such as the dura, cranial and upper cervical nerves, and bridging veins [14].

The incidence of post-LP headache seems higher in women; in patients with low body mass indices; in young adults, particularly those between 18 and 30 years; and in individuals with chronic or recurrent headache. While the reasons are unclear, it seems that the increased incidence in young adults may relate to a more elastic dura that prevents the hole from sealing quickly. Patients with purulent meningitis are at less risk of developing a post-LP headache, probably because the inflammatory reaction seals the dura mater hole, thus preventing the leaking of CSF. Headaches are typically bilateral and their cardinal feature is that they are positional: they occur in the upright position and are relieved by recumbence. They are generally severe enough to incapacitate the patient, often throbbing, worsened by coughing, and associated to nausea and tinnitus [15].

The incidence of post-LP headache is decreased by using small-bore needles (20 or 22 gauge), performing only one puncture, and by placing the bevel of the needle parallel to the long axis of the spine [16].

Most headaches resolve spontaneously in 1 week. Bed rest, forced hydration, caffeine, and nonsteroidal anti-inflammatory agents are used but are of questionable benefit [17]. When all these measures fail, a blood patch may be in order. It consists of an epidural injection of 15–20 mL of autologous blood at the puncture site. Presumably this maneuver produces an inflammatory reaction that seals the dural wound [18].

In some cases in addition to the post-LP headache, a low CSF volume syndrome is present; patients experience vertigo, tinnitus, nausea, and vomiting. The symptoms occur because of a loss of flotation, allowing the cerebrum to descend onto the brain stem. Traction on the cortical veins occurs, and rupture of stretched bridging veins can lead to a subdural hematoma or subarachnoid hemorrhage [19]. An MRI or CT scan would be necessary to diagnose this complication and occasionally surgery is required.

Brain MRI often reveals meningeal enhancement in these patients. The reason for this is unclear [20].

Infection After Lumbar Puncture

Streptococcus viridans are the most common cause of LP-related meningitis, particularly S. *salivarius*. Less common organisms include *Staphylococcus* species, *Pseudomonas* species, and *E. coli* [14]. Meningitis after a diagnostic LP is very rare, with an estimated frequency of 1/20.000 after spinal anesthesia [21]. The possible causes of post-LP bacterial meningitis include contamination of the instruments or the field by the oropharyngeal flora of the operator (clusters of meningitis have been associated with the same operator) [22], incomplete disinfection of the skin, contaminated instruments, or contamination of injected material in the case of spinal anesthesia. The latter possibility seems less likely in current medical practice with the use of commercially prepared trays and single-use vials; nevertheless, an outbreak of neutrophilic fungal meningitis has been reported recently after injection of intra-articular contaminated methylprednisolone [23].

Cranial Nerve Palsies

They occur as a consequence of low CSF pressure and traction on the cranial nerves. Diplopia due to sixth nerve palsy, decreased hearing, tinnitus, and a plugged or blocked sensation in the ears are the most frequent complaints [24].

Local Bleeding

After a so-called bloody tap, epidural, subdural, or subarachnoid bleeding at the point of puncture may occur [25]. A spinal hematoma may produce progressive radicular pain and represent a neurosurgical emergency. Figure 1.2 shows a patient without coagulation disorders or any other predisposing factors that developed a spinal cord hematoma following a diagnostic LP.

Back Pain

Back pain is due to local trauma and occurs in up to 35 % of patients. Rarely, the needle is inserted too far anteriorly and punctures the annulus fibrosis, resulting in disk herniation.

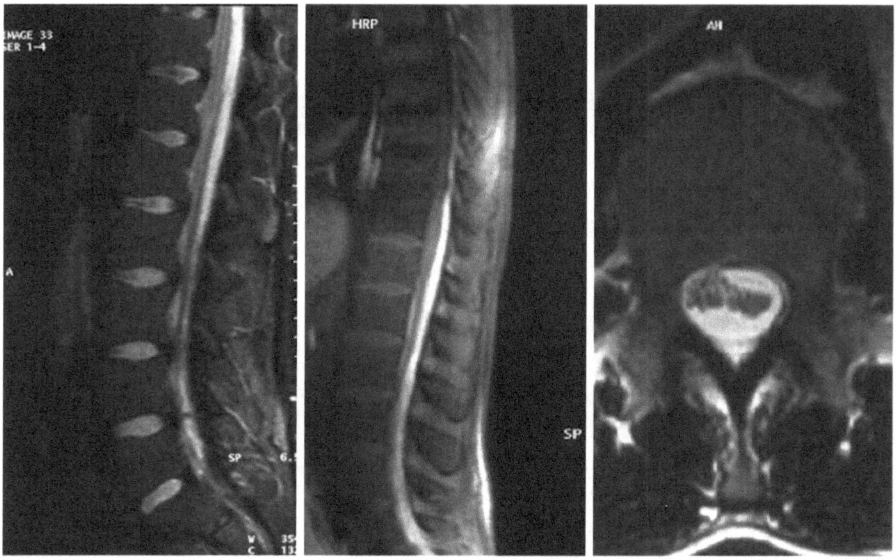

Fig. 1.2 Sagittal T1- (*left panel*) and T2-weighted MRI (*middle panel*) showing a hematoma extending from T10 to S2 vertebral bodies, most prominent at L1–L3 level, and displacing laterally the lumbosacral roots and the conus medullaris (*right panel*, axial view)

Spinal Epidural CSF Collection

Extensive dissection of CSF in the epidural space can occur after puncture of the dura from extravasation from the thecal sac and may spontaneously resolve in a few days [26].

Characteristic and Composition of the CSF

Pressure

CSF pressure is measured in recumbent position by attaching a manometer to the needle inserted into the subarachnoid space. The normal CSF pressure in adults is 80–180 mm of water and up to 250 mm of water for obese individuals. If the patient is seated, the pressure may increase to 300 mm of water. Children's normal pressure is 10–100 mm of water.

Disposable manometers measuring the CSF pressure in cm of water are available. Normal values in adult are between 7 and 20 cm.

With the needle properly placed in the subarachnoid space, the CSF pressure fluctuates with breath and pulse. Applying pressure on the cervical veins should increase the CSF pressure up to 200 mm of water (Queckenstedt's maneuver). A lack of pressure increase indicates a block in the CSF circulation. Low CSF pressure may occur with dehydration or in the presence of a CSF fistula [1].

Components of the CSF

The CSF contains ions, oxygen, sugars (glucose, fructose), lactate, proteins (albumin and globulins), amino acids, urea, ammonia, creatinine, lipids, neurotransmitters and its metabolites, hormones (insulin, gastrin), and vitamins. The regulation of these components is not known, but some of these substances are transported into the CSF by active diffusion and by a proteolytic transporter [3].

Macroscopic Appearance of the CSF

The normal CSF appears sparkling clear; any change in this characteristic is pathologic. The color may vary from red (erythrochromia) when there are >1,000 red blood cells per mm^3, to yellow (xanthochromia) if there is >150 mg/100 ml of proteins, and to cloudy if there is an increased number of white blood cells, usually >300 polynuclear cells per mm^3, or >500 lymphocytes per mm^3.

A traumatic tap is frequent and misleads the results of CSF analysis and is difficult to distinguish from a true hemorrhage. Comparing the redness of three subsequent CSF tubes (the three-tube test) may be helpful, since blood from a traumatic tap tends to clear in successive tubes. In contrast, in hemorrhages prior to the tap, blood mixes freely with the CSF and all the tubes display the same color.

When white blood cells (WBC) are present in the CSF of a traumatic tap, it must be decided whether these cells were introduced in the subarachnoid space by the spinal tap or they represent a real pleocytosis in a patient with meningitis. In an individual with a normal blood formula, 1 WBC per mm^3 for every 700 red blood cell (RBC) per mm^3 is subtracted. As an example, having 20 leucocytes with 14,000 RBCs in the CSF is considered normal and not an indication of meningitis.

Microbiological analysis of a bloody tap is unreliable, and therefore it is advisable to repeat the LP at a superior vertebral interspace or 48 h later. If the patient has significant anemia or leukocytosis, the following formula should be employed to accurately determine the true number of leucocytes in the CSF: CSF WBC = blood WBC × CSF RBC/blood RBC. To complicate the clinical decision, the presence of blood in the subarachnoid space produces a secondary inflammatory response that leads to a disproportionate increase in the number of WBCs, particularly 48 h after onset [13].

Microscopic Composition of the CSF

Cells

The normal total CSF leukocyte counts are <20/mm^3 for preterm infants, <15/mm^3 at 4–8 weeks, and no more than 5/mm^3 in older infants and adults. While cells in the CSF of adults are monocytic, polynuclears predominate (60 %) in newborns.

Table 1.2 Normal CSF values and tests for diagnosis

Test	Normal value
Cells	0–5 cells/μl (lymphocytes)
Glucose	40 mg/dl
	60 % of serum glucose
Proteins	
Lumbar	15–45 mg/dl
Cisternal	10–25 mg/dl
Ventricular	6–15 mg/dl
Gamma globulins	6–13 % of total CSF proteins
IgG	<8,4 mg/dl
IgM	37–374 ng/ml
IgG index	<0.77
Oligoclonal bands	0–1

Normal CSF does not contain polynuclears, eosinophils, plasma cells, or red blood cells, but may contain ependymal cells [4].

The normal total protein level of CSF ranges between 15 and 50 mg/dl.

Protein values are lower in the ventricles and cisterns than in the lumbar space.

Proteins

An elevated protein level is a nonspecific finding reflecting a pathologic increase in blood-brain barrier permeability, which occurs in many inflammatory, infectious, or neoplastic diseases, or with CSF blocks.

In acute bacterial meningitis, there is a brisk inflammatory response with protein level increasing up to 100–500 mg/dl. Proteins are moderately elevated in viral meningitis, usually <100 mg/dl (Table 1.2). To correct the CSF protein value in the presence of blood (bloody tap) subtract 1 mg for every 1,000 RBC; thus, if the red cell count on a CSF sample is 20.000 per mm^3 and the total protein is 120 mg/dl, the corrected protein level would be 100 mg per dl.

Although many proteins could be measured in the CSF, only an increase in immunoglobulins bears diagnostic importance. Such an increase is indicative of an infectious or inflammatory CNS disorder. Most CSF immunoglobulins derive from plasma, and only a small fraction is synthesized intrathecally. Their CSF concentration is <40 mg/L.

Immunoglobulin increase in CSF may be due to an increase in plasma, a blood-brain barrier impairment, or because an increase in intrathecal synthesis, which is the case of a chronic infection of the CNS. The integrity of the blood-brain barrier permeability is confirmed by a normal albumin index.

To verify if high immunoglobulin values correspond to intrathecal synthesis or they correspond to a blood-brain barrier leakage, the CSF IgG index is calculated. The normal CSF IgG index value is 0.65 and is calculated by the formula IgG (CSF) × albumin (serum)/IgG (serum) × albumin (CSF).

Isoelectric focusing allows the detection of CSF oligoclonal bands. The presence of ≥2 oligoclonal bands in the CSF that are absent in serum suggests intrathecal IgG synthesis. They are present in inflammatory CNS disorders, i.e., multiple sclerosis and in chronic infections.

Glucose

Glucose CSF concentration depends on serum glucose level, the carrier system that transfers glucose between blood and CSF, and the rate of glucose metabolism by the various cellular elements of the CSF. Normal CSF concentration is between 45 and 80 mg/dl, approximately 60 % of the serum glucose level [27]. Values <40 mg/dl are always pathological, regardless of serum values. Hypoglycorrhachia may be caused by bacterial, fungal, or tuberculous meningitis and less often by viral infections, particularly mumps [28], and is the result of glycolysis of the CSF white cells and the pathogen and impaired glucose transport. Noninfectious conditions, such as carcinomatous meningitis, subarachnoid hemorrhage, and hypoglycemia, also result in low glucose levels.

An isolated low glucose level in the CSF (i.e., normal cell count, proteins, and lactate) is highly suggestive of a genetic metabolic disorder known as a glucose transporter type 1 deficiency syndrome (GLUT1DS), in which glucose transport into the brain is disturbed [29]. It can be associated with epilepsy and movement disorders and requires specific diets.

A serum glucose determination should be obtained at the time of LP. Normal CSF values are summarized in Table 1.2.

Identification of Infectious Agents in the Cerebrospinal Fluid (Table 1.3)

Microbiological CSF analysis includes stains, aerobic and anaerobic cultures, serologic testing, nucleic acid amplification by polymerase chain reaction (PCR), bacterial antigen detection, and cryptococcal surface antigen detection [4, 9].

The use of PCR has revolutionized the diagnosis of CNS infection and allows for a demonstration of certain organisms regardless of prior antibiotic therapy.

PCR amplifies by at least one million-fold the abundance of defined microorganism nucleic acid present in the specimen. Its sensitivity and specificity for a specific organism are critical in correctly integrating the results. Negative results do not fully exclude infection and often depend on the timing of the spinal tap, as well as on the presence of bloody CSF [30].

Flow cytometry examination of the CSF represents a quantitative assay that identifies small cell populations with aberrant phenotypes and separates a few neoplastic cells within a population of normal lymphocytes. This technique may be useful for distinguishing between neoplastic and infectious meningitis [31].

Table 1.3 CSF findings in meningitis

	Pressure	Leukocytes (per μl)	Proteins (mg/dl)	Glucose (mg/dl)
Acute bacterial	Increased	>100 (mostly PMNs)	Increased (100–500)	Decreased (<40 or <60 % of serum value)
Viral	Normal to moderately increased	Five to few hundreds (lymphocytes; PMNs may predominate initially)	Mild increase (<100)	Normal Reduced in 25 % of cases of mumps and herpes simplex virus infection
Fungal	Increased (particularly with Cryptococcus)	0–800; mostly lymphocytes, rarely PMNs	Increased (20–500)	Decreased in most cases
Parasitic	Usually elevated. Low if dynamic block[a]	Increased mononuclear and PMNs with eosinophilia in 50 % of cases	Increased (50–200)	Decreased in 20 % of cases
Tumor	Normal or elevated	None to hundreds of mononuclear and malignant cells	Increased	Decreased in 75 % cases of carcinomatous meningitis
Tuberculous	Usually elevated may be low if dynamic block of CSF[a]	Rarely >500, mostly lymphocytes but PMNs the first days	Increased, 100–200 Much higher if dynamic block of CSF	Decreased in 75 % of cases

PMNs: polymorphonuclear cells
[a]Block: Due to inflammatory response in basal meninges, the CSF does not circulate properly and the pressure at lumbar levels is low.

CSF Profile in the Commonest Meningitis (Table 1.3)

Bacterial Meningitis

Classical CSF abnormalities include an increased opening pressure, the presence of polymorphonuclear pleocytosis (>100–500 WBCs/mm^3 in 90 % of patients), decreased glucose (<40 mg/dl), and increased proteins (>45 mg/dl in 90 % of patients).

Prior therapy with oral antibiotics will not alter the cell count or glucose concentration, but will decrease the likelihood of identifying the organism. Gram staining identifies the pathogen in 60–90 % of patients and relies on the CSF concentration of bacteria.

The commonest organisms of community-acquired meningitis may be detected by latex particle agglutination in the CSF, and their availability should be consulted with the laboratory. If the infecting organism is sensitive to the antibiotic prescribed, Gram and cultures should be negative in 24 h. CSF glucose concentration returns to normal in 3 days [9].

Viral Meningitis

With viral infections opening pressure is usually normal, and there is a lymphocytic pleocytosis with normal glucose concentration and normal to moderately increased proteins.

Enteroviruses (coxsackieviruses, echoviruses, and entoviruses 68–71) are the most common, followed by herpesviruses, human immunodeficiency virus, and arthropod-borne viruses.

Distinguishing between bacterial and viral meningitis may be difficult, particularly in patients with CSF abnormalities classic for bacterial meningitis but in whom the CSF Gram stain and culture are negative.

CSF lactate levels are nonspecific and can be elevated in both conditions. Increased serum procalcitonin levels is more consistent with bacterial meningitis but has not been universally adopted.

Fungal Meningitis

Fungal infections usually show normal or slightly elevated opening pressure (cryptococcal meningitis is notorious for significant pressure increase), lymphocytic pleocytosis (20–500 cells/mm^3), decreased glucose concentration, and elevated protein concentration. Aspergillus and related fungi result in neutrophilic meningitis. CSF should be sent for India ink and specific fungal culture. The cryptococcal antigen test is quite sensitive (90 %) and specific. When fungal meningitis is suspected, large volumes of CSF are needed to increase the yield.

Tuberculous Meningitis

The CSF shows an increased opening pressure, lymphocytic pleocytosis (10–500 cells/mm^3), decreased glucoses concentration, and elevated protein concentrations (100–500 mg/dl). Adenosine deaminase levels, an enzyme associated with disorders that induce cell-mediated responses, are increased in the CSF although false positives and negatives do occur in other infectious and neoplastic CNS disorders [32, 33].

The combination of chronic CSF lymphocytic (more than 4 weeks) pleocytosis or a persistent CSF neutrophilic pleocytosis with decreased glucose levels should raise the suspicion of TB meningitis.

Once specific therapy has begun, a so-called therapeutic paradox may occur and is characterized by clinical worsening and by a shift of the CSF lymphocytic pleocytosis into a polymorphonuclear response. It must not be interpreted as a failure in treatment [34]. CSF cultures are positive in 50–75 % but require 3–6 weeks. PCR is available but, at present, has insufficient sensitivity [35] and has not been properly standardized among different laboratories.

References

1. Rosenberg GA, et al. Brain Edema and disorders of the cerebrospinal fluid circulation. In: Daroff R. (eds.), Bradleys' neurology in clinical practice. Philadelphia: Elsevier Saunders; 2010.
2. Robert A Fishman. Composition of the cerebrospinal fluid. In: Robert A. Fishman (ed.), Diseases of the nervous system. Philadelphia: WB Saunders; 1992.
3. Cutler RW, Spertell RB. Cerebrospinal fluid: a selective review. Ann Neurol. 1982;11(1):1–10.
4. Biller J, Gruener G, Brazis P. Ancillary neurodiagnostic procedures-lumbar puncture and neuroimaging. In: Biller J, Gruener G, Brazis P, (eds), DeMyer's the neurological examination. A programmed text. New York: McGraw-Hill; 2011. p. 539–57.
5. Xie L, et al. Sleep drives metabolite clearance from the adult brain. Science. 2013;342(6156):373–7.
6. Grandgirard D, et al. The causative pathogen determines the inflammatory profile in cerebrospinal fluid and outcome in patients with bacterial meningitis. Mediators Inflamm. 2013;2013:312476.
7. Ellenby MS, et al. Videos in clinical medicine. Lumbar puncture. N Engl J Med. 2006;355(13):e12.
8. Tung CE. Education research: changing practice. Residents' adoption of the atraumatic lumbar puncture needle. Neurology. 2013;80(17):e180–2.
9. Roos KL, (ed.), Cerebrospinal fluid in principles of neurologic infectious diseases. New York: McGraw-Hill; 2005.
10. Berg K, et al. The development of a validated checklist for adult lumbar puncture: preliminary results. Am J Med Qual. 2013;28(4):330–4.
11. Joffe AR. Lumbar puncture and brain herniation in acute bacterial meningitis: a review. J Intensive Care Med. 2007;22(4):194–207.
12. Hasbun R, et al. Computed tomography of the head before lumbar puncture in adults with suspected meningitis. N Engl J Med. 2001;345(24):1727–33.
13. Kiwon F, (ed.), Lumbar puncture and cerebrospinal fluid examination in Merritt's neurology. Philadelphia: Lippincott Williams & Wilkins Wolters Kluwer; 2010.
14. Marra C. Neurologic infections. Hawaii: Course of the American Academy of Neurology; 2003.
15. Amorim JA, Gomes de Barros MV, Valenca MM. Post-dural (post-lumbar) puncture headache: risk factors and clinical features. Cephalalgia. 2012;32(12):916–23.
16. Hammond ER, et al. Needle type and the risk of post-lumbar puncture headache in the outpatient neurology clinic. J Neurol Sci. 2011;306(1–2):24–8.
17. Armon C, Evans RW. Addendum to assessment: prevention of post-lumbar puncture headaches: report of the Therapeutics and Technology Assessment Subcommittee of the American Academy of Neurology. Neurology. 2005;65(4):510–2.

18. Boonmak P, Boonmak S. Epidural blood patching for preventing and treating post-dural puncture headache. Cochrane Database Syst Rev. 2010(1):CD001791.
19. Lavie F, et al. Bilateral intracranial subdural hematoma following lumbar puncture: report of a case. Rev Neurol (Paris). 1998;154(10):703–5.
20. Schievink WI, et al. Diagnostic criteria for spontaneous spinal CSF leaks and intracranial hypotension. AJNR Am J Neuroradiol. 2008;29(5):853–6.
21. Trautmann M, Lepper PM, Schmitz FJ. Three cases of bacterial meningitis after spinal and epidural anesthesia. Eur J Clin Microbiol Infect Dis. 2002;21(1):43–5.
22. Baer ET. Iatrogenic meningitis: the case for face masks. Clin Infect Dis. 2000;31(2):519–21.
23. Kauffman CA, Pappas PG, Patterson TF. Fungal infections associated with contaminated methylprednisolone injections. N Engl J Med. 2013;368(26):2495–500.
24. Niedermuller U, Trinka E, Bauer G. Abducens palsy after lumbar puncture. Clin Neurol Neurosurg. 2002;104(1):61–3.
25. Sanchez-Menoyo JL, et al. Spinal cord hemorrhage complicating diagnostic lumbar puncture. Rev Neurol. 2009;48(8):418–20.
26. Ng WH, Drake JM. Symptomatic spinal epidural CSF collection after lumbar puncture in a young adult: case report and review of literature. Childs Nerv Syst. 2010;26(2):259–62.
27. Nigrovic LE, et al. Relationship between cerebrospinal fluid glucose and serum glucose. N Engl J Med. 2012;366(6):576–8.
28. Escalza-Cortina I, et al. Chronic mumps meningoencephalitis with low CSF sugar and acute hydrocephalus in an adult. Neurology. 2014;82;e41–e43.
29. Leen WG, et al. Child neurology: differential diagnosis of a low CSF glucose in children and young adults. Neurology. 2013;81(24):e178–81.
30. Aksamit AJ. Laboratory diagnosis of central nervous system infections. Philadelphia: Course of the American Academy of Neurology; 2001.
31. Galati D, Di Noto R, Del Vecchio L. Diagnostic strategies to investigate cerebrospinal fluid involvement in haematological malignancies. Leuk Res. 2013;37(3):231–7.
32. Garcia-Monco C, Berciano J. Sarcoid meningitis, high adenosine deaminase levels in CSF and results of cranial irradiation. J Neurol Neurosurg Psychiatry. 1988;51(12):1594–6.
33. Pettersson T, et al. Diagnostic value of cerebrospinal fluid adenosine deaminase determination. Scand J Infect Dis. 1991;23(1):97–100.
34. Garcia-Monco JC, Ferreira E, Gomez-Beldarrain M. The therapeutic paradox in the diagnosis of tuberculous meningitis. Neurology. 2005;65(12):1991–2.
35. Pai M, et al. Diagnostic accuracy of nucleic acid amplification tests for tuberculous meningitis: a systematic review and meta-analysis. Lancet Infect Dis. 2003;3(10):633–43.

Chapter 2
Acute Community-Acquired Bacterial Meningitis

Adarsh Bhimraj

Abstract Community-acquired bacterial meningitis is a significant cause of morbidity and mortality. The most common causative organisms are *Streptococcus pneumoniae* and *Neisseria meningitidis*. The incidence of *Listeria monocytogenes* infection increases over age 50 years and in those with compromised cell-mediated immunity. Symptoms and signs are not sensitive or specific enough to diagnose community-acquired bacterial meningitis. A lumbar puncture for cerebrospinal fluid is needed to reach the diagnosis, to identify the organism, and to determine antimicrobial susceptibilities. Computed tomography of the head is not necessary in all patients prior to a lumbar puncture, only in immunocompromised patients and in those who have features suggestive of or who are at risk of increased intracranial pressure. Appropriate empiric antimicrobials should be started as soon as possible.

Keywords Meningitis • Acute meningitis • Community-acquired bacterial meningitis • Central nervous system infection • *Streptococcus pneumoniae* • *Neisseria meningitidis* • *Listeria monocytogenes* • Kernig's sign • Brudzinski's sign • Jolt accentuation • Neck stiffness • CSF pleocytosis

Introduction and Epidemiology

Acute community-acquired bacterial meningitis (ACBM) is a condition whose rapid diagnosis and management is still important in clinical practice. Meningitis is inflammation of the pia and arachnoid (the inner two layers of the meninges). Acute community-acquired meningitis can develop within hours to days and is usually viral or bacterial. Viral meningitis usually has a good prognosis, whereas

A. Bhimraj, MD
Section of Neurologic Infectious Diseases, Department of Infectious Diseases,
Cleveland Clinic Foundation, 9500 Euclid Ave, Mail Stop G21, Cleveland, OH 44195, USA
e-mail: bhimraa@ccf.org

J.C. García-Moncó (ed.), *CNS Infections*,
DOI 10.1007/978-1-4471-6401-2_2, © Springer-Verlag London 2014

bacterial meningitis is associated with significant rates of morbidity and death, so it is critical to recognize and differentiate them promptly. Meningitis from fungi and mycobacteria, especially tuberculosis, can rarely present acutely, but generally tend to be subacute to chronic (weeks to months), and occurs in patients with specific risk factors for those diseases. Fungal and mycobacterial meningitis should be considered under those circumstances, but their discussion is beyond the scope of this chapter.

The incidence, mortality, and morbidity, from ACBM, have decreased significantly, especially in high-income countries, probably as a result of vaccination and better antimicrobial and adjuvant therapy, but the disease still has a high toll. Still, in the United States, mortality remains at 10–20 % [1, 2]. In the developing world, the mortality rates are as high as 50 % [3]. In the United States, meningitis from all causes accounts for about 72,000 hospitalizations and up to $1.2 billion in hospital costs annually [4]. However, the incidence of bacterial meningitis has declined from 3 to 5 per 100,000 per year a few decades ago to 1.3 to 2 per 100,000 per year currently [2]. In the early 1900s in the United States, the death rate from bacterial meningitis was 80–100 %. The use of intrathecal equine meningococcal antiserum during the first decades of the 1900s dramatically reduced the rate of death from meningococcal meningitis. With the advent of antimicrobial drugs in the 1930s and 1940s, the death rate from bacterial meningitis further declined [1].

The organisms that cause community-acquired bacterial meningitis differ somewhat by geographic region and by age. In a recent study based on surveillance data in the United States, from 1998 to 2007, the most common cause of bacterial meningitis among adults was *Streptococcus pneumoniae*. Among young adults, *Neisseria meningitidis* is nearly as common as *S. pneumoniae*. The incidence of *Listeria* infections increases with age in adults [2]. The relative incidence of these organisms is similar in most high-income countries.

The epidemiologic features of bacterial meningitis have changed dramatically over the past decades with the advent of the *Haemophilus influenzae* vaccine. In 1986, about half the cases of acute bacterial meningitis were caused by *H. influenzae*, but a decade later, the incidence of *H. influenzae* meningitis had been reduced by 94 % [4].

Pathogenesis

Most cases of CABM begin with colonization of the mucosal surface of the upper respiratory tract. In certain individuals, this leads to mucosal invasion and bacteremia. Not all organisms that cause bacteremia are capable of breaching the blood-cerebrospinal fluid barrier to enter the subarachnoid space to cause meningitis. Very few organisms have this capacity, but *Haemophilus influenzae*, *N. meningitidis*, and *S. pneumoniae*, especially those strains that have a capsule, do [5]. Some patients are at higher risk of meningitis because of an abnormal communication between the nasopharynx and the subarachnoid space due to either trauma or a congenital anatomic abnormality. The organisms in these instances can directly spread from the nasopharynx to the meninges. Patients without a spleen or with an immunoglobulin deficiency are also more prone to infections from encapsulated organisms such as pneumococci and meningococci. The opsonizing immunoglobulins coat the capsule, helping phagocytes in the spleen to remove them from the bloodstream. A patient presenting with multiple episodes of bacterial meningitis merits evaluation for these conditions. In contrast, *Listeria* spp. and, rarely, Gram-negative bacteria enter the bloodstream through the gastrointestinal tract and then spread to the meninges.

Once in the subarachnoid space, bacteria elicit a profuse inflammatory response, which can be damaging [5]. The inflammation in the subarachnoid space can extend along the Virchow-Robin spaces surrounding the blood vessels deep into the brain parenchyma. This perivascular inflammation can cause thrombosis in both the arterial and venous circulations. This inflammation can lead to intracranial complications such as hydrocephalous from blocking the arachnoid villi, cerebral edema, and strokes from thrombosis or vasculopathy involving the arterial or venous circulations [5, 6].

Organisms and Organism-Specific Risk Factors

Streptococcus pneumoniae is the most common cause of ACBM [2]. It can also cause a concomitant upper respiratory tract infection, pneumonia, and rarely endocarditis. Though it can affect any immunocompetent adult, those who are at a higher risk of infection are people without a spleen or/and with a primary or secondary immunoglobulin deficiency, including patients with multiple myeloma or human immunodeficiency virus infection.

Neisseria meningitidis is more common in young adults [5]. It is easily transmitted and is associated with crowding, as in school dormitories and military barracks. People with congenital deficiencies of components of complement are at greater risk for both meningococcal and gonococcal infections. Patients with recurrent episodes of *Neisseria* infection should be evaluated for complement deficiency. Meningococcal infection is more commonly associated with a rash. The most common rash of meningococcal meningitis is a very transient, maculopapular rash that appears early in the course of the disease. More pathognomonic is a petechial rash due to thrombocytopenia, which can very rapidly progress to purpura, ecchymosis, and disseminated intravascular coagulation. The petechial rash is evident in 60 % of adults and up to 90 % of children [7], and it is most likely to appear in dependent areas (such as the back of a patient lying down) and in areas of pressure, such as under the elastic band of underwear or stockings.

Listeria monocytogenes infection is usually acquired through contaminated food such as raw vegetables, unpasteurized milk, cheese, and deli meats. It spreads from the gastrointestinal tract to the bloodstream and then to the meninges. It is an intracellular pathogen; thus, people at greater risk are those with poor cell-mediated immunity due to immunosuppressant medications such as steroids or tumor necrosis factor inhibitors. The rate of *Listeria* meningitis starts to increase with age, especially after age 50, probably due to immune senescence or decreased immunity with age.

Aerobic Gram-negative enteric bacilli like *Escherichia coli* usually cause meningitis after head trauma or neurosurgery and are very uncommon causes of community-acquired meningitis. Disseminated strongyloidiasis should be suspected in any patient with community-acquired meningitis caused by enteric Gram-negative bacilli. *Strongyloides stercoralis* is a parasitic intestinal roundworm that is found in the tropics, in the subtropics, and in certain parts of the United States and Europe. The adult worm lives in the intestines where it lays eggs; the larvae are excreted in the stool. A small percentage of larvae penetrate the perianal skin and gut mucosa to cause an autoinfection. People may asymptomatically harbor the parasite for decades, then develop hyperinfection syndrome with dissemination to various organs when treated with immunosuppressive drugs such as steroids. In this syndrome, a significant proportion of the larvae penetrate the gut mucosa to enter the bloodstream and travel throughout the body, including the brain, carrying Gram-negative bacteria with them. The mortality rate of untreated hyperinfection syndrome can be greater than 70 % [8]; thus, it is important to identify and treat it in the context of Gram-negative bacillary meningitis.

Clinical Signs and Symptoms

The classic triad of acute meningitis is fever, neck stiffness, and altered mental status. Other signs and symptoms that have been described are photophobia, headache, nausea, vomiting, Kernig's sign (inability to allow full knee extension when the hip is flexed to a 90° angle), Brudzinski's sign (spontaneous flexion of the hips during attempted passive flexion of the neck), and jolt accentuation test (performed by asking a patient with a headache to quickly move his or her head twice horizontally; the result is positive if the headache worsens). The pathophysiologic rationale for the symptoms and signs is pia-arachnoid inflammation, raised intracranial tension, and irritation of cranial and spinal nerves from the inflammation.

Only a few studies of the diagnostic accuracy of signs and symptoms of acute meningitis have been done. Fourteen retrospective studies examined this issue, but they were heterogeneous with respect to patient age, immunosuppression status, and clinical presentation, as well as to how meningitis was diagnosed (via culture or cerebrospinal fluid analysis), making the results difficult to interpret and reach a consensus [9]. Retrospective studies are more prone to bias, as they lack a control group, and examiner bias is more likely. Based on retrospective data, the combination of fever, neck stiffness, and altered mental status has a sensitivity of only 0.46 [9].

Four prospective studies examined symptoms and signs. Thomas et al. [10] evaluated 297 patients with clinically suspected meningitis. In a study by Uchihara and Tsukagoshi [11], a single examiner was used to evaluate patients presenting with

Table 2.1 Diagnostic accuracy of signs in acute meningitis

	Sensitivity (%)	Specificity (%)	Positive likelihood ratio (+LR)	Negative likelihood ratio (−LR)
Neck stiffness				
Thomas et al. [10]	30	68	0.94	1.02
Uchihara and Tsukagoshi [11]	14.7	100	6.6	0.83
Waghdhare et al. [12]	39.5	70.3	1.33	0.86
Nakao et al. [13]	13	80	0.6	1.1
Kernig's sign				
Thomas et al. [10]	5	95	0.97	1
Uchihara and Tsukagoshi [11]	8.8	100	4.2	0.92
Waghdhare et al. [12]	14.1	92.3	1.84	0.93
Nakao et al. [13]	2	97	0.8	1
Brudzinski's sign				
Thomas et al. [10]	5	95	0.97	1
Waghdhare et al. [12]	11.1	93.4	1.69	0.95
Nakao et al. [13]	2	98	1	1
Jolt accentuation				
Uchihara and Tsukagoshi [11]	97.1	60	2.4	0.05
Waghdhare et al. [12]	6.06	98.9	5.52	0.95
Nakao et al. [13]	21	82	1.2	1

fever and headache, with only 54 patients in this series. Waghdhare et al.'s study included 190 patients with suspected meningitis, where the examiners were blinded to the CSF analysis results [12]. Nakao et al.'s study was a prospective study in 230 patients presenting to two inner city ER's with suspected meningitis [13].

A symptom, sign, or a test's diagnostic accuracy can be assessed with sensitivity, specificity, and positive and negative likelihood ratios. A test with a low value for negative likelihood ration (preferably less than 0.1) is good for ruling out a disease and that with a high positive likelihood ratio (greater than 10) is good for inclusion of a disease. For the prospective studies that evaluated symptoms, the 95 % confidence intervals (CIs) of the positive and negative likelihood ratios include the value 1 (a simple interpretation of that would be that the likelihood of finding these features is the same in patients with meningitis when compared with those without meningitis). Based on these prospective studies, the presence of nausea and vomiting, headache, or neck pain does not reliably rule in meningitis. Similarly, the absence of these does not rule it out.

The CIs of the positive and negative likelihood ratios for signs like those of the symptoms included the value 1 (see Table 2.1 for the exact values). Jolt accentuation looked promising in Uchihara and Tsukagoshi's study as a sensitive sign, but it did not perform that well in subsequent studies (see Table 2.1). In the physical examination, the presence or absence of fever, neck stiffness, Kernig's sign, Brudzinski's sign, or jolt accentuation could not reliably rule in or rule out acute meningitis. In summary, the history and physical examination are not sufficient to determine whether a patient has meningitis. If a patient is suspected of having meningitis, a lumbar puncture is needed.

Diagnostic Tests

Blood for cultures should be drawn before antimicrobial treatment is started [14–16]. Although they are positive only 19–70 % of the time, they can help identify the pathogen [17–19]. Lumbar puncture for CSF studies is essential to make the diagnosis, to identify the organism and its susceptibility to various antibiotics. If lumbar puncture can be performed immediately, it should be done before starting antibiotics, to maximize the yield of cultures. Pediatric studies show that after starting antibiotics, complete sterilization of the cerebrospinal fluid can occur within 2 h for *N. meningitides* and within 4 h for *S. pneumoniae* [16]. However, starting antimicrobials should not be delayed if a lumbar puncture cannot be done expeditiously as such a delay can adversely affect the prognosis [20, 21].

A computerized tomography of the brain is considered in the workup of acute meningitis as there are other mimicking conditions or complications of meningitis that can cause increased intracranial pressure and the possibility of brain herniation complicating a lumbar puncture. For ethical and practical reasons, it would be difficult to evaluate the need for a CT brain prior to LP in a randomized clinical trial. Hasbun et al. [22] performed a study to evaluate if any features on clinical presentation can predict abnormal findings on CT of the head suggestive of elevated intracranial pressure and thus the risk of herniation. The study included 301 adults with suspected meningitis. It found that abnormal findings on CT were unlikely if all of the following features were absent at baseline:

- Immunocompromised state
- History of central nervous system disease (mass lesion, stroke, or a focal infection)
- New onset of seizure (≤1 week from presentation)
- Specific abnormal neurologic findings (e.g., an abnormal level of consciousness, inability to answer two consecutive questions correctly or to follow two consecutive commands, gaze palsy, abnormal visual fields, facial palsy, arm drift, leg drift, abnormal language)

The absence of these baseline features made it unlikely that CT brain would be abnormal (negative likelihood ratio 0.1, 95 % CI 0.03–0.31) [22].

According to the guidelines from the Infectious Diseases Society of America (IDSA) [23], if none of those features is present, blood cultures and a lumbar puncture can be done immediately without performing a CT brain, followed by empiric antimicrobial therapy. If any of the features is present, blood cultures should be obtained first, and then empiric antimicrobial therapy started, followed by CT of the brain to look for contraindications to a lumbar puncture (Fig. 2.1 – modified from IDSA guidelines 1).

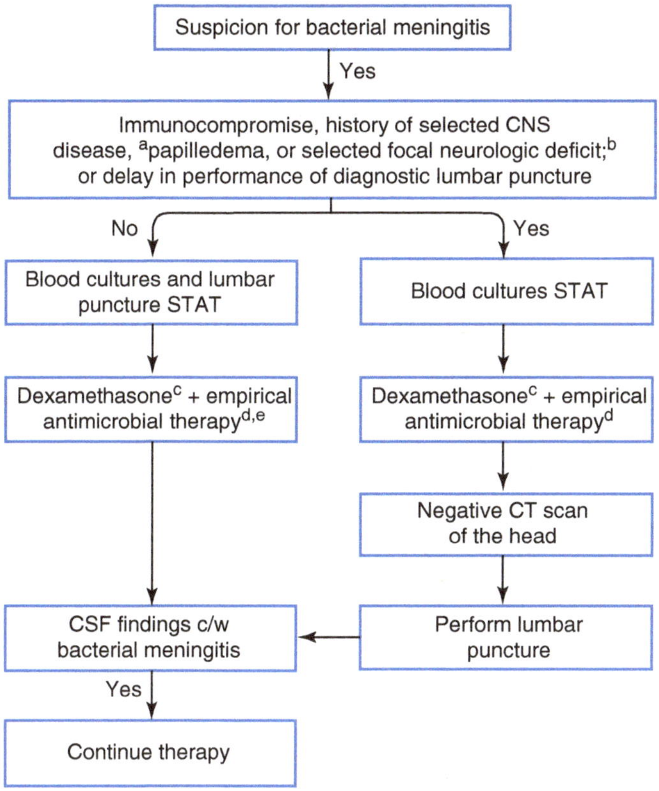

Fig. 2.1 Management algorithm for suspected bacterial meningitis (Adapted from Tunkel et al. [23])

Lumbar Puncture and CSF Studies

Results of lumbar puncture and CSF studies can help determine whether bacterial meningitis is present and, if so, whether the cause is likely bacterial or viral. *The opening pressure* is elevated (usually > 180 mm H_2O) in acute bacterial meningitis. The diagnostic accuracies (likelihood ratios) of the CSF tests were analyzed in a systematic review by Straus et al. using a positive CSF culture as a reference standard [24].

The CSF white blood cell count is raised and is predominantly neutrophilic, in acute bacterial meningitis. A CSF WBC count of 500/μL or higher increased the likelihood of meningitis (+ LR of 15; 95 % CI, 10–22), and a count of less than 500/μL lowered the likelihood (–LR 0.3, 95 % CI, 0.2–0.4) [24, 25].

The CSF glucose level is lower in bacterial meningitis than in viral meningitis. Because the glucose levels in the CSF and the blood equilibrate, *the ratio of CSF glucose to serum glucose* has better diagnostic accuracy than the CSF glucose level alone. The equilibration takes place within a few hours, so the serum glucose level should be ordered at the same time lumbar puncture is done. The CSF blood: Glucose ratio would be the preferred form is a better predictor of bacterial meningitis than the CSF white blood cell count. Bacterial meningitis is likely if the ratio is lower than 0.4. A CSF blood-glucose ratio of 0.4 or less increased the likelihood of bacterial meningitis (+LR 18; CI, 12–27), but a normal value lowered the likelihood (−LR 0.31; 95 % CI, 0.21–0.45) [24].

A CSF lactate level is not routinely done in many institutions, but is a good diagnostic test for evaluation of CABM. A CSF lactate level greater than 31.5 mg/dL (3.5 mmol/L) is predictive of meningitis (+LR 21; 95 % CI, 14–32), and a value lower than that makes the diagnosis unlikely (−LR, 0.12; 95 % CI, 0.07–0.23) [24]. *Protein* shows a mild to marked elevation in bacterial meningitis but is normal to elevated in viral meningitis and in a lot of other CNS diseases.

A Gram stain of the cerebrospinal fluid can be done quickly. *S. pneumoniae* is a Gram-positive diplococcus, and *N. meningitidis* is a Gram-negative diplococcic. *Listeria* is a Gram-positive rod and *E. coli* is a Gram-negative rod. If no bacteria are seen, the information is not helpful in ruling out bacterial meningitis (−LR 0.14; 95 % CI, 0.08–0.27). If it is positive, it is almost 100 % specific for bacterial meningitis due to the organism seen (+LR 735; 95 % CI, 230–2,295) [24].

Management

Antimicrobial Therapy

Empiric antimicrobial therapy must be started as soon as feasible. Most studies of the timing of antimicrobial drugs are retrospective and even when prospective included a very heterogeneous population [20, 21, 26]. Proulx et al. [21] in a retrospective study found that if antibiotics were given within 6 h of the time the patient presented to the emergency department, the case fatality rate was only 5–6 %. If treatment started 6–8 h after presentation, the death rate was 45 %, and if it started from 8 to 10 h after presentation, the death rate was 75 %. In a prospective, multicenter, observational study of 156 consecutive adults hospitalized for pneumococcal meningitis, an interval of greater than 3 h between hospital admission and administration of antibiotics was associated with an increase in 3-month mortality (odds ratio 14.12; 95 % CI, 3.93–50.9) [20]. Most experts would agree that starting antimicrobials early would be beneficial in an emergency like acute bacterial meningitis.

CSF concentrations of most antimicrobial drugs are considerably less than in the serum due to poor penetration of the blood-CSF barrier. Thus, the dose for treating meningitis is usually higher than the regular dose. For example, for the treatment of pneumococcal pneumonia, ceftriaxone is used at a dose of 1 g every 24 h, but for pneumococcal meningitis the dose is 2 g every 12 h.

Empiric treatment of community-acquired bacterial meningitis in immunocompetent adults up to 50 years of age consists of a third-generation cephalosporin such as cefotaxime 2 g intravenously every 4 h or ceftriaxone 2 g intravenously every 12 h, which covers most *S. pneumoniae* and *N. meningitides* strains [23]. The IDSA guidelines recommend adding vancomycin empirically in suspected *S. pneumoniae* meningitis when there are concerns about drug-resistant pneumococcal strains [23]. For vancomycin, 45–60 mg/kg intravenously per day divided into every-6-h or every-8-h doses would achieve better CSF concentrations [27]. In patients over age 50 or those with a cell-mediated immunodeficiency, empiric therapy should also include ampicillin 2 g intravenously every 4 h to cover *Listeria*. It is important to tailor therapy to the results of Gram stain, culture, and susceptibility as they become available.

Role of Corticosteroids

Glucocorticoids, especially dexamethasone, have been well studied as adjunctive therapies in bacterial meningitis. The rationale behind their use is that the profuse inflammatory response to the bacterial components in the CSF by itself has deleterious effects and steroids can reduce that.

In 2004, a Cochrane meta-analysis [28] of five randomized clinical trials, including 623 adults with bacterial meningitis, found a significant reduction in the death rate for patients who received steroids: the death rate was 12 % in patients who received steroids versus 22 % in those who did not (odds ratio 0.6; 95 % CI 0.40–0.81). This led to an IDSA practice guideline recommendation that in adults with suspected or proven pneumococcal meningitis, dexamethasone would be beneficial [23]. But since then, many more studies have emerged from Europe, South America, Malawi, and Vietnam. Another Cochrane meta-analysis [29] including these studies with 4,121 participants was published recently. In this analysis, corticosteroids were associated with a nonsignificant reduction in mortality (17.8 % versus 19.9 %; risk ratio (RR) 0.90, 95 % CI 0.80–1.01). They also had lower rates of severe hearing loss (RR 0.67, 95 % CI 0.51–0.88), any hearing loss (RR 0.74, 95 % CI 0.63–0.87), and neurologic sequelae (RR 0.83, 95 % CI 0.69–1.00). In subgroup analyses steroids reduced mortality in *S. pneumonia* meningitis, but not *N. meningitides* and *H. influenza* meningitis. The beneficial effects on morbidity were seen in high-income countries, but not in low-income countries. Based on these findings, the authors recommended the use of steroids in high-income countries, though the strength of the evidence was not optimal. The recommended steroid was dexamethasone 0.15 mg/kg intravenously and should be preferably started with or before the first dose of antimicrobials and administered every 6 h for 4 days [23].

References

1. Swartz MN. Bacterial meningitis – a view of the past 90 years. N Engl J Med. 2004;351(18):1826–8.
2. Thigpen MC, Whitney CG, Messonnier NE, et al. Bacterial meningitis in the United States, 1998-2007. N Engl J Med. 2011;364(21):2016–25.

3. van de Beek D, Farrar JJ, de Gans J, et al. Adjunctive dexamethasone in bacterial meningitis: a meta-analysis of individual patient data. Lancet Neurol. 2010;9(3):254–63.
4. Holmquist L, Russo CA, Elixhauser A. Meningitis-related hospitalizations in the United States, 2006: Statistical Brief #57. Healthcare Cost and Utilization Project (HCUP) Statistical Briefs. Rockville; 2006.
5. Mook-Kanamori BB, Geldhoff M, van der Poll T, van de Beek D. Pathogenesis and pathophysiology of pneumococcal meningitis. Clin Microbiol Rev. 2011;24(3):557–91.
6. Hughes DC, Raghavan A, Mordekar SR, Griffiths PD, Connolly DJ. Role of imaging in the diagnosis of acute bacterial meningitis and its complications. Postgrad Med J. 2010;86(1018):478–85.
7. Brouwer MC, Tunkel AR, van de Beek D. Epidemiology, diagnosis, and antimicrobial treatment of acute bacterial meningitis. Clin Microbiol Rev. 2010;23(3):467–92.
8. Lam CS, Tong MK, Chan KM, Siu YP. Disseminated strongyloidiasis: a retrospective study of clinical course and outcome. Eur J Clin Microbiol Infect Dis. 2006;25(1):14–8.
9. Attia J, Hatala R, Cook DJ, Wong JG. Does this adult patient have acute meningitis? In: Simel DL, Rennie D, editors. The rational clinical examination: evidence-based clinical diagnosis. New York: McGraw-Hill; 2009.
10. Thomas KE, Hasbun R, Jekel J, Quagliarello VJ. The diagnostic accuracy of Kernig's sign, Brudzinski's sign, and nuchal rigidity in adults with suspected meningitis. Clin Infect Dis. 2002;35(1):46–52.
11. Uchihara T, Tsukagoshi H. Jolt accentuation of headache: the most sensitive sign of CSF pleocytosis. Headache. 1991;31(3):167–71.
12. Waghdhare S, Kalantri A, Joshi R, Kalantri S. Accuracy of physical signs for detecting meningitis: a hospital-based diagnostic accuracy study. Clin Neurol Neurosurg. 2010;112(9):752–7.
13. Nakao JH, Jafri FN, Shah K, Newman DH. Jolt accentuation of headache and other clinical signs: poor predictors of meningitis in adults. Am J Emerg Med. 2014;32(1):24–8.
14. Geiseler PJ, Nelson KE, Levin S, Reddi KT, Moses VK. Community-acquired purulent meningitis: a review of 1,316 cases during the antibiotic era, 1954-1976. Rev Infect Dis. 1980;2(5):725–45.
15. Talan DA, Hoffman JR, Yoshikawa TT, Overturf GD. Role of empiric parenteral antibiotics prior to lumbar puncture in suspected bacterial meningitis: state of the art. Rev Infect Dis. 1988;10(2):365–76.
16. Kanegaye JT, Soliemanzadeh P, Bradley JS. Lumbar puncture in pediatric bacterial meningitis: defining the time interval for recovery of cerebrospinal fluid pathogens after parenteral antibiotic pretreatment. Pediatrics. 2001;108(5):1169–74.
17. Sigurdardottir B, Bjornsson OM, Jonsdottir KE, Erlendsdottir H, Gudmundsson S. Acute bacterial meningitis in adults. A 20-year overview. Arch Intern Med. 1997;157(4):425–30.
18. Aronin SI, Peduzzi P, Quagliarello VJ. Community-acquired bacterial meningitis: risk stratification for adverse clinical outcome and effect of antibiotic timing. Ann Intern Med. 1998;129(11):862–9.
19. Andersen J, Backer V, Voldsgaard P, Skinhoj P, Wandall JH. Acute meningococcal meningitis: analysis of features of the disease according to the age of 255 patients. Copenhagen Meningitis Study Group. J Infect. 1997;34(3):227–35.
20. Auburtin M, Wolff M, Charpentier J, et al. Detrimental role of delayed antibiotic administration and penicillin-nonsusceptible strains in adult intensive care unit patients with pneumococcal meningitis: the PNEUMOREA prospective multicenter study. Crit Care Med. 2006;34(11):2758–65.
21. Proulx N, Frechette D, Toye B, Chan J, Kravcik S. Delays in the administration of antibiotics are associated with mortality from adult acute bacterial meningitis. QJM. 2005;98(4):291–8.
22. Hasbun R, Abrahams J, Jekel J, Quagliarello VJ. Computed tomography of the head before lumbar puncture in adults with suspected meningitis. N Engl J Med. 2001;345(24):1727–33.
23. Tunkel AR, Hartman BJ, Kaplan SL, et al. Practice guidelines for the management of bacterial meningitis. Clin Infect Dis. 2004;39(9):1267–84.

24. Straus SE, Thorpe KE, Holroyd-Leduc J. How do I perform a lumbar puncture and analyze the results to diagnose bacterial meningitis? JAMA. 2006;296(16):2012–22.
25. Lindquist L, Linne T, Hansson LO, Kalin M, Axelsson G. Value of cerebrospinal fluid analysis in the differential diagnosis of meningitis: a study in 710 patients with suspected central nervous system infection. Eur J Clin Microbiol Infect Dis. 1988;7(3):374–80.
26. Radetsky M. Duration of symptoms and outcome in bacterial meningitis: an analysis of causation and the implications of a delay in diagnosis. Pediatr Infect Dis J. 1992;11(9):694–8; discussion 698–701.
27. Ricard JD, Wolff M, Lacherade JC, et al. Levels of vancomycin in cerebrospinal fluid of adult patients receiving adjunctive corticosteroids to treat pneumococcal meningitis: a prospective multicenter observational study. Clin Infect Dis. 2007;44(2):250–5.
28. van de Beek D, de Gans J, McIntyre P, Prasad K. Steroids in adults with acute bacterial meningitis: a systematic review. Lancet Infect Dis. 2004;4(3):139–43.
29. Brouwer MC, McIntyre P, Prasad K, van de Beek D. Corticosteroids for acute bacterial meningitis. Cochrane Database Syst Rev. 2013;(6):CD004405.

Chapter 3
Healthcare-Acquired Meningitis and Ventriculitis

Adarsh Bhimraj

Abstract Healthcare-associated meningitis and ventriculitis are infections that complicate craniotomies, CSF shunt, and drain surgeries. They are distinct clinical entities compared to community-acquired meningitis. Gram-positive cocci like *Staphylococcus epidermidis* and *S. aureus* are the most common pathogens, followed by Gram-negative rods and anaerobes like *P. acnes*. The diagnosis can be elusive as other noninfectious neurologic conditions and neurosurgeries can cause similar clinical and CSF findings. The management of these infections often requires surgical interventions and may need intraventricular or intrathecal administration of antimicrobials, as the organisms can be refractory to IV antimicrobials alone. Periprocedural antimicrobials and antimicrobial impregnated catheters have been shown to reduce infection rates.

Keywords Meningitis • Ventriculitis • VP shunt infections • External ventricular drain (EVD) infections • Ventriculostomy-related infections (VRI) • Craniotomy-related infections • Intraventricular antibiotics • Intrathecal antibiotics • Central nervous system (CNS) infections • Antimicrobial-impregnated catheters

Healthcare-associated ventriculitis or meningitis is a distinct entity, which differs considerably from community-acquired meningitis in epidemiology, pathogenesis, microbiology, and clinical features. They usually occur after surgeries like craniotomies, spine and otorhinologic surgeries where there is dural breach, cerebrospinal fluid (CSF) shunts (ventriculoperitoneal, lumboperitoneal, and ventriculoatrial shunts), or CSF drain (external ventricular drains and lumbar drains) surgeries. They can also occur after head trauma and rarely after lumbar punctures.

CSF shunts are permanent catheters, used for CSF diversion, with the proximal end in the cerebral ventricle or the lumbar subarachnoid space and the distal end in

---

A. Bhimraj, MD
Section of Neurologic Infectious Diseases, Department of Infectious Diseases, Cleveland Clinic Foundation, 9500 Euclid Ave, Mail Stop G21, Cleveland, OH 44195, USA
e-mail: bhimraa@ccf.org

J.C. García-Moncó (ed.), *CNS Infections*,
DOI 10.1007/978-1-4471-6401-2_3, © Springer-Verlag London 2014

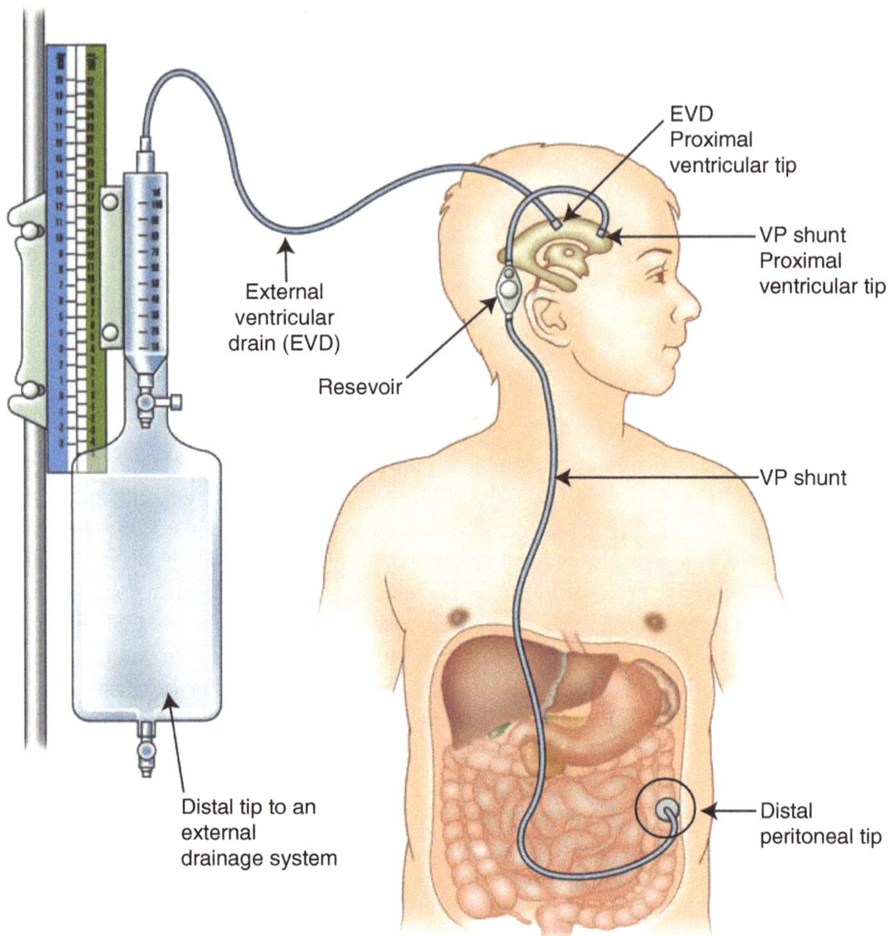

Fig. 3.1 CSF diversion catheters: ventriculoperitoneal shunt and external ventricular drain

the peritoneal cavity, pleural cavity, or right atrium of the heart. The most common type of shunt is the ventriculoperitoneal (VP) shunt. CSF drains are temporary catheters that divert the fluid externally. The proximal end is either in the cerebral ventricle (ventricular drain) or in the lumbar subarachnoid space (lumbar drain). The distal end of the catheter is connected to a collecting system, which has a drip chamber, sampling and injection ports, and a collection bag. Ventricular drains are mostly used for the temporary management of patients with elevated intracranial pressure (ICP) secondary to acute hydrocephalus caused by intracranial hemorrhage, neoplasms obstructing the CSF circulation, or trauma. Lumbar drains are mostly used in patients with CSF leaks after neurosurgery.

Often with CSF catheters whose proximal tips are in the ventricles, the resulting infection would be only ventriculitis without meningitis, and this does have implications on the clinical presentation and diagnostic testing (Fig. 3.1).

Epidemiology, Pathogenesis, and Microbiology

The incidence of CSF shunt infections reported in the literature has a wide range but in most studies rates around 10 % [1, 2]. Reported ventricular drain infection rates are also around 10 % [3]. Infections rates due to lumbar drains are 4.2 % [4].

The organisms that cause ventriculitis, after craniotomies, CSF shunt, and CSF drain surgeries are fairly similar. During these surgeries, the skull and meninges, which act as natural barriers to pathogens, are breached, making it possible for microorganisms that colonize the scalp and skin of the back, or those that live in the healthcare environment, to enter the subarachnoid space or ventricles and cause an infection. In patients with ventriculoperitoneal shunts, another less common route by which organisms enter the ventricles is spreading up along the catheter after a peritonitis. On the surface of catheters, these organisms can form biofilms, which are thick sticky polysaccharide layers making them resistant to antimicrobial action [5, 6]. The organisms that usually colonize the skin, especially the scalp, are coagulase-negative *Staphylococcus*, *Staphylococcus aureus*, and *Propionibacterium acnes*. The organisms that can be present in the healthcare environment are *Staphylococcus aureus* (both methicillin-resistant and methicillin-susceptible strains) and Gram-negative bacteria like *Escherichia coli* and *Klebsiella*, *Pseudomonas*, and *Acinetobacter* species (some of the strains can be multidrug resistant).

Staphylococcal species are the most common organisms causing infections, with *Staphylococcus epidermidis* (47–64 % of infections) being more common than *Staphylococcus aureus* (12–29 % of infections) [1, 3, 7]. Gram-negative bacteria account for 6–20 % of the infections [1, 3, 7, 8]. Diphtheroids (including *Propionibacterium acnes*) account for 1–14 % of the infection, but the reason for the low reported rates in some studies is probably an inadequate culture technique (i.e., anaerobic cultures with prolonged incubation are needed to detect *P. acnes*) [1–3, 9–11]. Fungi like *Candida*, though reported in the literature, are usually rare [12].

Clinical Symptoms, Signs, and Laboratory and CSF Parameters

The clinical presentation of healthcare-associated ventriculitis can vary from being acute and severe, if caused by virulent organisms like *Staphylococcus aureus* or Gram-negative bacteria, to more subtle and chronic, if due to less virulent organisms. Unlike the organisms that cause community-acquired bacterial meningitis, those causing CSF catheter-associated ventriculitis, like coagulase-negative staphylococci and *P. acnes*, are indolent, evoke minimal inflammation, and are usually pathogenic in the presence of prosthetic material [5, 6]. Often there may be ventriculitis without meningeal involvement or only mechanical blockage as a result of biofilm formation in or on the catheter [13]. In CSF shunt infections, fever can be present only in about half the time (52 %) [14]. Headaches (31 %) and changes in mental status (29 %) can be present less than half the time [14]. Meningismus is rarely found (4 %) [14] in these patients, and this is probably because this is mostly a ventriculitis than a meningitis.

Clinical signs and symptoms are even less reliable in ventricular and lumbar drain-related ventriculitis as symptoms like change in mental status, fever, or meningismus could be a manifestation of other neurologic diseases like intracranial hemorrhage or hydrocephalus from other causes. Fever in the neurocritical care unit can be due to intracranial hemorrhage, central fever, thrombotic episodes, and drug fevers [15] in addition to non-CNS infections like blood stream infections, hospital-acquired pneumonias, and urinary tract infections.

There are several studies that evaluated blood or serum markers like procalcitonin, C-reactive protein (CRP), and peripheral white blood cell counts in patients with healthcare-associated ventriculitis. In one open prospective study which recruited consecutive patients with ventricular drains, those with proven bacterial ventriculitis had significantly higher procalcitonin levels (4.7 ± 1.0 vs. 0.2 ± 0.01 ng/mL, $p < .0001$), CRP levels (134 ± 29 vs. 51 ± 4 mg/L, $p = .0005$), and peripheral white blood cell counts (16.1 ± 1.3 vs. 10.7 ± 0.3 10^9/L, $p = .0008$) [16]. In Martinez et al.'s study, a procalcitonin cutoff value of 1.0 ng/mL or more showed a specificity of 77 % and a sensitivity of only 68 % for ventriculitis, though it had better diagnostic accuracy in community-acquired bacterial meningitis [17]. In another study in children with suspected CSF shunt infections, the values for serum CRP in infected individuals were higher than in noninfected ones (91.8 ± 70.2 mg/L compared with 16.1 ± 28.3 mg/L, $p < 0.0001$) [18]. Despite the statistically significant p values in some studies, the confidence intervals for calculated sensitivities, based on traditional cutoffs, are wide. Though these markers are easy to obtain and are often presumed to be sensitive indicators of infections, we need further well-designed prospective studies to recommend their routine use in ruling out healthcare-associated ventriculitis, especially in infections with indolent organisms which cause minimal inflammation.

The diagnostic accuracy of CSF markers in healthcare-associated ventriculitis has been evaluated in several studies. Like the blood marker studies, they have design and methodological limitations. One of the major limitations in interpreting these studies is the heterogenous definition of the reference (gold) standard for the diagnosis of healthcare-associated ventriculitis. To evaluate the diagnostic utility of CSF parameters or any other test, an independent comparison to an acceptable reference standard is required. Often CSF cultures are used as a reference standard in many studies, but diagnosing ventriculitis by a single positive CSF culture will run the risk of a false-positive diagnosis due to colonization or contamination. More specific diagnostic criteria like the presence of multiple CSF cultures with CSF pleocytosis or hypoglycorrhachia with attributable clinical signs and symptoms (fever, headache, photophobia, neck stiffness, decreased level of consciousness) would be clinically meaningful, but using that as a reference standard to calculate diagnostic accuracy like sensitivity and specificity would be erroneous as they are part of the definition of the reference standard and are not independent.

In CSF drain-related ventriculitis, the diagnostic utility of CSF leukocyte count, glucose, and protein is limited, as noninfectious entities like intracranial hemorrhage and neurosurgical procedures can also cause abnormalities in these parameters.

Schade et al. [19] performed a prospective study in a cohort of 230 consecutive patients with ventricular drains. Results from analyses of 1,516 CSF samples showed no significant differences between the patients with EVD-related ventriculitis and a control group without EVD-related meningitis, with regard to CSF leukocyte count, protein concentration, glucose concentration, and CSF/blood glucose ratio. They evaluated the predictive and diagnostic value of the CSF parameters using ROC curves. For none of the CSF parameters could they establish a cutoff value with a sensitivity and specificity of at least 60 %. Pfisterer et al. [20] conducted a 3-year prospective study in patients with ventricular drains. Standard laboratory parameters, such as peripheral leukocyte count, CSF glucose, and CSF protein, were not reliable predictors for incipient ventricular catheter infection. The only parameter that significantly correlated with the occurrence of a positive CSF culture was an elevated CSF leukocyte count (unpaired t test, $p<0.05$). In a prospective study, Pfausler et al. [21] looked at the utility of cell index (CI), which is the ratio of leukocytes to erythrocytes in CSF and leukocytes to erythrocytes in peripheral blood, in predicting ventriculitis. The study was done in patients with intraventricular hemorrhage who had external ventricular drains. Diagnosis of bacterial ventriculitis by CI was possible up to 3 days prior to "conventional diagnosis" which was described as rise of CSF cell count, reduction of CSF/serum glucose, or a positive CSF culture.

There are few studies evaluating the diagnostic accuracy of CSF parameters in CSF shunt infections. In a retrospective study which compared children with VP shunt infection ($n=10$) to controls ($n=129$), a CSF leukocyte count over 100/mm^3 had a 96 % specificity and 60 % sensitivity. The CSF glucose of <40 mg/dL had a 93 % specificity and 60 % sensitivity. The reference standard (shunt infection) in this study was defined as "clinical signs and symptoms with a positive CSF culture" [22]. Often, less virulent organisms like *Staphylococcus epidermidis* and *P. acnes* might not cause significant inflammation, so a lower cutoff for CSF leukocyte count would have probably increased the sensitivity but that was not addressed in this study. However, CSF shunt infections can present with no CSF pleocytosis at times. In a retrospective analysis of CSF shunt infections in adults, the CSF white blood cell counts and lactate concentrations were normal in approximately 20 % of episodes [13]. The CSF parameter values might significantly differ depending on the site from which the CSF is obtained. In one study the leukocyte counts were significantly higher in CSF obtained by use of lumbar puncture (median leukocyte count, 573×10(6) cells/L; $p=.001$) and valve puncture (median leukocyte count, 484 × 10 (6) cells/L; $p=.016$) than in ventricular CSF (median leukocyte count, 8.5 × 10(6) cells/L) [13]. The site of sampling should be considered when interpreting the values as the CSF pleocytosis from ventricular fluid might not be very high even in patients with CSF shunt-related ventriculitis.

There are limited studies on the diagnostic accuracy of CSF parameters in post-craniotomy meningitis and ventriculitis. Often the surgery itself can cause "chemical meningitis" or postoperative meningitis, particularly posterior fossa surgeries. The CSF leukocyte and CSF glucose values can look very similar to infectious meningitis, making it hard to distinguish these entities based on these parameters. In one study only extreme values of CSF leukocyte count >7,500/μL (7,500 × 10(6)/L) and a glucose level of <10 mg/dL were able to distinguish post-neurosurgical chemical meningitis from bacterial meningitis [23]. Another caveat in post-neurosurgical patients is that the CSF pleocytosis and low CSF glucose might be a result of a bone flap infection, a subgaleal infection, or a deeper infection in the surgical bed like cerebritis or brain abscess.

CSF Microbiology Studies

CSF cultures are traditionally considered the gold standard for the diagnosis of meningitis and ventriculitis. In the context of community-acquired bacterial meningitis, positive CSF cultures for highly pathogenic organisms like pneumococcus or meningococcus are highly suggestive of meningitis and not contamination from skin colonizers. In the context of healthcare-associated meningitis, the common pathogenic organisms like *Staphylococcus epidermidis* and *P. acnes* are skin colonizers, and the possibility of contamination during specimen collection should be considered. Unlike organisms that cause acute community-acquired meningitis, those causing healthcare-associated meningitis are slow to grow on cultures and require anaerobic media. In a study on healthcare-associated ventriculomeningitis, a substantial number of positive CSF specimens grew bacteria after >3 days, with some requiring as long as 10 days [24].

The site of specimen collection for microbiology studies is also important, particularly for CSF shunt infections. The site of CSF collection for ventricular catheter infection is generally ventricular fluid; for LP shunts is lumbar subarachnoid fluid; for post-craniotomy infections is either lumbar subarachnoid fluid or intraoperative ventricular fluid and tissue cultures. For VP shunt infections, the options are CSF by a lumbar puncture, from a "shunt tap" (by accessing a subcutaneous reservoir underneath the scalp), or rarely intraoperatively during shunt surgery. In VP shunt infection studies, direct aspiration of the shunt yielded a positive culture in 91–92 %, whereas a lumbar puncture CSF culture was positive in only around 45–67 % [13, 25].

Polymerase chain reaction (PCR) might prove useful to detect organisms that are difficult or slow to grow by culture. In a study that used PCR to detect Gram-positive bacteria in 86 specimens, 42 were culture negative but PCR positive [26]. There were no positive culture results in patients with a negative CSF PCR, suggesting that a negative PCR result is predictive of the absence of infection. More studies are needed, however, before routine use of PCR can be recommended in this setting.

Diagnostic Approach

Given the limitations of symptoms, signs, and lab and CSF tests and the lack of a clear reference (gold) standard for healthcare-associated ventriculitis, it is often a difficult diagnosis to make. The diagnostic criteria and cutoffs suggested here are based on clinical experience rather than good evidence.

CSF Drain-Related Ventriculitis

Lozier et al. [27] proposed a classification system for ventriculitis with a hierarchy based on suspected probability of infection. The diagnostic classification proposed here is a modification of that. In addition to being clinically helpful for deciding when to use antimicrobials, such classification would hopefully establish standard criteria for future research and epidemiological purposes.

- *Contamination*: An *isolated* positive CSF culture or Gram stain, with expected CSF cell count and glucose with *NO attributable symptoms or signs*
- *Colonization*: *Multiple* positive CSF cultures or Gram stain, with expected CSF cell count and glucose with *NO attributable symptoms or signs*
- *Possible ventriculitis*: Progressive rise in cell index or progressive decrease in CSF/blood glucose ratio or an extreme value for CSF WBC count (>1,000/μL) or CSF/blood glucose ratio (<0.2), with attributable symptoms or signs, but NEGATIVE Gram stain and cultures
- *Probable ventriculitis*: CSF WBC count or CSF/blood glucose ratio MORE abnormal than expected, but NOT an extreme value (CSF WBC count >1,000/μL or CSF/blood glucose ratio <0.2) and STABLE (not progressively worsening) with attributable symptoms or signs and POSITIVE Gram stain and cultures
- *Definitive ventriculitis*: Progressive rise in cell index or progressive decrease in CSF/blood glucose ratio or an extreme value for CSF WBC count (>1,000/μL) or CSF/blood glucose ratio (<0.2), with attributable symptoms or signs and a POSITIVE Gram stain and cultures.

Contamination and colonization with skin colonizers generally do not need treatment. Antimicrobial treatment of contamination or colonization with virulent organisms is more controversial, but many clinicians might opt to treat positive CSF cultures for *Staphylococcus aureus* or Gram-negative rods. Antimicrobial treatment of a possible ventriculitis should also be individualized depending on the circumstances, as at times chemical meningitis from subarachnoid hemorrhage or neurosurgery could cause extreme CSF pleocytosis or hypoglycorrhachia, which a clinician might prefer not to treat. On the other instance, it might be classified as a possible ventriculitis if the CSF cultures are negative due to prior antimicrobial use or if the organism is slow to grow, when one might chose to treat with antimicrobials. Probable and definitive ventriculitis would be treated with antimicrobials by most clinicians (Fig. 3.2).

Post-craniotomy Meningitis

Post-craniotomy meningitis can also be classified as possible, probable, and definitive meningitis using the above criteria as the confounding comorbidities and organism causing meningitis are similar to CSF drain infections.

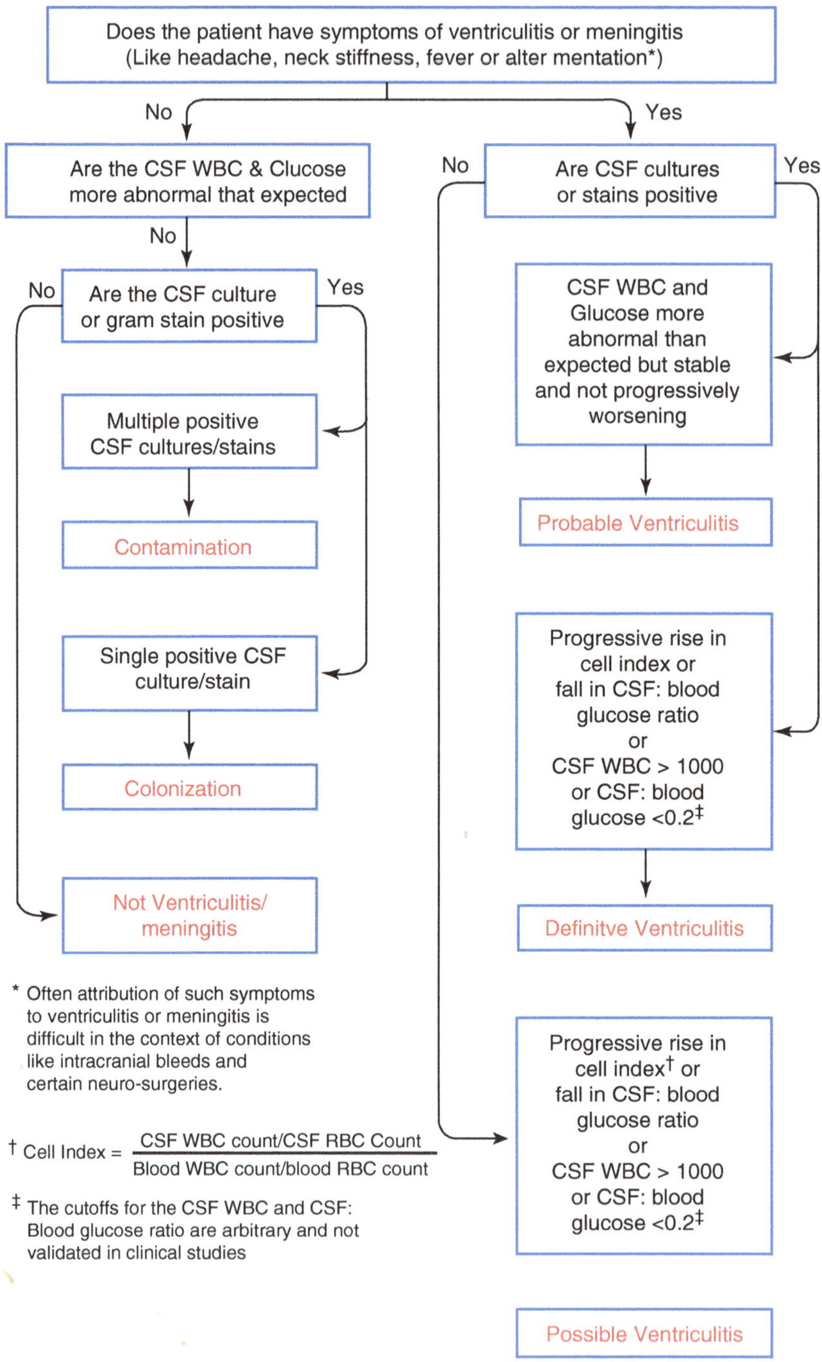

Fig. 3.2 Algorithmic approach to the diagnosis of CSF drain ventriculitis

CSF Shunt-Related Ventriculitis

A diagnosis of CSF shunt-related ventriculitis should be considered when the WBC count (from a shunt tap) is greater than 10/μL OR CSF/serum glucose ratio <0.4 with a positive CSF culture and attributable symptoms. The reason for using such a low cutoff for WBC count is because most often indolent organisms cause minimal inflammation, but the decision to treat based on this should be individualized.

Another instance would be when the WBC count and glucose values are normal, but there are multiple positive CSF cultures (from multiple shunt tap or explanted proximal shunt components) and attributable symptoms. CSF shunt infections can present as shunt blockage due to biofilms formed by organism without significant inflammation.

Principles of Management

Treatment of healthcare-associated ventriculitis is challenging for the following reasons:

1. It is difficult to achieve high CSF antimicrobial levels with intravenous antimicrobials because of the blood-CSF barrier.
2. Organisms like *Staphylococcus* spp. and Gram-negative rods tend to have higher MICs (minimum inhibitory concentrations) for antimicrobials than community-acquired organisms, making it harder to achieve therapeutically effective levels in the CSF.
3. Organisms often form biofilms on the catheters, which are mucoid layers into which antimicrobials do not penetrate well. This is especially an issue if the infected catheters are not removed.

Intravenous Antimicrobials

The recommendations for intravenous antimicrobials in patients with a normal renal clearance would be as follows:

Empiric Intravenous Antimicrobial Therapy

If ventriculitis is suspected, first, obtain CSF cultures and then start empiric treatment with vancomycin (for Gram-positive bacteria) as a continuous infusion or divided doses (2–3) of 60 mg/kg/day after a loading dose of 15 mg/kg with intravenous ceftazidime 2 g/8 h or cefepime 2 g/8 h (for Gram-negative bacteria).

In a penicillin-allergic patient, start empiric coverage with intravenous vancomycin (same dose as above) and aztreonam 2 g/6 h.

Organism-Specific Intravenous Antimicrobial Therapy

The following antibiotics can be started for specific organisms pending on antimicrobial susceptibilities, but knowledge of the local antibiogram and susceptibilities at each institution should direct therapy.

MRSA (methicillin-resistant *Staphylococcus aureus*) and MRSE (methicillin-resistant *Staphylococcus epidermidis*) with a vancomycin MIC $\leq$ 1 µg/Ml can be treated with vancomycin (same dose as above). If the catheter is retained, rifampin 300 mg IV q 12 h should be added.

MRSA and MRSE with a vancomycin MIC > 1 µg/mL or for patient with vancomycin allergy can be treated with linezolid 600 mg IV or PO q 12 h.

Specific treatment for MSSA (methicillin-susceptible *Staphylococcus aureus*) and MSSE (methicillin-susceptible *Staphylococcus epidermidis*) is nafcillin or oxacillin 2 g IV q 4 h.

Specific treatment for *Propionibacterium acnes* is penicillin G 2 MU IV q 4 h.

Specific treatment for *Pseudomonas* spp. is ceftazidime 2 g IV q 8 h or cefepime 2 g IV q 8 h or meropenem 2 g IV q 8 h.

Specific treatment for *E. coli* is ceftriaxone 2 g IV q 12 h or meropenem 2 g IV q 8 h (meropenem if there are epidemiological risk factors for prior colonization or infection with ESBL (extended-spectrum beta-lactamase) producers.

Specific treatment for *Enterobacter* spp. or *Citrobacter* spp. is cefepime 2 g IV q 8 h or meropenem 2 g IV q 8 h.

Intraventricular Antimicrobials

Intraventricular or lumbar intrathecal administration of antimicrobials might be needed when patients do not respond satisfactorily to intravenous treatment or when organisms have high MICs to antimicrobials that do not penetrate the CSF well. This route of administration bypasses the blood-CSF barrier, with controlled delivery directly to the site of infection. CSF pharmacokinetic modeling studies [28–31] show that for most Gram-negative bacteria if the MIC for some cephalosporins is greater than 0.5 µg/mL or for meropenem is greater than 0.25 µg/mL and for Gram-positive bacteria if the MIC for vancomycin is greater than 1 µg/mL, the target pharmacokinetic-pharmacodynamic (PK-PD) parameters in the CSF with intravenous antimicrobials may not be achieved.

Although no antimicrobial agent has been approved by the US Food and Drug Administration for intraventricular and intrathecal use, there have been several studies on their pharmacokinetics, safety, and efficacy, especially in adults [32–38]. CSF sterility and normalization of CSF parameters were achieved sooner with intraventricular and intravenous use when compared to intravenous use alone. However, the use of intraventricular antimicrobial agents was not recommended in infants based on data in a recent Cochrane review [39]. A clinical trial found a three times higher relative risk of mortality when infants with Gram-negative meningitis were treated with intraventricular gentamicin and intravenous antimicrobials, when compared to intravenous therapy alone, although one half of the infants in the intraventricular gentamicin group had received only one dose, raising doubts about the exact cause of death.

Antimicrobial agents administered by the intraventricular or intrathecal route should be preservative-free and should be prepared and given using strict sterile precautions. To avoid increasing the intracranial pressure prior to instilling the drug, a volume of CSF equal to the volume of drug diluent and saline flush should be aspirated and discarded. After administering the drug via a CSF drain, a saline flush can be used to minimize the amount of drug remaining in the draining catheter. When administered through a CSF drain, the drain should be clamped for 15–60 min to allow the antimicrobial solution to equilibrate in the CSF before opening the drain [40]. During and after the procedure, the patient's level of consciousness and ICP should be closely monitored. In treating CSF shunt ventriculitis, administration of the antimicrobials through the shunt reservoir may result in the agent draining distally into the peritoneal cavity; to avoid this issue, antimicrobials can be administered into the cerebral ventricles by placing a ventricular access device separate from the shunt reservoir [41].

Determining the correct dosing regimen is challenging as the CSF concentrations obtained for the same intraventricular dose in pharmacokinetic studies have been highly variable, probably due to the differences among patients in either the volume of distribution depending upon ventricular size or variable CSF clearance as a result of CSF drainage [32–37, 39]. A consensus guideline by the British Society for Antimicrobial Chemotherapy Working Party on Infections in Neurosurgery has recommended that the initial dose of an intraventricular antimicrobial be based on ventricular volume [42]. In adults, the recommended dose of vancomycin is 5 mg in patients with slit ventricles, 10 mg in patients with normal-sized ventricles, and 15–20 mg in patients with enlarged ventricles. Using the same rationale, the initial dosing of an aminoglycoside can also be tailored to ventricular size. The same Working Party recommended that the frequency of dosing be based on the daily volume of CSF drainage: once daily dosing if CSF drainage is >100 mL/day, every other day if the drainage is 50–100 mL/day, and every third day if drainage is <50 mL/day. The ranges of intraventricular or intrathecal dose/day for other antimicrobials are as follows:

Gentamicin: 4–8 mg
Tobramycin: 5–20 mg
Amikacin: 5–30 mg
Colistimethate sodium: 10 mg, which is 125,000 IU or 3.75 mg CBA (colistin base activity)
Daptomycin: 2–5 mg

Another approach, when drug levels can be monitored, is to base dosing on CSF drug concentrations, after the initial intraventricular dose. However, there are very few studies that have evaluated CSF therapeutic drug monitoring and given the variable CSF clearance of an antimicrobial agent; it is difficult to determine when to obtain CSF to measure peak and trough drug concentrations. A CSF drug concentration can be obtained 24 h after administration of the first dose, which can be presumed to be the trough CSF concentration. The trough CSF concentration divided by the minimal inhibitory concentration of the agent for the isolated organism is termed the *inhibitory quotient*, which should exceed 10–20 for consistent CSF sterilization [43, 44]. Although not standardized, this approach is reasonable to ensure that adequate CSF concentrations of the antimicrobial are obtained.

Operative Management

There is a wide range of management approaches to CSF shunt ventriculitis, in the published literature, ranging from conservative treatment with antimicrobials alone to removal of the entire shunt and later reimplanting a shunt after resolution of the ventriculitis [45, 46] There has only been one prospective, randomized trial that evaluated three different approaches to management of infected CSF shunts in 30 children (10 per each arm of the study) [47]. In the study, the arm that received antimicrobial therapy alone with no shunt removal had a 30 % cure rate, the arm with the one-stage shunt replacement (removal of the infected CSF shunt with replacement of a new shunt in the same surgery) had a 90 % cure rate, and the arm with the two-stage shunt replacement (removal of the infected CSF shunt with replacement of a new shunt in a second surgery after the ventriculitis cleared) had a 100 % cure rate. In a decision analysis [45] and a systematic review [46] which synthesized results from many studies, the outcomes were similar to that of the aforementioned trial. They showed that cure rates were better with a two-stage procedure (88–96 %) compared to a one-stage procedure (65 %), which were better than when treated with antimicrobials alone without removing the infected shunt (34–36 %) [45, 46]. In the two-stage approach, there might be a need for a temporary CSF drain, to treat raised ICP or hydrocephalus, while waiting for CSF cultures to clear before reimplanting a new CSF shunt. The optimal timing of shunt reimplantation has not been studied. Early placement may increase the risk of relapse, but a delay in reimplantation may increase the risk of secondary infection of the external ventricular drain. The timing of reimplantation should be individualized based on the isolated organism, severity of ventriculitis, and improvement of CSF parameters and CSF sterilization in response to antimicrobial therapy. Most experts in the field would wait for at least 7–10 days after the CSF cultures become sterile to reimplant a new shunt.

Conservative management without explanting infected prosthetic devices usually has lower cure rates as the organisms adhere to prostheses and form biofilms making them resistant to antimicrobial therapy. However, in one observational study of treatment with systemic and intraventricular antimicrobial agents (instilled via a separate ventricular access device), 84 % of 43 patients were cured, with a 92 % success rate for infections caused by bacteria other than *S. aureus* [41] suggesting that conservative management may be appropriate for selected patients with CSF shunt infections caused by less virulent microorganisms such as coagulase-negative staphylococci and *P. acnes*. In the treatment of CSF drain infections, removal of the infected drain would be a prudent approach.

Infection Prevention

Systemic Antimicrobial Prophylaxis

In addition to sterile technique and aseptic precautions during neurosurgeries such as craniotomies, the use of periprocedural systemic antimicrobial prophylaxis has been shown to decrease infection rates in most studies [48]. However, there are some studies that show that it does not prevent meningitis [49]. Systemic antimicrobial prophylaxis has also been shown to be effective in reducing CSF shunt infections. In a meta-analysis the infection rates were found to be decreased with the use of antibiotic prophylaxis for CSF shunt surgery (odds ratio 0.51; 95 % confidence interval 0.36–0.73) [50]. The antimicrobials that are generally used are first- or second-generation cephalosporins or vancomycin. Although periprocedural systemic prophylactic antimicrobials are used for CSF drains, the use of prolonged prophylactic systemic antimicrobials for the entire duration of external CSF drainage is more controversial. One study noted that the infection rate was 3.8 % in those who received prophylactic antibiotics for the duration of placement of the CSF drain and 4.0 % in those who received only periprocedural antibiotics [51], suggesting that prophylactic antibiotics throughout drainage did not significantly decrease the rate of ventriculitis. In contrast, another study demonstrated a lower infection rate with prophylactic antibiotics (2.6 % CSF infection rate vs. 10.6 % in those who only received periprocedural antibiotics; $P=.001$) [52], although the infections in those receiving prophylactic antimicrobials were caused by more drug-resistant, virulent pathogens and had a higher mortality rate (66 % vs. 41 %). In a systematic review [53] which pooled data from two randomized controlled trials and four observational studies, there was a relative risk reduction of 0.45 with the use of prophylactic prolonged systemic antimicrobials, although there were significant methodological limitations and heterogeneity in the pooled studies, the definitions of ventriculitis were variable, the type and dose of antimicrobials were different, adverse effects were not well studied, and most of the studies were retrospective and prone to bias. Given the availability of a safer efficacious alternative (i.e., antimicrobial-impregnated catheters; see below), it would be prudent to avoid the use of prophylactic prolonged systemic antimicrobials for the prevention of CSF drain infections.

Antimicrobial-Impregnated Catheters

The currently available antimicrobial-impregnated CSF drains and CSF shunts are typically impregnated with either minocycline or clindamycin, combined with rifampin. In a meta-analysis of 12 studies comparing antimicrobial-impregnated to non-antimicrobial-impregnated VP shunts, there was a statistically significant decrease in infections in patients who had received antimicrobial-impregnated shunts (RR 0.37; $P < .0001$) [54]. A similar reduction in infection rates have also been shown with the use of antimicrobial-impregnated external ventricular drains. A meta-analysis of five studies showed a statistically significant reduction in infections with antimicrobial-impregnated external ventricular drains (RR of 0.31; $P = .009$) [54]. The studies show that antimicrobial-impregnated CSF shunts and CSF drains are effective in preventing infections though larger prospective studies are needed to confirm this.

References

1. Tunkel A, Drake J. Cerebrospinal fluid shunt infections. In: Mandell G, Bennett J, Dolin R, editors. Principles and practice of infectious diseases. 7th ed. Philadelphia: Churchill Livingstone; 2009. p. –6.
2. Arnell K, Cesarini K, Lagerqvist-Widh A, Wester T, Sjolin J. Cerebrospinal fluid shunt infections in children over a 13-year period: anaerobic cultures and comparison of clinical signs of infection with Propionibacterium acnes and with other bacteria. J Neurosurg Pediatr. 2008;1(5):366–72.
3. Lozier AP, Sciacca RR, Romagnoli MF, Connolly Jr ES. Ventriculostomy-related infections: a critical review of the literature. Neurosurgery. 2008;62 Suppl 2:688–700.
4. Coplin WM, Avellino AM, Kim DK, Winn HR, Grady MS. Bacterial meningitis associated with lumbar drains: a retrospective cohort study. J Neurol Neurosurg Psychiatry. 1999;67(4):468–73.
5. Snowden JN, Beaver M, Smeltzer MS, Kielian T. Biofilm-infected intracerebroventricular shunts elicit inflammation within the central nervous system. Infect Immun. 2012;80(9):3206–14.
6. Braxton Jr EE, Ehrlich GD, Hall-Stoodley L, et al. Role of biofilms in neurosurgical device-related infections. Neurosurg Rev. 2005;28(4):249–55.
7. Wang KW, Chang WN, Shih TY, et al. Infection of cerebrospinal fluid shunts: causative pathogens, clinical features, and outcomes. Jpn J Infect Dis. 2004;57(2):44–8.
8. Sells CJ, Shurtleff DB, Loeser JD. Gram-negative cerebrospinal fluid shunt-associated infections. Pediatrics. 1977;59(4):614–8.
9. Brook I. Meningitis and shunt infection caused by anaerobic bacteria in children. Pediatr Neurol. 2002;26(2):99–105.
10. Rekate HL, Ruch T, Nulsen FE. Diphtheroid infections of cerebrospinal fluid shunts. The changing pattern of shunt infection in Cleveland. J Neurosurg. 1980;52(4):553–6.
11. Nisbet M, Briggs S, Ellis-Pegler R, Thomas M, Holland D. Propionibacterium acnes: an under-appreciated cause of post-neurosurgical infection. J Antimicrob Chemother. 2007;60(5):1097–103.
12. O'Brien D, Stevens NT, Lim CH, et al. Candida infection of the central nervous system following neurosurgery: a 12-year review. Acta Neurochir (Wien). 2011;153(6):1347–50.

13. Conen A, Walti LN, Merlo A, Fluckiger U, Battegay M, Trampuz A. Characteristics and treatment outcome of cerebrospinal fluid shunt-associated infections in adults: a retrospective analysis over an 11-year period. Clin Infect Dis. 2008;47(1):73–82.
14. Moores LE, Ellenbogen RG. Cerebrospinal fluid shunt infections. In: Hall WA, McCutcheon IE, AANS Publications Committee, editors. Infections in neurosurgery. Park Ridge, IL: American Assowwciation of Neurological Surgeons; 2000. p. –53.
15. Rabinstein AA, Sandhu K. Non-infectious fever in the neurological intensive care unit: incidence, causes and predictors. J Neurol Neurosurg Psychiatry. 2007;78(11):1278–80.
16. Berger C, Schwarz S, Schaebitz WR, Aschoff A, Schwab S. Serum procalcitonin in cerebral ventriculitis. Crit Care Med. 2002;30(8):1778–81.
17. Martinez R, Gaul C, Buchfelder M, Erbguth F, Tschaikowsky K. Serum procalcitonin monitoring for differential diagnosis of ventriculitis in adult intensive care patients. Intensive Care Med. 2002;28(2):208–10.
18. Schuhmann MU, Ostrowski KR, Draper EJ, et al. The value of C-reactive protein in the management of shunt infections. J Neurosurg. 2005;103(3 Suppl):223–30.
19. Schade RP, Schinkel J, Roelandse FW, et al. Lack of value of routine analysis of cerebrospinal fluid for prediction and diagnosis of external drainage-related bacterial meningitis. J Neurosurg. 2006;104(1):101–8.
20. Pfisterer W, Muhlbauer M, Czech T, Reinprecht A. Early diagnosis of external ventricular drainage infection: results of a prospective study. J Neurol Neurosurg Psychiatry. 2003;74(7):929–32.
21. Pfausler B, Beer R, Engelhardt K, Kemmler G, Mohsenipour I, Schmutzhard E. Cell index – a new parameter for the early diagnosis of ventriculostomy (external ventricular drainage)-related ventriculitis in patients with intraventricular hemorrhage? Acta Neurochir (Wien). 2004;146(5):477–81.
22. Lan CC, Wong TT, Chen SJ, Liang ML, Tang RB. Early diagnosis of ventriculoperitoneal shunt infections and malfunctions in children with hydrocephalus. J Microbiol Immunol Infect. 2003;36(1):47–50.
23. Forgacs P, Geyer CA, Freidberg SR. Characterization of chemical meningitis after neurological surgery. Clin Infect Dis. 2001;32(2):179–85.
24. Desai A, Lollis SS, Missios S, et al. How long should cerebrospinal fluid cultures be held to detect shunt infections? Clinical article. J Neurosurg Pediatr. 2009;4(2):184–9.
25. Noetzel MJ, Baker RP. Shunt fluid examination: risks and benefits in the evaluation of shunt malfunction and infection. J Neurosurg. 1984;61(2):328–32.
26. Banks JT, Bharara S, Tubbs RS, et al. Polymerase chain reaction for the rapid detection of cerebrospinal fluid shunt or ventriculostomy infections. Neurosurgery. 2005;57(6):1237–43; discussion 1237–43.
27. Lozier AP, Sciacca RR, Romagnoli MF, Connolly Jr ES. Ventriculostomy-related infections: a critical review of the literature. Neurosurgery. 2002;51(1):170–81; discussion 181–82.
28. Lodise TP, Nau R, Kinzig M, Drusano GL, Jones RN, Sorgel F. Pharmacodynamics of ceftazidime and meropenem in cerebrospinal fluid: results of population pharmacokinetic modelling and Monte Carlo simulation. J Antimicrob Chemother. 2007;60(5):1038–44.
29. Lodise Jr TP, Rhoney DH, Tam VH, McKinnon PS, Drusano GL. Pharmacodynamic profiling of cefepime in plasma and cerebrospinal fluid of hospitalized patients with external ventriculostomies. Diagn Microbiol Infect Dis. 2006;54(3):223–30.
30. Nau R, Prange HW, Kinzig M, et al. Cerebrospinal fluid ceftazidime kinetics in patients with external ventriculostomies. Antimicrob Agents Chemother. 1996;40(3):763–6.
31. Ricard JD, Wolff M, Lacherade JC, et al. Levels of vancomycin in cerebrospinal fluid of adult patients receiving adjunctive corticosteroids to treat pneumococcal meningitis: a prospective multicenter observational study. Clin Infect Dis. 2007;44(2):250–5.
32. Wang JH, Lin PC, Chou CH, et al. Intraventricular antimicrobial therapy in postneurosurgical Gram-negative bacillary meningitis or ventriculitis: A hospital-based retrospective study. J Microbiol Immunol Infect. 2012. pii: S1684-1182(12)00204-6. doi: 10.1016/j.jmii.2012.08.028. [Epub ahead of print]

33. Wilkie MD, Hanson MF, Statham PF, Brennan PM. Infections of cerebrospinal fluid diversion devices in adults: the role of intraventricular antimicrobial therapy. J Infect. 2013;66(3):239–46.
34. Ng K, Mabasa VH, Chow I, Ensom MH. Systematic review of efficacy, pharmacokinetics, and administration of intraventricular vancomycin in adults. Neurocrit Care. 2014;20(1):158–71. doi: 10.1007/s12028-012-9784-z.
35. Tangden T, Enblad P, Ullberg M, Sjolin J. Neurosurgical gram-negative bacillary ventriculitis and meningitis: a retrospective study evaluating the efficacy of intraventricular gentamicin therapy in 31 consecutive cases. Clin Infect Dis. 2011;52(11):1310–6.
36. Imberti R, Cusato M, Accetta G, et al. Pharmacokinetics of colistin in cerebrospinal fluid after intraventricular administration of colistin methanesulfonate. Antimicrob Agents Chemother. 2012;56(8):4416–21.
37. Ziai WC, Lewin 3rd JJ. Improving the role of intraventricular antimicrobial agents in the management of meningitis. Curr Opin Neurol. 2009;22(3):277–82.
38. Remes F, Tomas R, Jindrak V, Vanis V, Setlik M. Intraventricular and lumbar intrathecal administration of antibiotics in postneurosurgical patients with meningitis and/or ventriculitis in a serious clinical state. J Neurosurg. 2013;119(6):1596–602. doi: 10.3171/2013.6.JNS122126. Epub 2013 Aug 16.
39. Shah SS, Ohlsson A, Shah VS. Intraventricular antibiotics for bacterial meningitis in neonates. Cochrane Database Syst Rev. 2012;(7):CD004496.
40. Cook AM, Mieure KD, Owen RD, Pesaturo AB, Hatton J. Intracerebroventricular administration of drugs. Pharmacotherapy. 2009;29(7):832–45.
41. Brown EM, Edwards RJ, Pople IK. Conservative management of patients with cerebrospinal fluid shunt infections. Neurosurgery. 2006;58(4):657–65; discussion 657–65.
42. The management of neurosurgical patients with postoperative bacterial or aseptic meningitis or external ventricular drain-associated ventriculitis. Infection in Neurosurgery Working Party of the British Society for Antimicrobial Chemotherapy. Br J Neurosurg. 2000;14(1):7–12.
43. Ellner PD, Neu HC. The inhibitory quotient. A method for interpreting minimum inhibitory concentration data. JAMA. 1981;246(14):1575–8.
44. Tunkel AR, Hartman BJ, Kaplan SL, et al. Practice guidelines for the management of bacterial meningitis. Clin Infect Dis. 2004;39(9):1267–84.
45. Schreffler RT, Schreffler AJ, Wittler RR. Treatment of cerebrospinal fluid shunt infections: a decision analysis. Pediatr Infect Dis J. 2002;21(7):632–6.
46. Yogev R. Cerebrospinal fluid shunt infections: a personal view. Pediatr Infect Dis. 1985;4(2):113–8.
47. James HE, Walsh JW, Wilson HD, Connor JD, Bean JR, Tibbs PA. Prospective randomized study of therapy in cerebrospinal fluid shunt infection. Neurosurgery. 1980;7(5):459–63.
48. Barker 2nd FG. Efficacy of prophylactic antibiotics against meningitis after craniotomy: a meta-analysis. Neurosurgery. 2007;60(5):887–94; discussion 887–94.
49. Korinek AM, Baugnon T, Golmard JL, van Effenterre R, Coriat P, Puybasset L. Risk factors for adult nosocomial meningitis after craniotomy: role of antibiotic prophylaxis. Neurosurgery. 2006;59(1):126–33; discussion 126–33.
50. Ratilal B, Costa J, Sampaio C. Antibiotic prophylaxis for surgical introduction of intracranial ventricular shunts: a systematic review. J Neurosurg Pediatr. 2008;1(1):48–56.
51. Alleyne Jr CH, Hassan M, Zabramski JM. The efficacy and cost of prophylactic and periprocedural antibiotics in patients with external ventricular drains. Neurosurgery. 2000;47(5):1124–7; discussion 1127–9.
52. Poon WS, Ng S, Wai S. CSF antibiotic prophylaxis for neurosurgical patients with ventriculostomy: a randomised study. Acta Neurochir Suppl. 1998;71:146–8.
53. Sonabend AM, Korenfeld Y, Crisman C, Badjatia N, Mayer SA, Connolly Jr ES. Prevention of ventriculostomy-related infections with prophylactic antibiotics and antibiotic-coated external ventricular drains: a systematic review. Neurosurgery. 2011;68(4):996–1005.
54. Thomas R, Lee S, Patole S, Rao S. Antibiotic-impregnated catheters for the prevention of CSF shunt infections: a systematic review and meta-analysis. Br J Neurosurg. 2012;26(2):175–84.

Chapter 4
Acute Viral Meningitis

Virginia Pomar and Pere Domingo

Abstract Acute infections of the nervous system are among the most important problems in Medicine because early recognition, efficient decision making, and rapid institution of therapy can be lifesaving.

Although acute viral meningitis usually has a benign course, in some patients, it needs hospitalization. The development of the polymerase chain reaction (PCR) has enabled detection of viral genomes, facilitated a rapid diagnosis, and enabled the use of antiviral treatment when needed.

The prognosis is usually favorable.

Keywords Meningitis • Encephalitis • Aseptic meningitis • Cerebrospinal fluid • Central nervous system disease • Antiviral therapy

Acute Viral Meningitis Outline

1. Definition
2. Epidemiology
3. Clinical manifestations
4. Etiology
5. Diagnosis
6. Differential diagnosis

V. Pomar, MD
Infectious Diseases Unit, Hospital de la Santa Creu I Sant Pau, Barcelona, Spain

P. Domingo, MD, PhD (✉)
Infectious Diseases, Hospital de la Santa Creu I Sant Pau,
Av. Sant Antoni Mª Claret, 167, Barcelona 08025, Spain
e-mail: pdomingo@santpau.cat

J.C. García-Moncó (ed.), *CNS Infections*,
DOI 10.1007/978-1-4471-6401-2_4,

7. Specific viral etiologies
    - Enteroviruses
    - HSV
    - VZV
    - EBV and CMV
    - HIV
    - Mumps
    - LCMV (lymphocytic choriomeningitis virus)
    - Arbovirus
8. Treatment

Meningitis is an inflammation of the meninges, the thin membranes (especially the leptomeninges, i.e., pia mater and arachnoid) that surround the brain and spinal cord, most often caused by a bacterial or viral infection. The subarachnoid space lying between both meningeal layers contains the cerebrospinal fluid (CSF) and is also affected by inflammation. Since the subarachnoid space surrounds the brain and spinal cord, meningitis is by definition cerebrospinal.

Acute meningitis is defined as a syndrome characterized by the onset of meningeal symptoms over a period of hours to several days. Among them, headache is a prominent early symptom, often followed by a state of abnormal consciousness or coma, usually accompanied by signs of meningeal irritation.

Encephalitis is distinguished from meningitis, on a clinical basis, by the presence of an early decreased state of consciousness with minimal meningeal signs [1]. On a pathological basis, in encephalitis, the inflammatory process predominantly affects the brain parenchyma. However, secondary meningeal affection is usually present, and hence the term meningoencephalitis is applied.

Definition

Viral meningitis is an infection of the meninges and subarachnoid space (the covering of the brain and spinal cord) caused by a virus. The term is used interchangeably with aseptic meningitis, which refers to a meningitis with negative cultures and clear CSF. Aseptic meningitis, however, may also be caused by drugs and systemic disorders, among others.

Epidemiology

The exact incidence of viral meningitis is difficult to determine since most cases go unreported to public health authorities. In temperate climates, there is a substantial increase in cases during the summer and early autumn, reflecting the seasonal predominance of enteroviruses and arthropod-borne encephalitis virus (arboviruses) infections. In contrast, herpes simplex virus (HSV) and human immunodeficiency virus (HIV) have no seasonal predilection.

Table 4.1 Viruses causing acute meningitis

Common	Less common	Rare
Enteroviruses	HSV-1	Adenoviruses
Arboviruses	LCMV	CMV
HIV	VZV	EBV
HSV-2		Influenza A and B, parainfluenza, mumps, rubella

CMV cytomegalovirus, *EBV* Epstein-Barr virus, *HIV* human immunodeficiency virus, *HSV* herpes simplex virus, *LCMV* lymphocytic choriomeningitis virus, *VZV* varicella-zoster virus

Clinical Manifestations

Viral meningitis presents with fever, headache, and signs of meningeal irritation and may be accompanied by malaise, myalgia, anorexia, nausea and vomiting, abdominal pain, and/or diarrhea. Mild lethargy and drowsiness are not uncommon. The headache associated with viral meningitis is usually frontal or retro-orbital and often associated with photophobia and pain on moving the eyes.

The presence of more profound alterations in consciousness, such as stupor, coma, or marked confusion, should prompt the consideration of alternative diagnoses. Similarly, seizures or other focal neurological signs or symptoms suggesting involvement of the brain parenchyma do not usually occur in uncomplicated viral meningitis.

Nuchal rigidity (or neck stiffness) is present in most cases but may be mild and present only near the limit of the neck anteflexion. Other meningeal signs such as Kernig's and Brudzinski's signs are generally absent [2].

Etiology

Enteroviruses account for 85–90 % of aseptic meningitis cases in most series (see Table 4.1). Using a variety of diagnostic techniques including CSF real-time polymerase chain reaction (PCR) tests, culture, and serology, a specific viral etiology can be found in 75–90 % of cases of viral meningitis [2].

Diagnosis

Cerebrospinal Fluid Examination

The most important laboratory test in the diagnosis of viral meningitis is examination of the CSF. The typical CSF profile shows a lymphocytic pleocytosis (25–500 cells/mm^3), although neutrophils may predominate in the first 48 h of illness

Table 4.2 Cerebrospinal fluid (CSF) cyto-biochemical parameters associated with acute meningitis

	Normal CSF	Viral meningitis	Bacterial meningitis
White cells	<10/μl	100–500/μl	>1,000/μl
Neutrophils	–	<50 %	>50 %
Protein (mg/dl)	<30–40	<100	>100
Glucose (mg/dl)	>50	>50	<40
Gram's stain	Negative	Negative	Positive (60 %)

(they shift to lymphocytes in 24–48 h); mildly increased CSF proteins and normal or mildly decreased CSF glucose concentrations can also be found. Viral organisms are not seen on Gram's or acid-fast stain smears or India ink preparations (see Table 4.2).

Amplification of viral-specific DNA or RNA using real-time PCR has become the single most important method for diagnosing central nervous system viral infections. It allows a rapid and accurate diagnosis for enterovirus, herpes simplex virus (HSV), varicella-zoster virus (VZV), cytomegalovirus (CMV), and Epstein-Barr virus (EBV) infections and assists in clinical decision making, particularly regarding the potential use of antiviral therapy [3].

The overall results of viral CSF cultures for the diagnosis of viral infection are disappointing, presumably because of the generally low concentration of infectious virus present and the need to customize isolation procedures for individual viruses [2]. A delay in transporting or processing the sample further decreases the minimum number of viable viruses necessary to replicate in cell lines. However, the combination of both methods (PCR amplification and culture) remains useful [4].

Other Sources for Viral Isolation

Viruses may also be isolated from sites and body fluids other than the CSF, including the throat, stool, blood, and urine. Enteroviruses and adenoviruses may be found in feces; arboviruses, some enteroviruses, and lymphocytic choriomeningitis viruses (LCMVs) in blood; mumps and CMV in urine; and enteroviruses, mumps, and adenoviruses in throat washings. Nevertheless, the presence of enteroviruses in stool is not diagnostic and may result from residual shedding from a previous enteroviral infection [2].

Serologic Studies

Serology is the method of reference for meningitis caused by West Nile virus and LCMV, which are quite uncommon. Serum serologic studies are less useful for other viruses such as HSV, VZV, CMV, and VEB, for which the prevalence of

Table 4.3 Performance of the main methods for microbiological diagnosis of viral meningitis [4]

	CSF			Other sources		
Microorganisms	PCR	Culture	Serology	PCR	Culture	Serology
Enteroviruses	+++	++	–	+++ (throat, feces)	+++ (throat, feces)	+
Herpesviridae						
VHS	+++	–	+	–	–	–
VZV	+++	+/–	++	++ (vesicle)	++ (vesicle)	++
Mumps	+++	++	++	++ (urine, saliva)	++ (urine, saliva)	++
Arbovirus						
TOSV	+++	++	+	–	–	+++
WNV	++	+	++	++ (serum)	–	+++
LCMV	++	++	++	–	–	+++

CSF cerebrospinal fluid, *PCR* polymerase chain reaction, *HSV* herpes simplex virus, *VZV* varicella-zoster virus, *TOSV* Toscana virus, *WNV* West Nile virus, *LCMV* lymphocytic choriomeningitis virus

+++, high performance; ++, moderate; +, low; –, not recommended

antibody seropositivity among the general population is high. The demonstration of specific serum IgM to VZV, IgG seroconversion between serum of acute disease and the convalescent phase, or intrathecal production of specific antibodies can be useful for VZV meningitis (see Table 4.3) [4, 5].

Brain CT

Upon presentation, patients who are immunocompromised and have a prior history of central nervous system disease, papilledema, or focal neurological deficits should have a brain CT performed prior to lumbar puncture. However, the need for a brain CT should not mean delaying specific antimicrobial therapy if deemed necessary. This is especially important when bacterial etiologies are considered. The same is applicable in presumed cases of HSV encephalitis.

Differential Diagnosis

The most important issue in the differential diagnosis is the exclusion of nonviral causes that may mimic viral meningitis. The major categories of disease that should always be considered are [3]:

- Bacterial meningitis and other infectious meningitides (*Listeria monocytogenes*, *Mycobacterium tuberculosis*, *Treponema pallidum*, *Brucella*, *Cryptococcus*, *Coxiella*, and *Rickettsia*). However, in these cases, presentation is not acute, there are predisposing factors, or meningitis represents a complication of a pre-existing infection.

- Parameningeal infections or partially treated bacterial meningitis.
- Carcinomatous meningitis.
- Meningitis secondary to noninfectious, inflammatory diseases such as sarcoidosis, Behçet's disease, and the uveomeningitic syndrome.
- Some medications (i.e., NSAIDs).

Specific Viral Etiologies

Enteroviruses

They are the most common cause of viral meningitis (accounting for more than 85 % of all cases). They belong to one of the three types of the viral family *Picornaviridae* that cause disease in humans. Nearly 70 serotypes exist, and they are divided into three subgroups: echoviruses, coxsackieviruses A and B, and polioviruses [6].

They are highly contagious and most often spread from person to person through fecal contamination but may also be spread through respiratory secretions (saliva, sputum, or nasal mucus) of an infected person. Cases appear most often during the summer and autumn in temperate climates. However, sporadic cases are seen all year-round.

Patients typically present with an acute onset of fever, chills, headache, photophobia, and pain on eye movement. Nausea and vomiting are also common. Other clues to the presence of enteroviral disease include the presence of exanthemas, myopericarditis, conjunctivitis, pleurodynia, herpangina, and hand-foot-and-mouth disease [1, 2, 7].

Herpes Simplex Virus (HSV)

Two distinct epidemiologic and antigenic types of HSV exist: HSV type 1 and HSV type 2. HSV has worldwide distribution and direct contact with infected secretions is the principal mode of spread.

HSV-1 usually establishes latency in the trigeminal ganglion, and CNS infection typically results in an encephalitic illness, whereas HSV-2 establishes latency in the sacral sensory ganglia and typically causes meningitis [3]. Neurological disease after primary HSV-2 is seen most often in neonates.

Meningitis (usually by HSV-2) is usually characterized by a stiff neck and an acute onset of headache, fever, and photophobia; about 50 % of patients have transient neurological manifestations including seizures, hallucinations, diplopia, cranial nerve palsies, or altered consciousness. Meningitis appears in 36 % of women and 13 % of men at the time of an initial (primary) episode of genital herpes [1].

In some series, HSV-2 has been the most important cause of aseptic meningitis in adults, especially women, and overall, it is probably second only to enteroviruses as a cause of viral meningitis.

Of these patients, 20 % will develop a few or up to ten episodes of meningitis lasting 2–5 days followed by spontaneous recovery [8]. Almost all cases of recurrent HSV meningitis are due to HSV-2. Genital lesions may not be present, and most patients report no history of genital herpes.

Although HSV can be cultured from CSF during a first episode of meningitis, cultures are invariably negative during recurrences [9]. Diagnosis depends on amplification of HSV DNA from CSF by PCR.

Varicella-Zoster Virus (VZV)

Primary VZV infection, chicken pox (varicella), usually occurs during childhood as a mild-to-moderate disease. Latent VZV infection may occur in the cranial nerve ganglia, any dorsal root ganglia, and autonomic ganglia along the entire neuraxis. Years later, usually in association with a decline in cell-mediated immunity in elderly and immunocompromised individuals, VZV reactivates and causes a wide range of neurological disease; in fact, in recent years, VZV has been implicated with increasing frequency as a meningitis-producing agent and especially, meningoencephalitis with or without rash [10].

Epstein-Barr Virus (EBV) and Cytomegalovirus (CMV)

Both viruses can cause aseptic meningitis in association with mononucleosis syndrome, particularly in the immunocompromised host, but this occurs in less than 5 % of cases. EBV and CMV are almost never cultured from CSF, but DNA can be amplified in some patients [11].

Human Immunodeficiency Virus (HIV)

It has been estimated that HIV infection is the cause of 5 % of cases of aseptic meningitis. Aseptic meningitis may occur as part of the primary exposure to HIV (in up to 24 % of cases during or after the mononucleosis-like syndrome) or may be detected in an already infected patient (more commonly in patients with 200–500 CD4/mm^3 than in earlier stages) and can assume the form of chronic meningitis [12–14].

HIV meningoencephalitis may be the presenting form of HIV primary infection in around 8 % of patients. Cranial nerve palsies, most commonly involving cranial nerves V, VII, or VIII are more common in HIV meningitis than in other viral infections.

This syndrome usually resolves spontaneously within 2–4 weeks. The diagnosis of HIV meningoencephalitis is an accepted indication for starting antiretroviral therapy during primary HIV infection.

Mumps

Mumps is asymptomatic in nearly 30 % of children. Mumps meningitis has been reported in 1–10 % of persons with mumps and usually follows the onset of parotiditis, when present, by about 5 days. The most frequent clinical presentation is the triad of fever, vomiting, and severe headache, but only half of patients will have the salivary glands enlarged. Most patients have signs of meningitis but no evidence of cortical dysfunction. Mumps meningitis is usually self-limited, although cranial nerve palsies have occasionally led to permanent sequelae, particularly deafness [1, 15]. Hydrocephalus is frequent, particularly in children, and CSF analysis shows lymphocytic pleocytosis and increased proteins; in one-fourth of patients, glucose levels are decreased [16].

Recently, concern has been raised about vaccine failure and infection resurgence, with important outbreaks in the UK in 2005 and in the USA in 2006 [1, 2]. Prior to widespread vaccination, mumps was a main cause of aseptic meningitis. The vaccine with live attenuated virus is protective but imperfect, and outbreaks still occur even among vaccinated individuals [17].

Mumps meningitis should be considered during late winter or early spring, especially in males. Mumps infection confers lifelong immunity, so a documented history of previous infection excludes this diagnosis.

Diagnosis is typically made by isolation of virus from the CSF and/or demonstration of seroconversion between acute phase and convalescent sera [2].

Lymphocytic Choriomeningitis Virus (LCMV)

LCMV was one of the earliest and seemingly most significant viruses to be associated with human aseptic meningitis.

It is transmitted to humans by contact with rodents (rats, mice, hamsters, etc.) or their excreta; the greatest risk of infection is in laboratory workers, pet owners, and persons living in impoverished and unhygienic situations. Presumed routes of transmission are ingestion of food contaminated with animal urine and exposure of open wounds to dirt [1]. Person-to-person transmission has occurred only through maternal-fetal transmission (associated with congenital hydrocephalus, chorioretinitis, and mental retardation) and solid organ or hematopoietic transplantation [19–21].

Human cases are most common in autumn due to the result of seasonal population densities of rodents and the movement of mice into homes and barns during cold weather. Most LCMV infections occur among young adults, although persons of all ages have been affected [1].

LCMV illness occurs in most infected individuals usually 8–13 days after being exposed to the virus and it is usually nonspecific or influenza-like. Thirty-five percent of infected persons exhibit clinical evidence of CNS infection in a second phase (following a few days of recovery). There is an especially severe form of the disease in immunosuppressed patients because of solid organ or hematopoietic stem cell transplantation, in which LCMV may result in serious systemic infections and death [18]. The overall case fatality rate is less than 1 %, and people with complications including meningitis almost always recover completely. A more severe disease is likely to occur in people who are immunosuppressed. Mortality in these patients may be as high as 75 % [18–21].

Arbovirus Infections

The term arboviruses refer to viruses that have an arthropod vector, such as mosquitoes or ticks. These viruses are members of the togavirus (Eastern equine encephalitis, Western equine encephalitis, Venezuelan equine encephalitis, etc.), flavivirus (St Louis encephalitis, West Nile viruses, Japanese encephalitis, Murray Valley encephalitis, dengue and yellow fever viruses), and bunyavirus families (California encephalitis virus group, hantaviruses, Toscana virus).

For some arboviruses, distribution is universal, while for others, it is more geographically restricted since it is determined in large part by the range of their arthropod vectors. These infections appear most often during the summer and early autumn in temperate climates.

Most infections are asymptomatic, and the clinical picture, when it occurs, can range from a self-limited febrile syndrome to severe symptoms (meningitis or meningoencephalitis).

For the diagnosis, it is especially relevant to collect data about recent travel or insect bites; in the laboratory, the use of direct detection techniques such as CSF culture and/or PCR usually warrants etiologic diagnosis [22–24].

Treatment

Patients with a clinical picture suggestive of meningitis should be investigated for the possibility of bacterial and viral causes for the purpose of establishing the diagnosis and potential avoidance of unnecessary hospitalization and/or antibiotic treatment.

In the usual case of viral meningitis, treatment is symptomatic and hospitalization is not required.

Intravenous acyclovir may be of benefit in patients with meningitis caused by HSV-1 or HSV-2 (10 mg/kg per day in three divided doses for 14–21 days) and VZV (10–15 mg/kg per day in three divided doses for 10–14 days). Oral acyclovir (800 mg, five times a day), famciclovir (500 mg, twice a day), or valacyclovir (1,000 mg, twice a day) for the last week of the treatment may be used, although data on efficacy are lacking.

Antiviral therapy of enteroviral meningitis is limited. Pleconaril prevents viral replication by inhibiting viral uncoating and blocking viral attachment to host cell receptors. Pleconaril was tested in two placebo-controlled clinical trials and in both shortened the course of illness compared to placebo recipients, especially when given early in the course of the disease. However, the benefits were only modestly achieved in the subgroup of patients with more severe disease after adjusting for confounding variables [6]. Pleconaril has not achieved approval by the US Food and Drug Administration (FDA) because it induces CYP3A enzyme activity and has the potential for drug interactions. Antiretroviral therapy may be started for HIV meningoencephalitis.

References

1. Tunkel AR, van de Beek D, Scheld WM. Acute meningitis. In: Mandell GL, Bennet JE, Dolin R, editors. Principles and practice of infectious diseases. 7th ed. Philadelphia: Churchill Livingstone/Elsevier; 2010. p. 1189–229.
2. Roos KL, Tyler KL. Meningitis, encephalitis, brain abscess, and empyema. In: Kasper H, Braunwald L, Fauci J. Principles internal medicine. 16th ed. New York: McGraw Hill; 2005. p. 2471–90.
3. Jhekwaba UK, Kudesia G, McKendrick M. Clinical features of viral meningitis in adults: significant differences in cerebrospinal fluid findings among herpes simplex virus, varicella zoster virus, and enterovirus infections. Clin Infect Dis. 2008;47:783–9.
4. Navarro Mari JM, Pérez Ruiz M, Vicente Anza D. Diagnóstico de laboratorio de las meningitis linfocitarias. Enferm Infecc Microbiol Clin. 2010;28 Suppl 1:56–61.
5. Perez-Ruiz M, Vicente D, Navarro-Marí JM. Infecciones agudas del sistema nervioso central (meningitis y encefalitis) virales y bacterianas de origen autóctono. Enferm Infecc Microbiol Clin. 2008;26 Suppl 9:8–14.
6. Desmond RA, Accortt NA, Talley L, Villano SA, Soong SJ, Whitley RJ. Enteroviral meningitis: natural history and outcome of pleconaril therapy. Antimicrob Agents Chemother. 2006;50(7):2409–14.
7. Perez C, Oña M, Ballesteros S, Llaneza J, Lagunilla L, Perez S, Fernández C, Solis G. Meningitis por Enterovirus. Características epidemiológicas, clínicas y de laboratorio en una serie de 60 niños. An Esp Pediatr. 2001;55:11–4.
8. Shalabi M, Whitley RJ. Recurrent benign lymphocytic meningitis. Clin Infect Dis. 2006;43:1194–7.
9. Berger JR, Houff S. Neurological complications of herpes simplex virus type 2 infection. Arch Neurol. 2008;65:596–600.
10. Mueller NH, Gilden DH, Cohrs RJ, Mahalingam R, Nagel MA. Varicella zoster virus infection: clinical features, molecular pathogenesis of disease, and latency. Neurol Clin. 2008;26:675–97.
11. Steiner I, Budka H, Chaudhuri A, Koskiniemi M, Sainio K, Salonen O, Kennedy PGE. Viral meningoencephalitis: a review of diagnostic methods and guidelines for management. Eur J Neurol. 2010;17:999–1009.

12. Hanson KE, Reckleff J, Hicks L, Castellano C, Hicks CB. Unsuspected HIV infection in patients presenting with acute meningitis. Clin Infect Dis. 2008;47:433–4.
13. Schacker T, Coller AC, Hughes J, Shea T, Corey L. Clinical and epidemiological features of primary HIV infection. Ann Intern Med. 1996;125(4):257–64.
14. Zavasky D-M, Gerberding JL, Sande MA. Patients with AIDS. In: Wilson WR, Sande MA. Current diagnosis and treatment in infectious diseases. New York: McGraw Hill; 2001. p. 315–27.
15. Yung CF, Andrews N, Bukasa A, Brown KE, Ramsay M. Mumps complications and effects of mumps vaccination, England and Wales, 2002-2006. Emerg Infect Dis. 2011;17(4):661–7.
16. Escalza-Cortina I, Azkune-Calle I, Rodriguez-Sainz A, Gomez-Beldarrain M, Vicente-Olabarría I, Garcia-Monco JC. Pearls and Oy-sters: chronic mumps meningoencephalitis with low CSF glucose and acute hydrocephalus in an adult. Neurology. 2014;82: e41–3.
17. Hviid A, Rubin S, Muhlemann K. Mumps. Lancet. 2008;371:932–44.
18. Centers for Disease Control and Prevention (CDC). Brief report: lymphocytic choriomeningitis virus transmitted through solid organ transplantation. MMWR Morb Mortal Wkly Rep. 2008;57(29):799–801.
19. Fisher SA, Graham MB, Kuehnert MJ, et al. Transmission of lymphocytic choriomeningitis virus by organ transplantation. N Engl J Med. 2006;354(21):2235–49.
20. Amman BR, Pavlin BI, Albariño CG, et al. Pet rodents and fatal lymphocytic choriomeningitis in transplant meningitis. Emerg Infect Dis. 2007;13(5):719–25.
21. Kotton CN. Zoonosis in solid-organ and hematopoietic stem cell transplant recipients. Clin Infect Dis. 2007;44:857–66.
22. Drew WL. Viral infection of the central nervous system. In: Wilson WR, Sande MA, editors. Current diagnosis and treatment in infectious diseases. New York: McGraw-Hill; 2001. p. 315–27.
23. Solomon T. Flavivirus encephalitis. N Engl J Med. 2004;351:370–8.
24. Sánchez-Seco MP, Navarro JM. Infecciones por el virus de Toscana, el virus del Nilo Occidental y otros Arbovirus de interés en Europa. Enferm Infecc Microbiol Clin. 2005;23(9):560–8.

Chapter 5
Acute Viral Encephalitis: Herpesviruses and Enteroviruses

José Luis Sánchez-Menoyo and Javier Ruiz-Ojeda

Abstract Acute encephalitis is a syndrome of diverse etiology, mostly viral, which varies according to the time of the year and the geographic location. Etiology remains unidentified in many cases. The current outcome of viral encephalitis remains unsatisfactory with high mortality and morbidity rates in adults and children. Worldwide, herpes simplex type 1 encephalitis is the most common cause of sporadic encephalitis. Viral encephalitis represents a medical emergency that requires prompt diagnosis and therapy and a high index of suspicion. Early initiation of antiviral therapy is crucial while diagnostic test are being performed. Supportive care should be directed at the prevention and treatment of secondary complications, including cerebral edema and epilepsy.

Keywords Encephalitis • Herpesvirus • Herpes simplex • Herpes zoster • Cytomegalovirus • Enterovirus

Acute encephalitis is a syndrome of diverse etiology, mostly viral, which varies according to the time of the year and the geographic location (Table 5.1). In many instances, however, the etiology remains unidentified. A prospective Finnish study on encephalitis identified an etiologic agent in 36 % of the patients. The most common were herpes simplex type 1, varicella–zoster, and arboviruses [1]. In 2006, the California encephalitis project evaluated 1,570 patients with encephalitis and identified an infectious causative agent in one-third of them [2].

In this chapter the most common causes of viral sporadic encephalitis will be reviewed, with particular focus on the most frequent and severe herpes simplex encephalitis. Other herpesviruses, as well as enteroviruses and a type of arboviruses, tick-borne encephalitis, will be also discussed. Other arboviral infections are covered in Chap. 6.

J.L.Sanchez-Menoyo, MD (✉) • J.Ruiz-Ojeda, MD
Department of Neurology, Hospital de Galdakao-Usansolo,
Barrio Labeaga S/N, Galdakao, Bizkaia 48960, Spain
e-mail: joseluis.sanchezmenoyo@osakidetza.net

J.C. García-Moncó (ed.), *CNS Infections*,
DOI 10.1007/978-1-4471-6401-2_5, © Springer-Verlag London 2014

Table 5.1 Commonest agents of acute encephalitis

Etiologic agent	Comments
Herpesviruses	Throughout the year
Enteroviruses	Summer and fall
Arboviruses	Summer and fall Mosquito- or tick-borne

Herpes Simplex Virus Encephalitis

Herpes simplex encephalitis (HSE) is caused by herpes simplex virus (HSV) types 1 and 2 (HSV-1 and HSV-2), two DNA closely related, worldwide human pathogens that belong to the Herpesviridae family. They produce a wide variety of diseases, including mucocutaneous infections, central nervous system (CNS) infection, and infections of visceral organs. There are no animal vectors for HSV and humans are the only natural reservoir. Infection with HSV-1 is acquired more frequently and earlier than infection with HSV-2. More than 90 % of adults have antibodies to HSV-1 by the fifth decade of life. Antibodies to HSV-2 appear during puberty and correlate with initiation of sexual activity. Whereas HSV-1 typically causes encephalitis, HSV-2 is more often associated with aseptic meningitis and accounts for most cases of recurrent Mollaret's syndrome.

Epidemiology

HSE is the most common sporadic viral encephalitis worldwide, with an annual incidence of 1 in 250,000–500,000 [3]. In the United States, HSE accounts for approximately 10–20 % of the 20,000 annual viral encephalitis cases, with an incidence of approximately 2.3 cases per million [4]. In a nationwide study of HSV-1 encephalitis in Sweden over a 12-year period, the annual incidence of confirmed cases was 2.2 per million [5]. HSV is also the most commonly identified pathogen among hospitalized patients diagnosed with encephalitis in Australia [6, 7]. Cases are distributed throughout the year, and the age-specific incidence is bimodal, with peaks in the young (one-third of all cases occur in children and adolescents [8]) and in the elderly. Most HSE cases are due to HSV-1, but about 5–10 % are caused by HSV-2, particularly in immunocompromised individuals and neonates [9].

Pathogenesis

HSV often causes a mild disease restricted to the skin and mucosa and much less commonly a severe encephalitis. While HSV-1 is typically transmitted via the orolabial route, HSV-2 is the cause of most cases of genital herpes [10]. Primary infections, acquired through close contact from an infected individual, are mostly asymptomatic in adults but result in gingivostomatitis in 10 % of infected children. They occur during the first three decades of life, while reactivation occurs at any time. After initial replication in the skin and mucosa, the virus infects the sensory nerve endings innervating the infected territory and migrates by retrograde axonal flow toward the neuronal nuclei of the trigeminal ganglia where it remains latent. Latency is defined by the presence of the viral genome in host tissue without the production of infective particles [11].

Reactivation gives rise to mucocutaneous recurrence confined to the anatomic distribution of a single dorsal root ganglion and is not accompanied by permanent sensory deficit, a marker of neuronal death. Reactivations can be symptomatic (recrudescence) or, more frequently, asymptomatic with inadvertent transmission.

The mechanisms whereby HSV-1 penetrates the nervous system, evades the immune response, and causes encephalitis are incompletely understood. HSV could enter into the brain by reactivation of the viral genome in the trigeminal ganglion with axonal spread via the trigeminal nerve into the frontal and temporal lobes [12]. Also, in situ reactivation of the latent virus from central nervous system (CNS) tissue can occur [13], as well as primary CNS infection. These options are not mutually exclusive. HSE may occur either during primary HSV infection, a situation more common in children and adolescents, or during reactivation in HSV-seropositive adult patients. Only 10 % of patients present symptoms of cutaneous or mucous HSV infection at the time of encephalitis. However, a study showed that the viral strain recovered from the brain differed from the strain recovered from the lip or pharynx in 3 out of 8 HSE cases, suggesting that encephalitis can occur after reinfection as well as after primary infection or reactivation [14].

Several studies implicate the immune response to HSV-1 in causing widespread CNS disease, but the exact cause of the extensive destruction of the CNS is unknown. Multiple cell populations, including natural killer cells, macrophages, T lymphocytes, and lymphokines, play a role in host defense against HSV infection [15]. T cells play a major role in viral containment and prevention of lethal disseminated disease, although antibodies also help reduce viral titer in neural tissue [16]. Widespread local extension and dissemination occur in patients with inadequate cell-mediated immunity, including infants, organ transplant recipients, and HIV-infected persons [15]. Defects in the innate immune response have been associated with severe viral infections in humans as in animal models [17], suggesting that the outcome of viral infection depends on a balance between the host immune response and counteracting viral factors [18]. Genetic defects impairing recognition of pathogens by the innate immune system have been identified. Deficiency of an intracellular protein, UNC-93B, causing impaired cellular interferon α/β and λ antiviral responses, was associated with HSE [19].

Neonatal infection acquired through the mother's genital tract during delivery implicates both HSV-2 and HSV-1. In the newborn, encephalitis may be caused by hematogenous spread with multiorgan involvement and diffuse brain necrosis. It occurs during the first week of life and is the only manifestation of 25 % of neonatal HSV infections. Most often, encephalitis develops after the second week of life and presents a focal cerebral involvement resembling the transneuronal spread of older patients [20].

The highest risk to the neonate (30–50 % risk of transmission) is primary maternal infection close to delivery [21] leading to a high viral load in the absence of HSV antibodies passed to the neonate. The risk of transmission from mothers with recurrent infection on delivery is much lower (<3 %). Primary and recurrent infections are often asymptomatic in pregnant women. Neonatal HSV-1 infections may also be acquired through postnatal contact with people with orolabial HSV-1 infection. Thus, nursery personnel and other adults with HSV external lesions should avoid intimate contact with the newborn. Neonates (infants younger than 6 weeks) have the highest frequency of visceral and CNS infection of any HSV-infected population. Congenitally infected infants have been reported, but they were almost invariably born to mothers with primary HSV-1 or HSV-2 infection during pregnancy [22]. Clinical features included microcephaly, hydrocephalus, and chorioretinitis.

Clinical Features

Symptoms and signs of HSE include headache, fever, nausea and vomiting, and sometimes neck stiffness associated with signs of brain dysfunction such as abnormal consciousness, behavioral changes (hypomania, hallucinations, agitation), focal neurological signs (dysphasia, hemiparesis, hemianopia), cognitive disturbances (memory, speech, and orientation disturbances), and seizures. There may be prodromal symptoms of upper respiratory tract infection and neurological dysfunction of the frontotemporal lobes, sometimes mimicking acute psychiatric conditions.

Behavior disorders may also include excessive animation, decreased need for sleep, inflated self-esteem, and hypersexuality [23]. There are atypical cases with milder and less severe forms of encephalitis without the classical frontotemporal syndrome [24]. These include low-grade fever, speech disturbances (dysphasia and aphasia), and behavioral changes, which can be mistaken for psychiatric illness or the consequences of drugs or alcohol [25]. Disease presentation is acute, usually less than a week. Fever and headache are present in the vast majority (up to 90 %) at the time of presentation, and their absence should cast doubts upon the diagnosis.

In the clinical series of the pre-PCR era, personality changes, confusion, and disorientation were present in about three-quarters of the patients, seizures in half, and focal neurological signs in one-third of all patients [26].

In AIDS and others immunocompromised patients, the presentation of HSE might vary and become a clinical challenge. Patients may present with behavioral abnormalities without prodromal symptoms, fever, or even headache or focal neurological deficits [27, 28].

Immunosuppressed patients present with less prodromal symptoms and focal deficits and more extensive CNS involvement, including the brainstem and cerebellum, sometimes in the absence of temporal lobe involvement. Normal CSF cell counts are not unusual and their morbidity and mortality is substantially higher [28].

Neurological examination shows findings related to the presence of meningeal irritation and brain dysfunction. Signs of autonomic and hypothalamic disturbances may be present (diabetes insipidus, syndrome of inappropriate antidiuretic hormone secretion).

Only 10 % of patients present symptoms of cutaneous or mucous HSV infection at the time of encephalitis [18]. The finding of labial herpes has no diagnostic specificity for HSV encephalitis and may be merely a marker of critical illness [25]. The very young and the very old display the most extensive and serious signs of encephalitis [29].

Neonatal HSV infection occurs in approximately 1 in 3,200 deliveries [21] and may present with a combination of (a) involvement of skin, eyes, mouth, or a combination; (b) neurological infection; and (c) disseminated infection [20, 30]. Neonates have the highest frequency of CNS infection of any HSV-infected population. If untreated, neonatal herpes undergoes dissemination or develops into CNS infection in more than 70 % of cases with an overall rate of death of 65 %; less than 20 % of survivors with CNS infection develop normally. Skin lesions may be absent in infants until well into the course of disease [31]. In the pediatric population, HSE most commonly occurs under the age of 3, particularly in children aged 3–12 months [32, 33].

The classical clinical presentation of HSE in children consists of fever (>38.5 C), altered level of consciousness, and focal seizures. Focal febrile seizures in the context of a nonspecific febrile disease and soon turning into status epilepticus are the first neurological symptoms in most children under the age of 3 (Rozenberg 2013). Subacute or milder forms of HSE are common in children.

The acute opercular syndrome, characterized by a disturbance of voluntary control of the facio-linguo-glosso-pharyngeal muscles leading to orofacial palsy, dysarthria, and dysphagia, may be the initial neurological manifestation of HSE in children [34, 35]. Its occurrence in children is probably due to the high frequency of extra-temporal brain lesions occurring in this patient group [36].

Diagnosis

HSE is a medical emergency that requires prompt diagnosis and therapy; yet, both are often delayed for several reasons. First, clinical presentation is nonspecific and may be mistaken for stroke, epilepsy, nonspecific delirium, or a primary psychiatric disorder. Most patients have serological evidence of prior infection with HSV-1, consistent with reactivation disease. Furthermore, CSF cell count is normal in 5–10 % of patients, particularly in children, and early in the infection neuroimaging may be normal and DNA detection negative [37].

We will review the diagnostic aids for HSE.

Electroencephalography (EEG)

The EEG shows background slowing and frequent periodic lateralized epileptiform discharges (PLEDs) over the temporal lobe (Fig. 5.1). PLEDs are not specific for HSE and are present from day 2 to day 14 after disease onset [38]. The severity of EEG abnormalities correlates with prognosis. EEG is also useful to identify non-convulsive seizures, which occur in both HSE and other encephalopathies [39]. EEG has a high sensitivity (84 %) but low specificity (32 %) for the diagnosis of herpes simplex encephalitis [40].

Neuroimaging

Initial computed tomography (CT) scan of the brain shows changes consistent with HSE in 25–80 % of patients, mostly over the temporal and frontal lobes (Fig. 5.2a). They include contrast-enhancing, hypodense lesions with mass effect, scattered hemorrhages. Follow-up scans demonstrate more widespread abnormalities with contralateral temporal lobe, insulae, and cingulate gyrus involvement [29, 41]. Early CT scan also helps in detecting mass lesions that could represent a risk for lumbar puncture and in indicating an alternative diagnosis. One study showed that 2 of 21 patients (10 %) with suspected encephalitis had a cerebrovascular event detected by CT scan [42].

Magnetic resonance imaging (MRI) is more sensitive and specific than CT and is the choice in patients with suspected HSE [43] (Fig. 5.2b). Ninety percent of patients with PCR-proven HSE have MRI abnormalities [41].

Early findings include gyral edema (T1-weighted sequences) and high signal intensities over the medial temporal lobe and cingulate gyrus (T2, FLAIR, and diffusion-weighted (DWI) sequences), often with foci of hemorrhage. Bilateral, asymmetrical temporal lobe and cingulate gyrus involvement is nearly pathognomonic of HSE but is a late development [43]. DWI sequences are very sensitive to early changes [44, 45].

Neonatal HSV-2 encephalitis causes more widespread abnormalities than HSV-1 encephalitis, with periventricular white matter involvement and sparing of the medial temporal and inferior frontal lobes [46].

Cerebrospinal Fluid (CSF)

CSF analysis is essential in diagnosing encephalitis, and lumbar puncture only be delayed in the presence of formal contraindications, in which case antiviral therapy should be empirically started.

In adults with HSE, the CSF opening pressure is moderately elevated, and there is a lymphocytic CSF pleocytosis (10–500 cells per mm^3, average 100 cells per mm^3), mildly increased proteins, and normal glucose [41]. Occasionally, polynuclear cells predominate, particularly in immunocompromised and children.

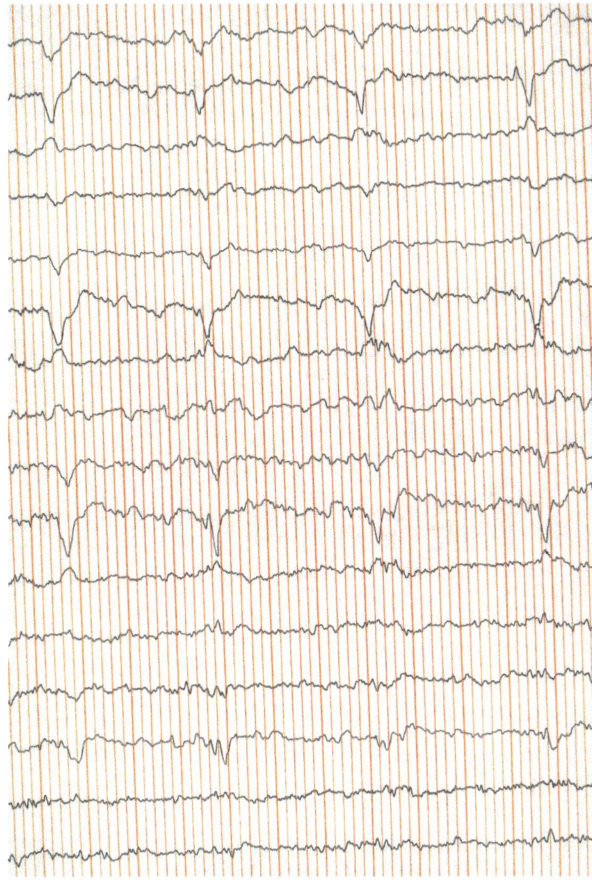

Fig. 5.1 EEG of a patient with herpes simplex type 1 encephalitis. Note the presence of slow right temporal lobe discharges over a moderately slow background activity. The same patient as in Fig. 5.2

Pleocytosis is absent in 5–10 % of adults with proven HSE [29, 41], particularly early in the illness, in infants, in immunocompromised, and in patients taking tumor necrosis factor (TNF-alpha) inhibitors [47]. When the initial CSF is normal, a subsequent sample 24–48 h later is likely to be abnormal [29, 41]. Red blood cells are present in the CSF of 50 % of patients reflecting the hemorrhagic nature of HSE. Low glucose is uncommon and may suggest an alternative diagnosis [48].

Virological Diagnosis

The gold standard for diagnosis is the detection of herpes simplex virus DNA in the CSF by polymerase chain reaction (PCR). CSF PCR for HSV between days 2 and10 of illness has an overall sensitivity and specificity >95 % in immunocompetent adults [49]. Although HSV PCR may be negative in the first few days of illness, a second CSF taken 3–7 days later will often be positive, even with acyclovir treatment [50], and remains detectable for at least 2–4 weeks. The use of PCR has

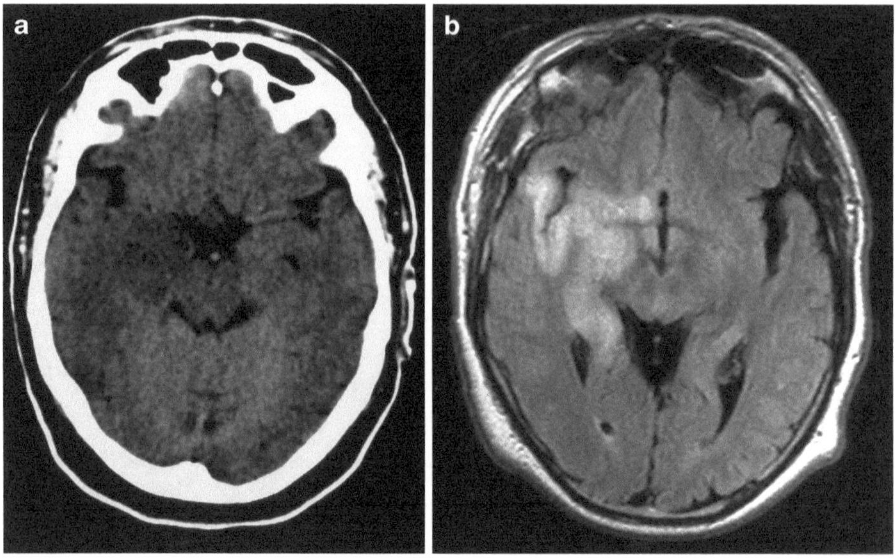

Fig. 5.2 Neuroimaging of a patient with herpes simplex type 1 encephalitis. Note the hyperintense lesion involving the right temporal lobe. Brain CT scan (*left panel* **a**) and brain MRI (FLAIR sequence, *right panel* **b**)

allowed the identification of atypical forms of HSE, including brainstem encephalitis, myelitis, and diffuse encephalitis without temporal lobe involvement [49]. Negative PCR results have been associated with CSF containing <10 cells/mm^3 and low protein levels, a situation more frequent in the pediatric population [32], where PCR sensitivity is 75–100 %.

Quantification of viral load in the CSF has been estimated between10^2 and 10^7 HSV genomes/ml, with no apparent correlation between initial load and prognosis [51], though a lack of decline in the viral load after treatment correlates with a poor outcome [5].

Intrathecal synthesis of anti-HSV IgG also has diagnostic value [10], particularly in patients in whom an earlier CSF was not taken or was not tested for HSV by PCR and in atypical forms of the disease. Intrathecal synthesis of HSV-specific IgG antibodies is detected after 10–14 days of illness, peaks after 1 month, and persists for years. Although titers of CSF and serum antibodies to HSV increase in most cases of HSE, they rarely do before 10 days of illness and thus are not helpful in early diagnosis [52]. Intrathecal immune responses may be abrogated by early antiviral therapy.

Viral culture of CSF is rarely positive in patients with brain biopsy-proven HSV encephalitis and is not a useful diagnostic tool.

Brain Biopsy

Prior to the availability of PCR testing, brain biopsy was the only accurate diagnostic test but nowadays, it is rarely performed. It may be useful in patients with suspected HSE who are PCR negative and in those who deteriorate despite acyclovir.

In dubious cases, it can identify potentially treatable mimickers of encephalitis. In one series, brain biopsy revealed an alternative diagnosis (treatable in 50 % of cases) in one-fifth of patients with suspected HSE [53].

The histopathological basis of HSE is the association of damage to the parenchyma, reactive gliosis, and inflammatory cellular infiltration. Macroscopically, the brain shows necrotic bilateral, asymmetrical lesions of the temporal and orbital cortices. Microscopically, necrosis is associated with diffuse inflammation and perivascular lymphocytic infiltration [54]. Viral intranuclear inclusions are inconstant, and viral antigens are detectable only at early stages [55]. Later, gliosis and microglial proliferation develop. Viral DNA is detectable in brain tissue [56].

Differential Diagnosis

Many infectious and noninfectious conditions can mimic HSE. In a retrospective study of 432 patients who underwent brain biopsy for a presumed diagnosis of HSE, 45 % had a final diagnosis of HSE, 22 % had other identifiable causes of their symptoms, and 33 % remained undiagnosed [53]. Infectious encephalitis cannot be separated on clinical grounds. Among cases with biopsy-proven HSE, there are no distinguishing clinical characteristics with other encephalitis.

HSV-1, varicella–zoster virus, Epstein–Barr virus, mumps virus, measles virus, and enteroviruses are responsible for most cases of sporadic viral encephalitis in immunocompetent individuals [1]. This also depends on geographic and environmental factors: West Nile virus has become an important cause of viral encephalitis in the USA. Nonviral infectious causes of encephalitis include tuberculosis, rickettsial disease, and trypanosomiasis. Epidemiological and demographic features, such as prevalent or emergent infections in the community, occupation, a history of travel, and animal contacts, may provide helpful clues.

There are postinfectious and noninfectious encephalitis that occur without direct brain infection. Acute disseminated encephalomyelitis is an example of postinfectious encephalitis, more frequent in the young. Noninfectious causes include antibody-associated encephalitis, often paraneoplastic [40].

Encephalitis should be differentiated from encephalopathy, the latter defined as a diffuse disruption of brain function without a direct structural or inflammatory process. It can be caused by drug intoxication, systemic organ dysfunction (e.g., liver, kidney, pancreas), or systemic infection. In contrast to encephalitis, CSF values are usually normal and there is no parenchyma inflammation on neuroimaging.

Treatment

Acyclovir remains the therapy of choice for HSE since two randomized trials in the 1980s showed that it reduced the mortality to <20–30 % while vidarabine had a mortality rate in excess of 70 %. The functional status was significantly better in the acyclovir-treated patients [57, 58].

Acyclovir is an acyclic nucleoside analog that is a substrate for HSV-specified thymidine kinase and is selectively phosphorylated by HSV-infected cells to acyclovir monophosphate and then by cellular enzymes to acyclovir triphosphate, a competitive inhibitor of viral DNA polymerase. Acyclovir triphosphate is incorporated into the growing DNA chain of the virus causing chain termination. Acyclovir has potent in vitro activity against both HSV-1 and HSV-2. Because acyclovir is only effective in stopping viral replication, it should be given early to prevent extensive replication and CNS damage. Patients with advanced age, a reduced Glasgow coma score, or delay of >48 h between admission and treatment [41] have the worst outcome.

Acyclovir dosing in the randomized trials was 10 mg/kg/8 h a day for 10 days. However, relapses after 10 days of treatment may occur [59], likely due to immune-mediated, inflammatory reaction to the infection [57, 59, 60]. Nonetheless, there is evidence for continuing viral replication in some cases, including the appearance of new lesions distant from the initial site of HSE and positive CSF PCR [18, 41, 60]. The presence of choreoathetoid movements during relapses conveys a poor prognosis and might be due to an immune-mediated process [61].

Thus, most clinicians extend its use to 14–21 days in confirmed cases, and some advocate repeating a CSF examination at 14–21 days, and continuing treatment until the CSF PCR becomes negative [25]. Later relapses occasionally occur [41]. The duration of therapy for immunosuppressed patients is 21 days [29]. Dosing for neonatal HSE is 60 mg/kg/day. Pediatric HSE suffers clinical relapses in 30 % of cases.

Interestingly, it has recently been reported that relapses of HSV-1 encephalitis may trigger an autoimmune-mediated encephalitis against NMDA receptor that will respond to steroid therapy and not to acyclovir [62].

Because CSF levels of acyclovir average only 30–50 % of plasma levels, the dose of acyclovir used for treatment of CNS infection (30 mg/kg/day) is double than that used for the treatment of mucocutaneous or visceral disease (15 mg/kg/day). Given orally, acyclovir does not achieve adequate CSF levels; however, its valine ester, valacyclovir, has good oral bioavailability and is converted to acyclovir after absorption [63]. Valacyclovir may have a role in patients with HSV detectable in the CSF after 2–3 weeks [9].

Acyclovir should be empirically started upon suspicion of HSE and continued until a definite alternative diagnosis is established. Otherwise, it may be continued for 10 days, even if PCR is negative. One case of HSE with normal cerebral MRI scan has been reported, where the diagnosis of HSE was made by PCR from a CSF sample obtained on the day of admission that became negative after 8 days of acyclovir therapy [64].

Acyclovir is excreted unchanged in the urine, so renal impairment can precipitate acyclovir toxicity, and in turn high-dose acyclovir may result in renal failure. Transient renal insufficiency is the main side effect, usually caused by crystallization of the compound in the renal parenchyma. It manifests after 4 days of intravenous therapy and occurs in 20 % of patients [65]. Slow drug administration (>1 h) and good hydration can partly avoid it.

Occasionally, acyclovir induces a toxic encephalopathy that causes confusion with the encephalitis itself. Concomitant renal dysfunction may point to this side effect. Other rare adverse events include hepatitis and bone marrow failure.

Acyclovir resistance occurs in the immunosuppressed, organ transplant recipients, and HIV patients. It affects 5–25 % of immunocompromised patients receiving long-term prophylactic treatment with acyclovir [66]. Foscarnet, an inhibitor of viral DNA polymerases by binding to the pyrophosphate binding site, is recommended in acyclovir-resistant HSE (60 mg/kg intravenously infused over 1 h every 8 h for 3 weeks). Foscarnet can cause a dose-related, reversible renal impairment, electrolyte wasting, nausea, paresthesias, and seizures. Cidofovir, a nucleoside analog that is phosphorylated to its active compound by cellular enzymes [67], is the second-line alternative. Cidofovir can be administered once weekly, is nephrotoxic, and should be administered with probenecid to decrease nephrotoxicity. However, acyclovir-resistant HSE has not been reported in immunocompetent patients, and second-line drugs should be used only in patients with clinically suspected HSE who continue to deteriorate despite acyclovir therapy with a reactive CSF in whom alternative possibilities have been excluded [29].

Corticosteroids are often used, especially in patients with marked cerebral edema, brain shift, or raised intracranial pressure, but their role remains controversial because of their potential to facilitate viral replication. A retrospective analysis of 45 patients with HSE showed that older age, lower Glasgow coma score on admission, and lack of administration of corticosteroids were significant independent predictors of a poor outcome [68].

Surgical decompression for HSE may be indicated in selected cases for impending herniation or increased intracranial pressure refractory to medical management, improving the outcome in individual cases [69]. Intracerebral hematoma as a complication of HSE is rare, with less than 25 cases reported in the literature. Early surgical decompression can lead to a good neurological outcome [70, 71].

Supportive therapy is also essential in the management of HSE patients, who should have access to intensive care unit equipped with mechanical ventilators. Careful attention must be paid to seizure control, respiratory function, cardiac rhythm, fluid balance, prevention of deep vein thrombosis and aspiration pneumonia, and medical management of raised intracranial pressure and secondary bacterial infections.

Prognosis

Despite acyclovir therapy, the current outcome of HSE remains unsatisfactory with high mortality and morbidity rates in adults and children [5, 33, 72]. Almost half of HSE survivors are left with serious disability [73]. Early treatment, immunocompetent state, young age, and normal level of consciousness associate with improved outcome [28].

HSE sequelae include epileptic seizures, neuropsychiatric deficits, mood and behavioral disorders, developmental and learning delay in children, and residual motor or visual deficits. They often result in hospital readmission [5].

Long-term follow-up of treated patients may show residual neurological deficits [74], including dysnomia and impaired learning of verbal and visual material, despite normal performances on standard mental status examination [75].

Postencephalitic epilepsy is often refractory to medical treatment, contributing to an unfavorable clinical outcome. Seizures during acute disease represent the main risk for the development of postencephalitic epilepsy. They occur in 40–65 % of patients with HSE and may be the presenting symptom [39]. This high rate is in part due to the predilection of HSV for areas highly epileptogenic such as the mesial temporal lobes and the orbitofrontal cortex. Epilepsy surgery is a potential treatment option but only in a subgroup of patients suffering from unilateral mesiotemporal lobe epilepsy and congruent neuropsychological impairment.

Rehabilitation

Although there are few studies on the outcome of rehabilitation following encephalitis [29], all patients should have access to rehabilitation services. A multidisciplinary assessment and rehabilitation are desirable, including specialists in neuropsychology, neuropsychiatry, speech and language therapy, physical therapy, and occupational therapy. Access to specialists in brain injury rehabilitation is key to recovery in many cases. The support provided by voluntary sector organizations is helpful for these patients and their families [9].

Varicella–Zoster Virus (VZV)

Primary infection with VZV causes varicella (chickenpox), and once the illness resolves, the virus remains latent in the dorsal root ganglia, usually for a long period of time. The virus can reactivate later, often with advanced age or immunosuppression, coinciding with a decline in viral immunity, resulting in a painful dermatomal rash (shingles). Zoster may be complicated by postherpetic neuralgia as well as meningoencephalitis, myelitis, retinal necrosis, and vasculopathy, including a multifocal VZV vasculopathy with temporal artery infection [76, 77].

Hematogenous VZV dissemination gives rise to small- or large-vessel vasculitis. The latter is a granulomatous angiitis that occurs weeks or months after the appearance of zoster vesicles in the first branch of the trigeminal nerve (zoster ophthalmicus) in immunocompetent individuals and may result in ischemic or hemorrhagic stroke. Small-vessel vasculitis appears in immunosuppressed subjects without a preceding skin lesion and causes small ischemic, hemorrhagic, and demyelinating lesions located on the gray–white matter interface of the brain. Finally, periventriculitis in immunosuppressed patients may occur as a consequence of ventricular viral dissemination or of ischemic or demyelinating lesions in the periventricular region and is often associated to hydrocephalus [78].

The clinical manifestations in zoster encephalitis are similar to other viral encephalitis. CSF examination shows a mild lymphocytic pleocytosis (around 100 cells per mm^3) with increased proteins and normal glucose. Diagnosis is confirmed by the detection of viral genome in the CSF by PCR or by demonstrating the presence of specific IgM in the CSF or of an increase in the ratio of viral antibodies in the CSF to that in the blood [76]. Shingles episodes are often accompanied by asymptomatic CSF pleocytosis, as revealed by lumbar punctures performed for other reasons, and this likely reflects a more frequent CNS involvement than clinically suspected in varicella–zoster virus infection.

The incidence of varicella–zoster virus encephalitis is estimated in 1–2 individuals per every 10,000 cases of varicella. The risk of viral reactivation increases with age, immunosuppressive states, and HIV infection [79, 80]. Despite a lack of randomized therapy trials, the use of intravenous acyclovir (10 mg/kg/8 h) is recommended for 14–21 days. When vasculitis is present, steroids are usually added.

Cytomegalovirus

Cytomegalovirus (CMV), another member of the Herpesviridae family, causes encephalitis in immunosuppressed patients, particularly with HIV infection. In fact, CMV is the commonest opportunistic infection in AIDS patients. Patients with CNS complications by CMV often had prior CMV infection, most commonly retinitis, but encephalitis can be the presenting CNS manifestation in AIDS. More commonly, CMV causes a lower-limb ascending polyradiculopathy with marked involvement of the cauda equina and lumbosacral nerve roots. It also results in meningoencephalitis with evidence of ventriculitis with subependymal enhancement as shown by MRI. Presentation as a Wernicke's encephalopathy-like syndrome has been reported [81].

Therapy is often disappointing and includes intravenous ganciclovir (5 mg/12 h) for 2 weeks followed by a maintenance dose of 5 mg/kg/day for one more week. Some experts recommend adding foscarnet (60 mg/kg every 8 h or 90 mg/kg intravenously every 12 h) during the first 2 weeks. Therapy in immunosuppressed patients should continue for 6 weeks.

Enterovirus

They are RNA viruses of the Picornaviridae family transmitted by the fecal–oral route and through respiratory secretions and are the agents of hand-foot-and-mouth disease, skin rash, myocarditis and pericarditis, and pleurodynia, among others.

As for the CNS complications, they are responsible for 10–20 % of encephalitis cases in which an etiologic agent is identified [1]. They more commonly cause aseptic meningitis in the summer.

The initial classification divided them into five subgenera: polioviruses, group A coxsackieviruses, group B coxsackieviruses, echoviruses, and newer enteroviruses. A classification based on RNA homology within the capsid divides the nonpolioviruses into four classes, designated A through D.

Of the 96 current human serotypes, the most commonly implicated in encephalitis are echoviruses (6, 9, and18) and coxsackieviruses (A9, B2, and B5). They usually cause a benign disorder with nonspecific clinical manifestations, although infection in agammaglobulinemia patients may be severe (echovirus 11 is usually responsible). CSF examination reveals a moderate lymphocytic pleocytosis (usually < 1,000 cells per mm^3) with normal glucose and slightly elevated proteins. Brain MRI is often normal or shows meningeal contrast enhancement. Confusion with partially treated bacterial meningitis is frequent, so antibiotics should be maintained until CSF culture results are obtained.

Epidemics of infection due to enterovirus 71 have been identified in Taiwan and other Southeast Asian countries, Eastern Europe, and the USA [82].

Enterovirus 71 has also been associated with severe neurological syndromes, such as acute flaccid paralysis and bulbar and brainstem encephalitis that may be fatal. Children with EV71 infection and CNS involvement often have long-term neurological sequelae and delayed neurodevelopment [83].

Arboviruses: Tick-Borne Encephalitis

Arboviruses (arthropod-borne virus) are transmitted by ticks or mosquitoes and cause heterogeneous clinical presentations that include asymptomatic infection, febrile syndrome, hemorrhagic fevers, and meningoencephalitis [84]. Although most arbovirus infections are mild or asymptomatic, they represent the most frequent cause of epidemic encephalitis worldwide. After replicating in the vectors, arboviruses spread to salivary glands and are inoculated by vector bite.

Arboviral infections occur in sporadic or epidemic zoonoses that involve birds and rodents as reservoirs. Humans are accidentally infected and are usually dead-end hosts. There are over 150 arboviruses that are pathogenic to humans and belong to different RNA virus families that include the Togaviridae, Reoviridae, Bunyaviridae, and Flaviviridae (Table 5.2).

The neurological complications of arboviral infections include aseptic meningitis or encephalitis, and the diagnosis is mainly based on the serological demonstration of specific antibodies in serum and CSF. The presence of specific IgM or a rise in the titer of IgG is highly suggestive of active infection in paired serum specimens. Viral genome can be detected by PCR in the CSF of patients with certain arboviruses [85]. Viral isolation is possible in laboratory animals or in tissue culture depending on the viral load in the blood. There is no specific therapy for arboviral

Table 5.2 Differential diagnosis of herpesvirus encephalitis

Acute viral encephalitis	
Sporadic	
Herpesviruses	Varicella–zoster virus
	Epstein–Barr virus
	Cytomegalovirus
	Human herpesvirus 6
	Human herpesvirus 7
Enteroviruses	Enterovirus 70
	Enterovirus 71
	Poliovirus
	Coxsackieviruses
	Echoviruses
	Parechovirus
Paramyxovirus	Measles virus
	Mumps virus
Others	Influenza virus
	Adenovirus
	Erythrovirus B19
	Rubella virus
	Choriomeningitis virus
	HIV
Arthropod-borne and zoonotic	
Flaviviruses	West Nile virus
	Japanese encephalitis virus
	Tick-borne encephalitis virus
	Dengue viruses
Alphaviruses	Western equine encephalitis virus
	Eastern equine encephalitis virus
	Venezuelan equine encephalitis virus
	Chikungunya virus
Others	Lacrosse virus
	Colorado tick fever virus
	Rabies virus
	Chandipura virus
	Nipah virus
	Toscana virus
Nonviral encephalitis	
Bacteria	
Mycoplasma pneumoniae	
Rickettsiae	
Coxiella burnetii	
Tropheryma whipplei	
Bartonella henselae	
Brucella spp.	
Listeria monocytogenes	
Treponema pallidum	
Borrelia burgdorferi	
Nocardiosis	
Actinomycosis	

(continued)

Table 5.2 (continued)

Parasites	
Trypanosoma brucei	
Naegleria fowleri	
Balamuthia mandrillaris	
Angiostrongylus spp.	
Fungi	
Coccidioidomycosis	
Histoplasmosis	
Blastomycosis	
Para-/postinfectious encephalitis	
Acute disseminated encephalomyelitis (ADEM)	
Acute hemorrhagic leukoencephalopathy (AHLE)	
Acute necrotizing encephalitis (ANE) in children	
Bickerstaff's encephalitis	
Noninfectious causes	
Vascular	Systemic lupus
	Primary angiitis of the central nervous system
	Subarachnoid hemorrhage
	Subdural hematoma
	Ischemic stroke
	Behcet's disease
Neoplastic	Paraneoplastic encephalitis
Metabolic encephalopathy	Hepatic encephalopathy
	Renal encephalopathy
	Hypoglycemia
	Toxics (alcohol, drugs)
	Septic encephalopathy
	Mitochondrial diseases
Antibody-mediated encephalitis	VGKC complex
	NMDA encephalitis
	Encephalitis lethargica
Others (*may mimic the clinical picture*)	
Cysticercosis	
Trichinosis	
Cryptococcosis	
Trichinosis	
Neurosarcoidosis	
Reye's syndrome	
Primary brain tumor	
Brain metastases	
Mycobacterium tuberculosis	
Brain abscess	
Brain empyema	
Parameningeal infections	
Endocarditis	

Modified from Ref. [9]

infections, and arthropod-bite prevention and vaccination when possible are the most effective measures.

Flaviviruses are particularly important to human disease, since they include many pathogenic agents, including West Nile virus, Japanese encephalitis virus, and Dengue virus. All these infections are discussed together with other tropical encephalitis in Chap. 6. We will center here on tick-borne encephalitis, which is also caused by a flavivirus frequent in Europe, particularly in Russia, Austria, and other countries of Central and Western Europe.

Tick-borne encephalitis virus is transmitted by Ixodes ticks, the same vector that transmits the spirochetal agent of Lyme disease. Infection occurs most often in summer, when tick activity is high and exposure (leisure activities) is more frequent.

The disease follows a biphasic course. After an incubation period of about 8 days (range 4–28 days) following the tick bite, viremia occurs and is accompanied by fever, headache, and malaise. Tick bite can go unnoticed and serology at this point is negative, complicating the diagnostic suspicion. After an asymptomatic period of 1 week, encephalitis develops, sometimes accompanied by flaccid paralysis. At this point specific, IgM against the virus should be present in the serum, and IgG starts to rise. A serum sample taken 4 weeks later will show a three- to fourfold rise in the IgG titer. The CSF shows a moderate pleocytosis (usually less than 100 cells/mm^3), initially polymorphonuclear and later lymphocytic, with normal glucose and increased proteins.

Brain MRI shows abnormalities in 20 % of patients, more often in the cerebellum, thalamus, caudate nuclei, and brainstem. The electroencephalogram shows nonspecific abnormalities.

Some patients develop a flaccid paralysis that bears some resemblance to poliomyelitis, although in this case, upper limbs are preferentially involved in contrast to poliovirus infection.

There are successful vaccines, although their effectiveness has not been shown in controlled studies.

Postinfectious Encephalitis or Encephalomyelitis (PE)

This condition is characterized by CNS inflammation and demyelination after viral infection but without the evidence of viral presence or persistence that characterizes viral encephalitis. It also occurs after vaccination and less commonly after infection with other pathogens [86]. In the California Encephalitis Project, which evaluated over 1,500 patients with encephalitis, 8 % were thought to represent a postinfectious disease process [2].

PE is supposed to be caused by an abnormal immune reaction against CNS self-antigens in response to the eliciting pathogen, and therefore, no evidence of viral presence in the CNS by CSF PCR can be demonstrated. An etiologic agent is only seldom identified, usually serological or clinical demonstration of prior viral infection.

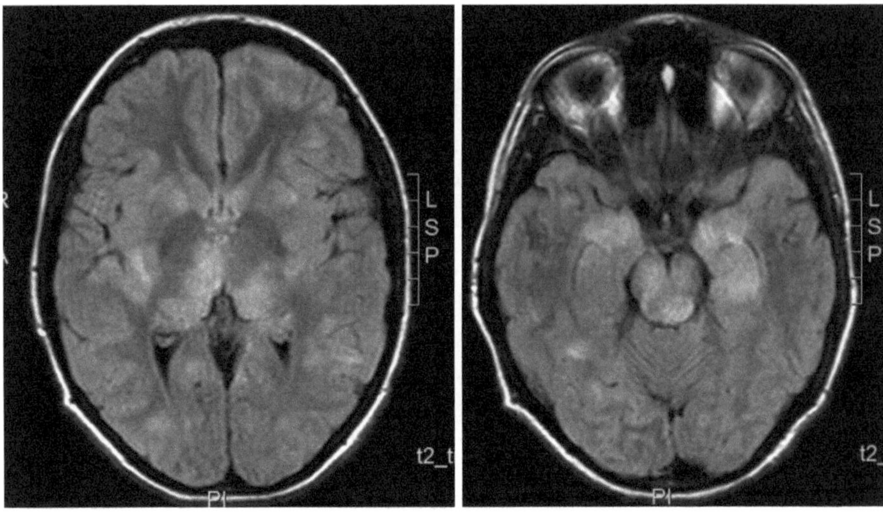

Fig. 5.3 Brain MRI (T2-weighted sequences) from a 16-year-old girl with acute demyelinating encephalomyelitis following a nonspecific upper respiratory infection. There was an extensive involvement of the gray and white matter both supra- and infratentorial. She presented with fever, seizures and decreased level of consciousness, and CSF lymphocytic pleocytosis. The clinical picture and MRI abnormalities normalized over several months after initial intensive steroid therapy

PE is most frequent in children, often associated to childhood exanthematic diseases, and its clinical spectrum is protean, encompassing acute disseminated encephalomyelitis or acute hemorrhagic leukoencephalitis. Importantly, adult patients with PE often present with typical features of acute infection of the CNS.

The CSF in PE shows slightly increased protein levels, normal CSF glucose levels, and sterile cultures. It shows normal values in up to one-third of patients. MRI shows diffuse areas of abnormal signal involving the brain, brainstem, and spinal cord (Fig. 5.3).

Treatment of severe cases includes pulses of methylprednisolone (1 g daily for 3–5 days) followed by oral steroids (starting 1 g/kg daily and tapering for 4–6 weeks) [86].

PE appears as a complication of rubella and mumps, usually as a reversible encephalitis, and less often in the form of Guillain–Barré syndrome or myelitis. Measles complications are discussed in Chap. 6.

Varicella–zoster infection in children can be complicated by an immune-mediated acute cerebellar ataxia, which occurs in approximately 1 in 4,000 infections. Ataxia appears after the cutaneous lesion and has no specific therapy.

Human herpesvirus 6 infections are responsible for febrile seizures in infancy and rarely can be complicated with encephalitis.

Epstein–Barr virus infection occasionally complicates with acute disseminated encephalomyelitis, Guillain–Barré syndrome, or cerebellitis, among other neurological problems.

Rotavirus infection can also be complicated with encephalitis, seizures, and cerebellitis.

Neurological complications of influenza appear more often in young children, particularly from Asia, and include myelitis, seizures, Guillain–Barré syndrome, and encephalitis.

Reversible Splenial Lesion Syndrome

The presence of transient lesions involving the splenium of the corpus callosum (SCC) has been recently described in patients with encephalitis or encephalopathy of varied etiology, including infections, high-altitude cerebral edema, metabolic disorders (hypoglycemia and hypernatremia), or antiepileptic drug withdrawal [87].

Most patients with this disorder are children or young adults from Japan. When identified, the most common infectious agents were influenza virus, Epstein–Barr virus, rotavirus, and a miscellaneous of less common bacterial pathogens.

It is characterized by the presence of round, nonenhancing lesions involving exclusively the splenium of the corpus callosum as revealed by magnetic resonance imaging. The lesions are hyperintense on T2-weighted, FLAIR, and DWI sequences, and hypointense on T1 sequences and on the ADC map, findings consistent with cytotoxic edema.

The pathophysiology is unclear, and it represents a benign disorder except in those patients with an underlying severe disorder.

References

1. Kupila L, Vuorinen T, Vainionpaa R, Hukkanen V, Marttila RJ, Kotilainen P. Etiology of aseptic meningitis and encephalitis in an adult population. Neurology. 2006;66:75–80.
2. Glaser CA, Honarmand S, Anderson LJ, et al. Beyond viruses: clinical profiles and etiologies associated with encephalitis. Clin Infect Dis. 2006;43:1565–77.
3. Whitley RJ. Herpes simplex encephalitis: adolescents and adults. Antiviral Res. 2006;71:141–8.
4. Olson LC, Buescher EL, Artenstein MS, Parkman PD. Herpesvirus infections of the human central nervous system. N Engl J Med. 1967;277:1271–7.
5. Hjalmarsson A, Blomqvist P, Skoldenberg B. Herpes simplex encephalitis in Sweden, 1990-2001: incidence, morbidity, and mortality. Clin Infect Dis. 2007;45:875–80.
6. Huppatz C, Durrheim DN, Levi C, et al. Etiology of encephalitis in Australia, 1990-2007. Emerg Infect Dis. 2009;15:1359–65.
7. Huppatz C, Kelly PM, Levi C, Dalton C, Williams D, Durrheim DN. Encephalitis in Australia, 1979-2006: trends and aetiologies. Commun Dis Intell Q Rep. ;33:192–7.
8. Whitley RJ, Kimberlin DW. Herpes simplex encephalitis: children and adolescents. Semin Pediatr Infect Dis. 2005;16:17–23.
9. Solomon T, Michael BD, Smith PE, et al. Management of suspected viral encephalitis in adults – Association of British Neurologists and British Infection Association National Guidelines. J Infect. 2012;64:347–73.

10. Nahmias AJ, Lee FK, Beckman-Nahmias S. Sero-epidemiological and -sociological patterns of herpes simplex virus infection in the world. Scand J Infect Dis Suppl. 1990;69:19–36.
11. Steiner I, Kennedy PG. Herpes simplex virus latent infection in the nervous system. J Neurovirol. 1995;1:19–29.
12. Davis LE, Johnson RT. An explanation for the localization of herpes simplex encephalitis? Ann Neurol. 1979;5:2–5.
13. Fraser NW, Lawrence WC, Wroblewska Z, Gilden DH, Koprowski H. Herpes simplex type 1 DNA in human brain tissue. Proc Natl Acad Sci U S A. 1981;78:6461–5.
14. Whitley R, Lakeman AD, Nahmias A, Roizman B. Dna restriction-enzyme analysis of herpes simplex virus isolates obtained from patients with encephalitis. N Engl J Med. 1982; 307:1060–2.
15. Koelle DM, Corey L. Recent progress in herpes simplex virus immunobiology and vaccine research. Clin Microbiol Rev. 2003;16:96–113.
16. Kapoor AK, Buckmaster A, Nash AA, Field HJ, Wildy P. Role of neutralizing antibodies and T-cells in pathogenesis of herpes simplex virus infection in congenitally athymic mice. Immunol Lett. 1982;5:259–65.
17. Sancho-Shimizu V, Zhang SY, Abel L, et al. Genetic susceptibility to herpes simplex virus 1 encephalitis in mice and humans. Curr Opin Allergy Clin Immunol. 2007;7:495–505.
18. Rozenberg F. Acute viral encephalitis. Handb Clin Neurol. 2013;112:1171–81.
19. Casrouge A, Zhang SY, Eidenschenk C, et al. Herpes simplex virus encephalitis in human UNC-93B deficiency. Science. 2006;314:308–12.
20. Kimberlin DW. Neonatal herpes simplex infection. Clin Microbiol Rev. 2004;17:1–13.
21. Brown ZA, Wald A, Morrow RA, Selke S, Zeh J, Corey L. Effect of serologic status and cesarean delivery on transmission rates of herpes simplex virus from mother to infant. JAMA. 2003;289:203–9.
22. Kimura H, Futamura M, Kito H, et al. Detection of viral DNA in neonatal herpes simplex virus infections: frequent and prolonged presence in serum and cerebrospinal fluid. J Infect Dis. 1991;164:289–93.
23. Fisher CM. Hypomanic symptoms caused by herpes simplex encephalitis. Neurology. 1996;47:1374–8.
24. Fodor PA, Levin MJ, Weinberg A, Sandberg E, Sylman J, Tyler KL. Atypical herpes simplex virus encephalitis diagnosed by PCR amplification of viral DNA from CSF. Neurology. 1998;51:554–9.
25. Solomon T, Hart IJ, Beeching NJ. Viral encephalitis: a clinician's guide. Pract Neurol. 2007;7:288–305.
26. Steiner I. Herpes simplex virus encephalitis: new infection or reactivation? Curr Opin Neurol. 2011;24:268–74.
27. Grover D, Newsholme W, Brink N, Manji H, Miller R. Herpes simplex virus infection of the central nervous system in human immunodeficiency virus-type 1-infected patients. Int J STD AIDS. 2004;15:597–600.
28. Tan IL, McArthur JC, Venkatesan A, Nath A. Atypical manifestations and poor outcome of herpes simplex encephalitis in the immunocompromised. Neurology. 2012;79:2125–32.
29. Steiner I, Budka H, Chaudhuri A, et al. Viral meningoencephalitis: a review of diagnostic methods and guidelines for management. Eur J Neurol. 2010;17:999–e57.
30. Corey L, Wald A. Maternal and neonatal herpes simplex virus infections. N Engl J Med. 2009;361:1376–85.
31. Whitley R, Arvin A, Prober C, et al. Predictors of morbidity and mortality in neonates with herpes simplex virus infections. The National Institute of Allergy and Infectious Diseases Collaborative Antiviral Study Group. N Engl J Med. 1991;324:450–4.
32. De Tiege X, Heron B, Lebon P, Ponsot G, Rozenberg F. Limits of early diagnosis of herpes simplex encephalitis in children: a retrospective study of 38 cases. Clin Infect Dis. 2003;36:1335–9.
33. Elbers JM, Bitnun A, Richardson SE, et al. A 12-year prospective study of childhood herpes simplex encephalitis: is there a broader spectrum of disease? Pediatrics. 2007;119:e399–407.

34. De Tiege X, Rozenberg F, Burlot K, Gaudelus J, Ponsot G, Heron B. Herpes simplex encephalitis: diagnostic problems and late relapse. Dev Med Child Neurol. 2006;48:60–3.
35. Garcia-Ribes A, Martinez-Gonzalez MJ, Prats-Vinas JM. Suspected herpes encephalitis and opercular syndrome in childhood. Pediatr Neurol. 2007;36:202–6.
36. De Tiege X, Rozenberg F, Heron B. The spectrum of herpes simplex encephalitis in children. Eur J Paediatr Neurol. 2008;12:72–81.
37. Sabah M, Mulcahy J, Zeman A. Herpes simplex encephalitis. BMJ. 2012;344:e3166.
38. Lai CW, Gragasin ME. Electroencephalography in herpes simplex encephalitis. J Clin Neurophysiol. 1988;5:87–103.
39. Misra UK, Tan CT, Kalita J. Viral encephalitis and epilepsy. Epilepsia. 2008;49 Suppl 6:13–8.
40. Tuzun E, Dalmau J. Limbic encephalitis and variants: classification, diagnosis and treatment. Neurologist. 2007;13:261–71.
41. Raschilas F, Wolff M, Delatour F, et al. Outcome of and prognostic factors for herpes simplex encephalitis in adult patients: results of a multicenter study. Clin Infect Dis. 2002;35:254–60.
42. Bell DJ, Suckling R, Rothburn MM, et al. Management of suspected herpes simplex virus encephalitis in adults in a U.K. teaching hospital. Clin Med. 2009;9:231–5.
43. Marchbank ND, Howlett DC, Sallomi DF, Hughes DV. Magnetic resonance imaging is preferred in diagnosing suspected cerebral infections. BMJ. 2000;320:187–8.
44. Kuker W, Nagele T, Schmidt F, Heckl S, Herrlinger U. Diffusion-weighted MRI in herpes simplex encephalitis: a report of three cases. Neuroradiology. 2004;46:122–5.
45. McCabe K, Tyler K, Tanabe J. Diffusion-weighted MRI abnormalities as a clue to the diagnosis of herpes simplex encephalitis. Neurology. 2003;61:1015–6.
46. Hinson VK, Tyor WR. Update on viral encephalitis. Curr Opin Neurol. 2001;14:369–74.
47. Bradford RD, Pettit AC, Wright PW, et al. Herpes simplex encephalitis during treatment with tumor necrosis factor-alpha inhibitors. Clin Infect Dis. 2009;49:924–7.
48. Razavi B, Razavi M. Herpes simplex encephalitis – an atypical case. Infection. 2001;29:357–8.
49. DeBiasi RL, Kleinschmidt-DeMasters BK, Weinberg A, Tyler KL. Use of PCR for the diagnosis of herpesvirus infections of the central nervous system. J Clin Virol. 2002;25 Suppl 1:S5–11.
50. Davies NW, Brown LJ, Gonde J, et al. Factors influencing PCR detection of viruses in cerebrospinal fluid of patients with suspected CNS infections. J Neurol Neurosurg Psychiatry. 2005;76:82–7.
51. Schloss L, Falk KI, Skoog E, Brytting M, Linde A, Aurelius E. Monitoring of herpes simplex virus DNA types 1 and 2 viral load in cerebrospinal fluid by real-time PCR in patients with herpes simplex encephalitis. J Med Virol. 2009;81:1432–7.
52. Aurelius E, Johansson B, Skoldenberg B, Forsgren M. Encephalitis in immunocompetent patients due to herpes simplex virus type 1 or 2 as determined by type-specific polymerase chain reaction and antibody assays of cerebrospinal fluid. J Med Virol. 1993;39:179–86.
53. Whitley RJ, Cobbs CG, Alford Jr CA, et al. Diseases that mimic herpes simplex encephalitis. Diagnosis, presentation, and outcome. NIAD Collaborative Antiviral Study Group. JAMA. 1989;262:234–9.
54. Sobel RA, Collins AB, Colvin RB, Bhan AK. The in situ cellular immune response in acute herpes simplex encephalitis. Am J Pathol. 1986;125:332–8.
55. Esiri MM. Herpes simplex encephalitis. An immunohistological study of the distribution of viral antigen within the brain. J Neurol Sci. 1982;54:209–26.
56. Lellouch-Tubiana A, Fohlen M, Robain O, Rozenberg F. Immunocytochemical characterization of long-term persistent immune activation in human brain after herpes simplex encephalitis. Neuropathol Appl Neurobiol. 2000;26:285–94.
57. Skoldenberg B, Forsgren M. Acyclovir versus vidarabine in herpes simplex encephalitis. Scand J Infect Dis Suppl. 1985;47:89–96.
58. Whitley RJ, Alford CA, Hirsch MS, et al. Vidarabine versus acyclovir therapy in herpes simplex encephalitis. N Engl J Med. 1986;314:144–9.

59. Dennett C, Klapper PE, Cleator GM. Polymerase chain reaction in the investigation of "relapse" following herpes simplex encephalitis. J Med Virol. 1996;48:129–32.
60. VanLandingham KE, Marsteller HB, Ross GW, Hayden FG. Relapse of herpes simplex encephalitis after conventional acyclovir therapy. JAMA. 1988;259:1051–3.
61. Valencia I, Miles DK, Melvin J, et al. Relapse of herpes encephalitis after acyclovir therapy: report of two new cases and review of the literature. Neuropediatrics. 2004;35:371–6.
62. Leypoldt F, Titulaer MJ, Aguilar E, et al. Herpes simplex virus-1 encephalitis can trigger anti-NMDA receptor encephalitis: case report. Neurology. 2013;81:1637–9.
63. Lycke J, Malmestrom C, Stahle L. Acyclovir levels in serum and cerebrospinal fluid after oral administration of valacyclovir. Antimicrob Agents Chemother. 2003;47:2438–41.
64. Hollinger P, Matter L, Sturzenegger M. Normal MRI findings in herpes simplex virus encephalitis. J Neurol. 2000;247:799–801.
65. Pacheco LR, Tavares HM, Moyses Neto M, et al. Acute renal failure related to intravenous acyclovir. Rev Assoc Med Bras. 2005;51:275–8.
66. Chen Y, Scieux C, Garrait V, et al. Resistant herpes simplex virus type 1 infection: an emerging concern after allogeneic stem cell transplantation. Clin Infect Dis. 2000;31:927–35.
67. Cundy KC. Clinical pharmacokinetics of the antiviral nucleotide analogues cidofovir and adefovir. Clin Pharmacokinet. 1999;36:127–43.
68. Kamei S, Sekizawa T, Shiota H, et al. Evaluation of combination therapy using aciclovir and corticosteroid in adult patients with herpes simplex virus encephalitis. J Neurol Neurosurg Psychiatry. 2005;76:1544–9.
69. Yan HJ. Herpes simplex encephalitis: the role of surgical decompression. Surg Neurol. 2002;57:20–4.
70. Lo WB, Wilcock DJ, Carey M, Albanese E. Herpes encephalitis complicated by cerebral haemorrhage. J Neurol Neurosurg Psychiatry. 2013;84(12):1404–6.
71. Rodriguez-Sainz A, Escalza-Cortina I, Guio-Carrion L, et al. Intracerebral hematoma complicating herpes simplex encephalitis. Clin Neurol Neurosurg. 2013;115:2041–5.
72. Riancho J, Delgado-Alvarado M, Sedano MJ, Polo JM, Berciano J. Herpes simplex encephalitis: clinical presentation, neurological sequelae and new prognostic factors. Ten years of experience. Neurol Sci. 2013;34(10):1879–81.
73. Whitley RJ. Viral encephalitis. N Engl J Med. 1990;323:242–50.
74. Arciniegas DB, Anderson CA. Viral encephalitis: neuropsychiatric and neurobehavioral aspects. Curr Psychiatry Rep. ;6:372–9.
75. Gordon B, Selnes OA, Hart Jr J, Hanley DF, Whitley RJ. Long-term cognitive sequelae of acyclovir-treated herpes simplex encephalitis. Arch Neurol. 1990;47:646–7.
76. Gilden D, Cohrs RJ, Mahalingam R, Nagel MA. Varicella zoster virus vasculopathies: diverse clinical manifestations, laboratory features, pathogenesis, and treatment. Lancet Neurol. 2009;8:731–40.
77. Nagel MA, Gilden D. The challenging patient with varicella-zoster virus disease. Neurol Clin Pract. 2013;3:109–17.
78. Gilden DH, Kleinschmidt-DeMasters BK, LaGuardia JJ, Mahalingam R, Cohrs RJ. Neurologic complications of the reactivation of varicella-zoster virus. N Engl J Med. 2000;342: 635–45.
79. Cohen EJ. Prevention of herpes zoster: we need to do better. JAMA Ophthalmol. 2013;131:396–8.
80. Cohen JI. Clinical practice: herpes zoster. N Engl J Med. 2013;369:255–63.
81. Torgovnick J, Arsura EL, Lala D. Cytomegalovirus ventriculoencephalitis presenting as a Wernicke's encephalopathy-like syndrome. Neurology. 2000;55:1910–3.
82. Ho M, Chen ER, Hsu KH, et al. An epidemic of enterovirus 71 infection in Taiwan. Taiwan Enterovirus Epidemic Working Group. N Engl J Med. 1999;341:929–35.
83. Chang LY, Huang LM, Gau SS, et al. Neurodevelopment and cognition in children after enterovirus 71 infection. N Engl J Med. 2007;356:1226–34.
84. Rust RS. Human arboviral encephalitis. Semin Pediatr Neurol. 2012;19:130–51.

85. Huang C, Chatterjee NK, Grady LJ. Diagnosis of viral infections of the central nervous system. N Engl J Med. 1999;340:483–4.
86. Sonneville R, Klein IF, Wolff M. Update on investigation and management of postinfectious encephalitis. Curr Opin Neurol. 2010;23:300–4.
87. Garcia-Monco JC, Cortina IE, Ferreira E, et al. Reversible splenial lesion syndrome (RESLES): what's in a name? J Neuroimaging. 2011;21:e1–14.

Chapter 6
Tropical Viral CNS Infections

Sanjeev K. Handique and Mausumi Barthakur

Abstract Viral infections of the CNS in the tropics and Indian subcontinent are not only different from that encountered in the western world, but many types are constantly emerging. While age-old scourges like polio have recently been contained in these geographical areas to a great extent, thanks to effective vaccination programs, others like Japanese encephalitis, rabies, and measles in the form of subacute sclerosing panencephalitis have been inadequately controlled. In recent times some viruses causing predominant CNS symptoms such as West Nile, Chandipura, and Nipah have emerged. Emerging viruses also include others that may occasionally cause CNS symptoms such as enterovirus, dengue, and chikungunya. The CNS manifestations of most of these viruses may be in the form of aseptic meningitis, encephalitis, or myelitis either in isolated form or in combination. Many of these viruses such as Japanese encephalitis cause large-scale epidemics with high mortality and morbidity. This chapter discusses the current status of many of these viral infections of the CNS predominant in these geographical areas.

Keywords Viral encephalitis • Myelitis • Meningitis • Tropics • Japanese encephalitis • West Nile • Dengue • Enterovirus • Nipah virus • Rabies • Measles • Chandipura • Chikungunya • CNS infection

Viral infections of the central nervous system (CNS) in the tropics are different than those seen in the western developed countries. This is due to different climatic conditions and environment, different insect and animal vectors, different host immunity, and different social and agricultural practices with contribution from inadequate

S.K. Handique, MD (✉)
Department of Radiology, GNRC Hospitals, Six Mile, Guwahati, Assam 781022, India
e-mail: sanjeevhandique1@gmail.com

M. Barthakur, MD
Department of Clinical Neurophysiology, GNRC Hospitals, Guwahati, Assam India

J.C. García-Moncó (ed.), *CNS Infections*,
DOI 10.1007/978-1-4471-6401-2_6, © Springer-Verlag London 2014

health-care and sanitation facilities in many tropical countries. Climatic and environment changes in recent times have led to the emergence of many other viruses that can cause either altered or fresh CNS disease or spread into new geographical destinations.

The CNS is protected from viral invasion by anatomic barriers and virus-specific and nonspecific host immunity. When viruses do invade the CNS, they can infect the brain, meninges, spinal cord, or cranial nerves either in isolation or in combination, very often with devastating consequences. This is due to the fact that virus-specific treatment does not exist in most instances and adequate supportive treatment cannot be given on time. The silver lining to this scenario is the existence of effective preventive measures chiefly in the form of vaccines that have been used by some countries to control these infections.

This chapter discusses the prevalent viral infections of the CNS in the tropics and the challenges of emerging viral infections of the CNS in the tropics with emphasis to the Indian subcontinent.

Viral Meningitis

Viruses can infect the meninges leading to acute viral meningitis (VM), the most common cause of aseptic meningitis. The responsible causative agents in more than half the cases are enteroviruses (Coxsackie viruses, echoviruses, and polioviruses). Other responsible viruses include the arboviruses, herpes family viruses, and respiratory viruses such as adenoviruses, mumps, and HIV [1]. The etiological profile and incidence of VM in tropical countries like India are unknown because cost of diagnosis, lack of diagnostic facilities, and the benign nature of the disease lead to underreporting. However, epidemics of enterovirus (EV) meningitis in children have been reported from India [2]. Increased incidence of benign neurological illness possibly due to meningitis is seen in patients especially in children during epidemics of Japanese encephalitis (JE) in India [1]. Mumps meningitis is still prevalent in India, possibly due to inadequate vaccination [1]. While all age groups can be affected by the disease, children and elderly are more susceptible to VM. Both EV and mumps meningitis are more common in males.

Some clinical features are common to all VM, and these include headache, fever, myalgia, malaise, chills, sore throat, abdominal pain, nausea, vomiting, photophobia, stiff neck, and drowsiness. Altered consciousness, focal neurological deficits, and seizures suggest associated encephalitis. Meningeal signs can be elicited, and some VM are accompanied by a rash. Parotitis accompanies mumps meningitis, while EV is reported to be associated with hand, foot, and mouth disease; encephalitis; and flaccid paralysis in India as elsewhere. Most cases are self-limiting and recover completely within 5–14 days. Persistent severe illness should prompt exclusion of other causes which may be difficult [1].

Diagnosis is by characteristic changes in the cerebrospinal fluid (CSF). CSF pressure is usually increased. There is initial increase in polymorphonuclear leukocytes followed by a mononuclear or lymphocytic pleocytosis, usually less than 500/cumm. CSF protein is elevated, while glucose may be normal or decreased. Definitive diagnosis is by virus isolation or demonstration of virus-specific IgM in the CSF. In recent times the polymerase chain reaction (PCR) test has become available for specific viral agents. Rise of specific antibody in convalescent serum of more than fourfold can provide a diagnosis, but is time-consuming [1]. Imaging by computed tomography (CT) and magnetic resonance imaging (MRI) usually fails to show abnormalities. Meningeal enhancement on MRI was reported in 9 out of 23 patients in one study from China [3, 4]. However it is prudent to do imaging as it may help differentiate VM from other clinical mimics such as tubercular meningitis and pickup complications such as hydrocephalus.

Treatment is supportive, symptomatic, and aimed at preventing complications. Analgesics, antipyretics, and antiemetics may be given and fluid balance maintained. Those with more severe disease, altered sensorium, or seizures need more aggressive treatment with hospitalization. Specific treatment with antivirals is indicated if the causative agent is HSV, varicella, or cytomegalovirus. There is available effective vaccination for viruses like measles, mumps, varicella, rubella, and JE and should be used for prevention [1].

Viral Encephalitis

Viral encephalitis (VE) refers to infection of the brain by a virus causing usually a diffuse inflammatory process. Acute VE commonly presents with fever and altered sensorium with or without focal neurological deficit. It may be accompanied by meningeal inflammation as well when the term meningoencephalitis is used. VE may less commonly present as a slower indolent process when the term slow viral infection is used. VE has to be distinguished from acute disseminated encephalomyelitis (ADEM) which is an altered immune response to viral illness or vaccination. This chapter discusses acute viral encephalitides that are endemic to the South Asian region and the Indian subcontinent. It also discusses the problem of emerging viruses of the region with CNS invasiveness. Table 6.1 gives a list of common viruses that are known to cause viral encephalitis in the Indian subcontinent.

The true incidence of VE is difficult to determine as in most cases a viral etiology cannot be confirmed. The term acute encephalitic syndrome (AES) which is defined as acute-onset fever with altered mental status with or without seizures is considered for surveillance purposes. Most AES is due to viral encephalitis. In a review of 25 studies of AES, 28–85 % of cases did not have a confirmed viral etiology. There was a wide range of reported incidences varying from 0.9 to 185 per 100,000 in different age groups from both tropical and western settings. In two robust prospective studies of AES, the reported incidence was 6.34 and 7.4 in a tropical and western setting, respectively [5]. In a recent study from Central India, the incidence of AES reported was 16 per 100,000 [6]. In the Indian subcontinent, the etiological profile of AES has been changing over the years. While most studies reported from India

Table 6.1 Common causes of viral encephalitis in the Indian subcontinent

Herpes viruses – HSV 1, 2, varicella zoster, CMV, EBV, HHV6
Adenoviruses
Influenza (including H1N1)/parainfluenza
Enteroviruses – poliovirus, echovirus, Coxsackie, EV 71, 75, 76, 89
Mumps, measles, rubella
Rabies
Arboviruses – JE, WNV, dengue, Kyasanur Forest disease, Chikungunya, Chandipura
Paramyxoviruses – Nipah

Abbreviations: *HSV* herpes simplex virus, *EV* enteroviruses, *JE* Japanese encephalitis, *WNE* West Nile encephalitis

during the period of 1975 to 1999 identified Japanese encephalitis virus (JEV) as the main cause of AES, studies published after 2000 have identified Chandipura and EV as the most common causes, in both outbreaks and surveillance studies. This may be due to vaccination campaigns against JEV, unmasking of other etiological agents after incidence of JE has come down, and advancement of diagnostic techniques over the years [7].

Most viruses gain entry into the CNS through the hematogenous route (e.g., JEV) and less commonly through the neuronal route (e.g., HSV). Despite the variety of viruses that can cause encephalitis, there is some uniformity in the pathology they produce in the immunocompetent host. All encephalitides are accompanied by cell death or "neuronophagia" involving destruction of neurons with disruption in their cell membranes and to some extent the glial cells. The dead cells disappear, and the remnants are surrounded by microglial cells and lymphocytes forming so-called glial stars, nodules, clusters, or knots. The rate at which cells undergo neuronophagia varies and can take no more than a few days in acute encephalitis to months to years in slow viral infections. The scale of neuronophagia also varies between different encephalitides. A second type of cell death without lysis is called apoptosis and is seen in some encephalitides. Another common feature of viral encephalitis is the development of inflammatory response to the viral infection. This occurs within few days in the site of infection and is accompanied by variable degree of edema. The perivascular spaces are filled with inflammatory cells, mostly mononuclear cells, macrophages, lymphocytes, and plasma cells forming so-called perivascular cuffs. While necrosis occurs in all encephalitides, the distribution of necrotic lesions within the CNS depends on the selective vulnerability of a particular cell to the invading virus, chiefly due to the requirement of virus-specific receptors that must be present in the cell for it to be susceptible to the virus. For example, poliovirus invades the anterior horn cells binding to the CD155 receptor protein. Not all instances of anatomic distribution of lesions of viral encephalitis can be explained on the basis of this, however. The temporal lobe specificity of lesions of HSE may have more to do with the neuronal route of spread than viral tropism, as the receptor for the HSV exists in all neurons. Healing of the encephalitic lesions and edematous areas occurs by glial reaction which may continue for weeks to months after the infection. Focal or diffuse atrophy, shrinkage of white matter, and healing of encephalitic and edematous areas by glial reaction are late sequels of the disease [8]. The targeted involvement of some areas of the CNS and associated inflammatory changes are reflected on imaging especially on MRI which is a more sensitive investigation due to its superior contrast resolution in comparison to computed tomography (CT). Late sequels can be picked up on MRI as well.

Japanese Encephalitis

Japanese encephalitis (JE) is a mosquito-borne flaviviral encephalitis that is the most important cause of VE worldwide. It was first recognized in Japan since the 1870s, and despite the fact that JE is vaccine preventable, in the present day it has spread across Southern and Eastern Asia and the Pacific Rim. The erstwhile term of Japanese B encephalitis was used to distinguish it from von Economo's encephalitis lethargica which was known as Japanese A encephalitis. The term "B" was later dropped. The Nakayama strain of JEV was isolated from a brain of a fatal case in 1935 [9]. In the later part of the 1980s, it was estimated that 50,000 new cases of JE occurred annually in 2.4 billion population in 16 countries affected by JE at that time with an annual incidence of 2 per 100,000 overall [10]. A recent study estimates 68,000 cases to occur annually in 24 JE endemic countries with an incidence of 1.8 per 100,000 overall. Seventy-five percent of the cases occur in children with an annual incidence of 5.4 per 100,000 in this group [11]. About one-third of patients die while half of those that survive have severe neuropsychiatric sequels [9]. The true incidence of JE is however difficult to establish as the disease is underreported because of variable intensity of surveillance and availability of laboratory diagnostic facility in affected countries.

The JEV is a member of the genus *Flavivirus* and family Flaviviridae. The JEV virion consists of a single strand of positive-sense RNA of approximately 11 kilobase in length. It is wrapped in a nucleocapsid with a surrounding glycoprotein-containing envelope. The virion consists of three structural proteins (core [C], premembrane [PrM], and envelope [E]) and seven nonstructural (NS) proteins (NS1, NS2A, NS2B, NS3, NS4A, NS4B, and NS5) [12]. Five genotypes of the virus have been described from different geographical areas [13–15]. Genotypes IV and V are the most divergent and have remained confined to their region of origin in Indonesia-Malaysia while the newer genotypes I through III have spread across Asia.

JE is a zoonotic disease where man is incidentally infected and a dead-end host. The JEV cycle is maintained in nature between waterbirds and vertebrate hosts through the mosquito vector. Ardeid waterbirds such as herons and egrets serve as reservoirs and amplifiers of the virus and may be responsible for the spread of the disease across continents [9]. Among the vertebrate hosts that have been implicated in the spread of JE, pigs are the most important hosts responsible for transmission to man as they can have high and prolonged viremia, are in close proximity to man, and reproduce in plenty providing hitherto uninfected hosts [9]. The virus is transmitted by culicine mosquitoes between birds and pigs. *Culex tritaeniorhynchus* is the principal vector responsible for transmission of JE in South, East, and Southeastern Asia. It breeds in stagnant water such as in rice fields. *C. annulirostris* is the main vector in North Australia. Many other species of Culex, Mansonia, and Anopheles mosquitoes are responsible vectors in India [16, 17]. Man becomes incidentally infected when bitten by an infected mosquito. Only 1 in 25 to 1 in 1,000 infections with the JEV are clinically apparent [18]. This is a dead-end infection as man-to-man transmission does not occur due to transient and mild viremia. Human activity such as rice cultivation and pig farming, conditions that are abundant in Asia contribute to maintenance and spread of the disease.

JE is predominantly a disease of children and young adults. However, when it occurs in an area for the first time as has been reported from Sri Lanka, India, and Nepal, adults may be equally affected. Nonimmune travelers to endemic areas stand at risk of acquiring the disease [9]. Two epidemiological patterns of JE have been described. JE tends to occur in epidemic forms in the northern part of the tropical zone of Asia such as in China, Japan, Nepal, Northern and Northeastern India, Korea, North Vietnam, and Thailand. In southern tropical zones of Asia such as in Southern Vietnam, South Thailand, Indonesia, Malaysia, the Philippines, Sri Lanka, and Southern India, JE is endemic with peak cases occurring after the rainy season [19]. This pattern is possibly related to temperature rather than amount of rainfall or the strain of JEV [20].

The geographical area of JE prevalence has been steadily increasing in the past 70 years or so (Fig. 6.1). Though the mechanism of spread of JE into new areas is not fully known, changing land usage and agricultural practice, deforestation, increasing rice growing, windblown mosquitoes, bird migration, and movement of infected hosts are factors that possibly contribute to the spread [21]. Mass childhood vaccination programs in several countries like Japan, Korea, and Taiwan have virtually eliminated JE in them in the recent years. In other Asian countries that have been slow in implementing such programs, the disease still persists. Currently approximately half of the reported JE cases of the world are from China [11]. However the annual incidence of JE in China is decreasing in the recent years. During the period of 2000 and 2005, the annual incidence of JE decreased from 0.9/100,000 to about 0.4/100,000 [22]. The other big contributor to JE cases of the world is India. During 2006–2009, out of approximately 27,000 cases of JE reported to the World Health Organization, 86 % were from India and China [11]. Approximately 4,000–8,000 new cases occurred during the period 2007–2012 across several Indian states [23]. These figures may be an underestimate as many JE cases in India go unreported.

After the JEV gains entry into the human body through the bite of the infected mosquito, it multiplies locally and in the regional lymph nodes. Thereafter it spreads to secondary lymphoid organs before entering the blood circulation. There is a transient viremia which spreads the virus to peripheral organs such as the kidney, liver, and spleen after which the virus spreads to the CNS by crossing the blood-brain

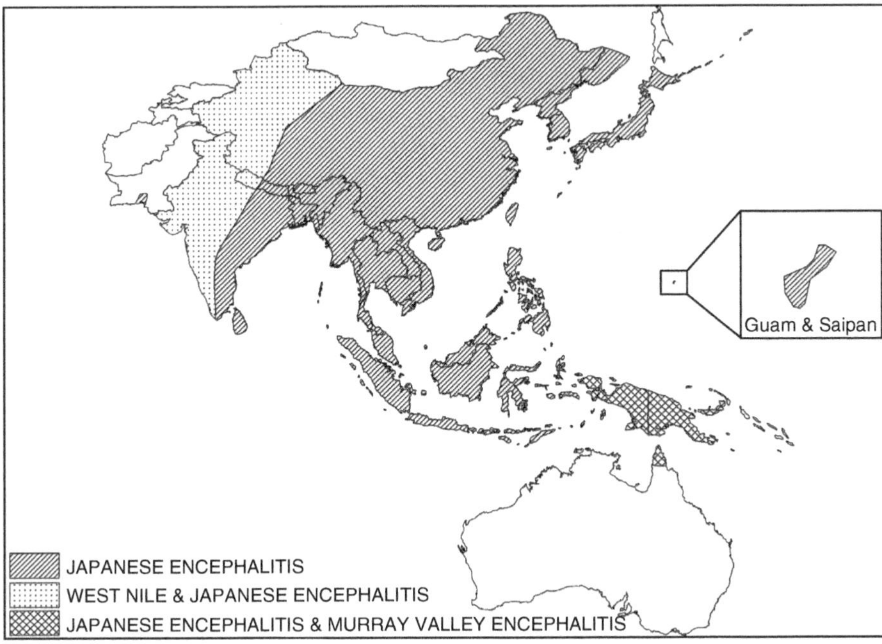

Fig. 6.1 Map showing distribution of Japanese encephalitis

barrier (BBB) [24]. JEV may cross the BBB by passive transport across the vascular endothelium, by an active replication process in the vascular endothelial cells or by a "Trojan horse" mechanism by which it is carried across by inflammatory cells [25]. The pathological changes in the brain in fatal JE cases include leptomeningeal haziness, vascular congestion, cerebral edema, and brain swelling. Histologically there is leptomeningeal mononuclear inflammation extending into the perivascular spaces with formation of perivascular cuffs. Two types of characteristic lesions are seen: the cell-rich gliomesenchymal nodule and the cell-poor necrolytic lesion. The gliomesenchymal nodule is formed by aggregates of microglial cells and lymphocytes around degenerating neurons. These lesions are seen in the medulla, thalamus, substantia nigra, pontine and reticular nuclei of the brainstem, cerebral cortex, dentate nuclei and Purkinje cells of the cerebellum, and Ammon's horn of the hippocampus. The necrolytic lesion is seen in the cerebral cortex, thalamus, corpus striatum, midbrain, and pons [26–28].

Clinically apparent JEV infection can present as encephalitis, aseptic meningitis, or acute flaccid paralysis. The incubation period of JE is 5–15 days [21]. The disease can occur in an acute or less commonly in a subacute form. The course of the disease can be divided into three stages: a prodromal stage, an encephalitis stage, and a convalescent stage. The prodromal phase precedes CNS features and is characterized by constitutional symptoms such as malaise, fever which may be high grade and accompanied by chills, headache, nausea and vomiting, and diarrhea which is more common in children. This is followed by the encephalitic stage in 3–5 days. This is characterized by altered sensorium, convulsions, focal neurological deficits, behavioral changes, movement disorders, and associated meningitis. Focal neurological deficit may include motor paralysis and cranial nerve deficits. Behavioral changes may present in the form of restlessness, disorientation, delirium, and irrelevant talk. Movement disorders include head nodding, dystonia, coarse tremors, choreoathetosis, and parkinsonian features such as masklike facies, rigidity, and oculogyric crisis. Most deaths occur during the first 5 days of illness. The encephalitic stage may persist from a week to a few weeks if there are complications. Those that survive this stage either regain complete neurological function or may be left with residual neurological deficits in the convalescent stage that lasts from a few weeks to months [28]. Only one-third of the patients recover completely, while majority are left with mild to severe residua. Residual deficits include intellectual impairment, speech defects, and motor deficits. Secondary infections are frequent complications during convalescence [29]. Clinical features that have been associated with a poor outcome include short prodromal stage, deep coma, abnormalities in tone and breathing, decerebrate posturing, and seizures [9, 30].

Other than the classical encephalitic form of presentation of JE, few atypical presentations have been reported. JE can present with aseptic meningitis. Febrile seizure-like presentation has been reported in children. Adolescents can present with abnormal behavior as an initial presentation [29]. Acute flaccid paralysis has been reported in a subgroup of patients either as the lone presentation or with progression to subsequent encephalitis [31]. A biphasic illness pattern of JE has been reported where there is relapse of meningoencephalitic symptoms. In the second phase, symptoms may be different but still conform to the known features of JE, and MRI may show fresh areas of involvement, also conforming to JE lesions [32, 33].

Peripheral blood examination in JE may show polymorphonuclear leukocytosis. CSF examination shows elevated opening pressure. Increased CSF cell counts usually less than 1,000/cumm. may be seen with lymphocytic predominance and at times with increased polymorphs. CSF protein is elevated in two-thirds of the patients [28]. Abnormal electroencephalographic (EEG) findings may be seen which include diffuse theta and delta waves, burst suppression, epileptiform activity, and alpha pattern coma. These findings are nonspecific and do not correlate with clinical status and outcome [34].

Imaging studies by CT or MRI reflect the pathological changes in the brain. The typical imaging findings are lesions in the thalami, substantia nigra, basal ganglia, and hippocampi (Fig. 6.2). Lesions can also be seen less commonly in the cerebral cortex, midbrain, pons, medulla, cerebellum, and white matter. MRI is more sensitive in picking up these lesions and should be the investigation of choice. Bilateral or unilateral, asymmetric thalamic lesions are the hallmark of JE and can be seen in 87–94 % patients with abnormal MRI. JE lesions are hyperintense on T2-weighted imaging and fluid-attenuated inversion recovery (FLAIR) sequences and slightly hypointense to normal brain on T1-weighted images. Acute lesions have some amount of local brain swelling. Evidence of hemorrhage may be seen.

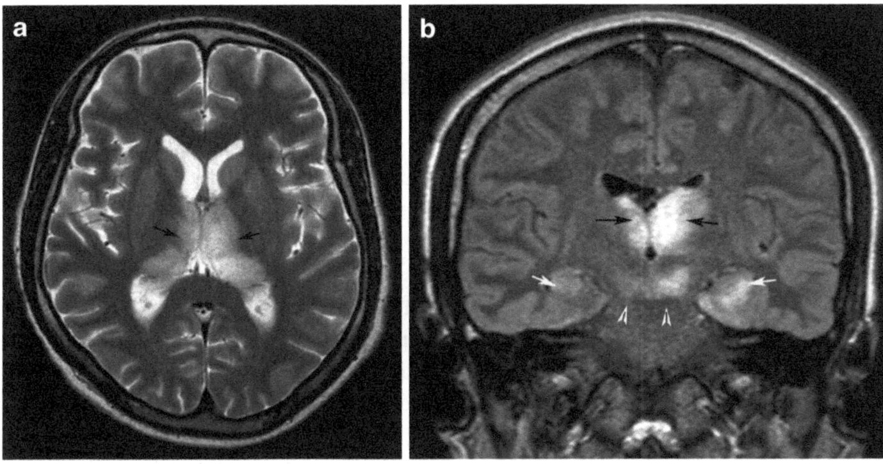

Fig. 6.2 A 50-year-old male with Japanese encephalitis. (**a**) T2-weighted axial MRI image showing bilateral thalamic lesions (*black arrows*). (**b**) Coronal fluid-attenuated inversion recovery sequence showing bilateral thalamic (*black arrows*), hippocampal (*white arrows*), and substantia nigra (*white arrowheads*) lesions. The lesions are asymmetric, even though they are bilateral and have local mass effect

The lesions do not enhance on post-gadolinium-enhanced images [3, 35–37]. A characteristic pattern of hippocampal involvement with the involvement of the tail and body and usual sparing of the rest of the temporal lobes with associated lesions of JE differentiates it from herpes simplex encephalitis (HSE) [37]. In an endemic area, the presence of thalamic lesions in a patient of AES is 100 % specific and 23 % sensitive for the diagnosis of JE with positive and negative predictive values of 100 and 42.1 %, respectively [38]. When using a current generation 1.5 T MRI, sensitivity and specificity were 90.9 and 50 %, respectively, in the first week of onset of JE which is comparable to the commonly used test for detection of JE, specific immunoglobulin (IgM) detection by immunoassay capture in the CSF (CSF Mac-ELISA) [3]. The presence of thalamic lesions on MRI can therefore be a rapid, sensitive, and fairly specific test for establishing a diagnosis of JE in AES in an endemic area. The JE lesions tend to be more conspicuous on conventional MRI sequences than on diffusion-weighted (DW) sequences [3]. No correlation between the radiological features of JE and clinical outcome has been found (Handique SK, Barua S, 2013) [39]. However, a significant association of thalamic lesions on imaging was found with development of dystonia [39].

The definitive diagnosis of JE is either by (1) virus isolation or (2) by demonstration of virus-specific antigen or antibody in the CSF/blood. JEV isolation can be done by intracerebral inoculation of clinical specimens in suckling mouse brain. Viral cell cultures used more recently include primary chick or duck embryo cells and lines of Vero. JEV antigen detection tests in the CSF include reverse passive hemagglutination, immunofluorescence, and staphylococcal coagglutination tests using polyclonal or monoclonal antibodies [29]. JEV antibody detection by Mac-ELISA is currently the most widely used test to demonstrate the antibody in the CSF or blood [40]. However, it is to be noted that this test may be positive in the CSF in the first week of onset of the disease in only 50 % of patients, although it is invariably positive beyond the first week [28]. Many newer modifications of this test are currently available which are simpler and more convenient to use especially in rural hospitals [9]. Viral genomic mapping by reverse transcriptase-polymerase chain reaction (RT-PCR) tests has been developed in recent times.

There is no definitive treatment of JE. A number of antiviral agents such as INF alfa-2a [41] and diethyldithiocarbamate [42] have been tried but have not shown any improvement of outcome of JE. Corticosteroids have not shown any benefit either [43]. A drug that has shown promise in experimental models is minocycline which has currently been approved for trials in India [44]. Another drug that has been shown to be effective in vitro is N-methylisatin-beta-thiosemicarbazone [45]. Current treatment is supportive and is aimed at reduction of intracranial pressure, optimization of blood pressure to maintain adequate cerebral perfusion, and prevention of secondary infection [29].

Vaccination of the population at risk has been an effective means of controlling JE since the 1940s. There are three vaccines that are currently being widely used. These include the inactivated mouse brain-derived vaccine from the Nakayama or Beijing 1 strains, inactivated primary hamster kidney cell vaccine from the P3 strain, and live attenuated primary hamster kidney cell vaccine from the SA-14-14-2 strain. Efficacy of these vaccines varies from 85 to 95 % [29]. Besides vaccination other measures such as prevention of exposure to mosquito bites, vector control measures, separation of piggeries from human dwellings, and vaccination of pigs have been used effectively for JE control.

West Nile Encephalitis

West Nile virus (WNV) is a positive-stranded RNA virus of the family *Flaviviridae* that is closely related to other flaviviruses such as JEV, Murray valley encephalitis virus, and the St. Louis encephalitis virus. A closely related virus, the Kunjin virus, has now been classified as a subtype of WNV. Five lineages of WNV have been described out of which only lineage 1 is known to cause neuroinvasive disease [46]. WNV is transmitted to humans by mosquitoes. Various species of Culex mosquitoes have been implicated in the spread of WNV to man. In India, the vector implicated primarily is *Culex vishnui* besides other Culex species [47]. Man is a dead-end host like in JE due to low viremia which prevents further transmission of the virus. In nature, the virus is maintained in a cycle involving birds and mosquitoes. Several species of birds have been implicated as vertebrate carriers and amplifiers in different WNV prevalent geographical areas. In India ardeid birds like pond herons and cattle egrets have been implicated [47, 48]. Man-to-man transmission does not occur. However, the virus can spread transplacentally and by breast-feeding to newborns or by blood transfusion [46].

WNV was first isolated in the West Nile district of Uganda in 1937. It is today the most widespread flavivirus across the world and is distributed throughout Africa, the Middle East, Europe, many parts of Asia, Australia, and America. Outbreaks have occurred in several countries in the past 50 years with the largest outbreaks reported from Greece, Israel, Romania, Russia, and the USA [49]. In India, WNV was first reported in 1952 [50]. The virus has since been reported in Southern, Central, Western, and Northeastern India [46, 51]. Despite the abundant presence of the mosquito vectors of WNV and the neurovirulent strain of the virus, large-scale epidemics in the lines of those seen in the Western Hemisphere, Europe, and the Middle East are not seen in the Indian subcontinent. Though the cause for this is not known, the presence of other flaviviruses may offer cross protection for the WNV or dual infections of the vectors with JE, and WNV may lead to interference. Also, the WNV vectors are zoophilic and do not prefer to feed on birds which may decrease the efficacy of the WNV transmission cycle [48]. However, epidemics of febrile illness and encephalitis due to WNV have been reported from Western India [47]. It is now being recognized in India that patients presenting with AES in the summer may also be due to WNV encephalitis. In one study of AES from Northeastern India where JE is endemic, 11 % of patients were due to WNV [51].

Animal models suggest that the WNV replicates locally at the site of inoculation with subsequent spread to draining lymph nodes with resultant viremia and infection of the peripheral organs such as the spleen and kidney. Although it is likely that the CNS is invaded through the hematogenous route, other routes of entry are possible such as through the olfactory bulb, through passive transport through choroid plexus epithelial cells, through infected immune cells, or through retrograde axonal transport from infected peripheral neurons [52]. Fatal cases of WNV encephalitis show evidence of encephalitis and meningoencephalitis. Histologically there is evidence of perivascular inflammatory change with microglial nodule formation with neuronophagia involving the gray and white matter. The brainstem is typically involved with involvement of the temporal lobes, basal ganglia, cerebellum, and cortex. Spinal cord and cranial nerve root involvement may be seen [53, 54].

The incubation period in humans is approximately 2–15 days [46]. Most (80 %) WNV infections are asymptomatic. Most symptomatic patients develop West Nile fever which is usually a self-limited disease characterized by fever, headache, fatigue, malaise, muscle pain, and weakness. GI symptoms and an upper trunk and extremity macular rash may sometimes manifest. CNS disease is seen in less than 1 % of patients. This may manifest as aseptic meningitis, encephalitis, acute flaccid paralysis, or Guillain-Barré syndrome [46, 52].

CSF examination usually shows increased cells (mostly lymphocytes) with increased protein and normal glucose. Virus-specific Mac-ELISA test to detect IgM antibody in the CSF within 8 days of disease onset is the most efficient diagnostic test for WNV encephalitis as the antibody does not cross the blood-brain barrier [55].

CT usually does not show any abnormalities, whereas a third to more than half of MRI scans in WNV encephalitis are abnormal [55–57]. Leptomeningeal involvement may be seen as FLAIR hyperintensities or meningeal enhancement. White matter involvement mimicking demyelinating lesions may be seen in 10–50 % of the patients.

On MRI anatomic areas involved are the basal ganglia, thalami, mesial temporal lobe, midbrain, pons, and cerebellum [56, 57]. Diffusion-weighted imaging (DWI) abnormalities may be seen in the gray and white matter in as many as half of the patients. Patients with abnormalities on both DWI and T2-weighted imaging seem to have a poorer outcome when compared to patients with normal scans or with lesions seen only on DWI [56]. Anterior horn cell involvement with nerve root enhancement has been seen in patients with acute flaccid paralysis [56, 57].

Treatment of the disease is mainly supportive and symptomatic as no specific treatment exists. There is anecdotal evidence of efficacy of intravenous immunoglobulin in the treatment of WNV CNS invasive disease (see section on viral myelitis below). No approved vaccine is available for humans. Vector control methods described for control of Culex mosquitoes have been suggested in countries like India for the control of the disease [47].

Dengue

Dengue is the most rapidly spreading arboviral disease in the world. An estimated 50 million dengue cases occur annually. About 2.5 billion people live in dengue-endemic areas, out of which about 70 % live in Southeast Asia and Western Pacific region which bear about 75 % of the disease burden of dengue. In countries of the South Asian region such as India, Bangladesh, and Maldives, cyclic epidemics are being seen with increasing frequency with spread of the disease into new geographical areas like Bhutan and Nepal. The dengue virus is a Flavivirus transmitted to man by the bite of the infected *Aedes* mosquito. It is a single-stranded RNA virus consisting of four serotypes (DEN 1–4) [58].

Most infections may be asymptomatic. Symptomatic infections may manifest as dengue fever, dengue hemorrhagic fever, or dengue shock syndrome [59]. Atypical manifestations may involve the CNS, gastrointestinal, renal, cardiac, respiratory, musculoskeletal, or lymphoreticular systems [60]. CNS complications can occur in 0.5–6.2 %. These may be due to a neurotropic effect of the virus, immune mediated or related to systemic complications of the infection. There is increasing evidence of a neurotropic effect of the dengue virus which may result in encephalitis, myelitis, or aseptic meningitis. This is supported by virus isolation from the CSF, detection of the virus in the brain, lymphocytic pleocytosis, and demonstration of virus-specific IgM [61]. Dengue virus serotypes 2 and 3 have been reported to cause CNS invasive disease [60]. MRI has been reported to show JE-like lesions in the thalami, globus pallidus, temporal lobe, and pons in dengue encephalitis. These lesions are focal suggesting possible encephalitis rather than encephalopathy which shows more global change. Spinal cord lesions have also been reported on MRI in patients with myelitis [62]. Postinfectious immune-mediated effects on the CNS include acute disseminated encephalomyelitis (ADEM), Guillain-Barré syndrome, and mono- and polyneuropathies. Encephalopathy may result from the systemic complications of dengue infection. Multiple factors such as cerebral edema, hemorrhage, hyponatremia, hepatic or renal failure, and cerebral hypoxia may contribute to the pathophysiology of encephalopathy. MRI has been reported to show cerebral edema, scattered focal lesions, and hemorrhage. Hemorrhagic stroke may result from vasculopathy, thrombocytopenia, and platelet dysfunction in dengue infection. Ischemic stroke can also be seen due to coagulopathy and vasculopathy [61].

Enterovirus

Enteroviruses (EVs) belong to a genus of single-stranded RNA viruses that include Coxsackie viruses, echoviruses, polioviruses, and newer enteroviruses. In the past, poliomyelitis was the most significant CNS disease caused by EVs. With extensive intervention by way of vaccination in recent times, there has been a significant submergence of the virus with only three countries (Afghanistan, Pakistan, and Nigeria) remaining endemic to polio in 2013 [63]. Extensive use of live attenuated vaccine for polio eradication has led to the emergence of circulating vaccine-derived polioviruses (cVDPV) in nature which have caused outbreaks in several parts of the world notably in Southeast Asia. Poliomyelitis-like disease has been reported in children with cVDPV with fever and asymmetric paralysis. With the submergence of the poliovirus, newer EVs with the ability to cause CNS disease like aseptic meningitis, encephalitis, and acute flaccid paralysis have emerged in the recent past. Notable among these is EV71 which is an emerging virus that has significantly expanded its geographical range. It causes hand, foot, and mouth disease (HFMD) in children. There have been several outbreaks of EV71 disease in Southeast Asia and Pacific region since 1997 [64]. In China the disease was first seen in 1981, and in India, the first outbreak was reported in 2004. Many small-scale outbreaks have been reported from India after the first outbreak [65]. Over the past decade EV along with Chandipura virus has emerged as the most common cause of AES in India [7]. Severe outbreaks are followed by milder attacks and periods of decreased disease activity and vice versa as has been seen in China and Taiwan [65]. Occurrence of CNS disease in EV71 infections is variable. The reason for this is not well understood but could be due to high spontaneous mutation rate of the virus and presence of numerous subtypes. EVs are transmitted by the feco-oral route although respiratory oral spread and spread through fomites are possible. Invasion of the CNS is through hematogenous route following viremia. Up to 30 % of patients with EV71 infections may show CNS disease. This commonly includes aseptic meningitis, encephalitis, and acute flaccid paralysis and may also include cerebellitis, brainstem encephalitis, opsoclonus-myoclonus syndrome, Guillain-Barré syndrome, and transverse myelitis [64]. Laboratory confirmation of the disease can be done by virus isolation (from the throat, ulcer, rectal swabs, serum, or CSF) or by detection of virus-specific antibody. The latter can be done by IgM ELISA which is fast and a cost-effective technique. Reverse transcriptase-PCR tests are able to detect serotypes of the virus [65]. MRI of EV71 encephalitis from Taiwan has shown brainstem involvement in the posterior medulla and pons and in the midbrain. Cerebellar dentate nuclei, thalami, putamina, and cervical cord were also involved [66]. In a study from North India, brainstem (midbrain and pons) lesions were the most common. Other lesions were seen in the thalami, cerebellum, cortex, basal ganglia, and substantia nigra [67]. Other EVs that have been reported to cause outbreaks of encephalitis in India include EV76 and 89 from North India and EV 75 from South India [68, 69]. Numerous other non-polio EVs have been identified in association with acute flaccid paralysis in India [70]. No specific treatment or vaccination exists for EV infections at present. Basic prevention for the feco-oral spread should be practiced, and these include personal hygiene such as hand washing, cleaning of utensils, and prevention of contact with infected patients [65].

Nipah Virus Encephalitis

Nipah virus encephalitis (NVE) is an emerging zoonosis that was first reported from Malaysia and Singapore in 1998. The Nipah Virus (NV) is closely related to the Hendra virus. Both viruses are species of the genus *Henipavirus*, a new class of virus in the Paramyxoviridae family. It has the ability to cause potentially fatal encephalitis in humans with case fatalities of 40–75 %. Other domestic animals such as pigs are also susceptible to the virus. Fruit bats of the Pteropodidae family are the natural hosts of the virus but do not suffer from NV disease. Farm animals possibly get infected from bat urine or saliva. In the first outbreaks reported from Malaysia, the disease was transmitted to man from contact with infected pigs or their contaminated tissues. Most of the initial outbreaks occurred in pig farm workers or residents of pig-farming villages. Transmission may have occurred through respiratory droplets, contact with throat or nasal secretions of pigs, or contact with a sick animal. Following the initial attacks in Southeast Asia, outbreaks of NVE have occurred in the sub-Himalayan region of the state of West Bengal in India and in the adjoining areas of West Central Bangladesh since 2001. In India and Bangladesh, consumption of fruit or fruit juices such as raw date palm juice contaminated by bat urine or saliva was the possible source of infection. Direct human-to-human transmission has been documented in Bangladesh and India possibly through close contact with patient secretions and excretions. In North Bengal, transmission of NVE was reported in a health-care setting with 75 % cases occurring in hospital staff or visitors. Approximately half of the reported cases from Bangladesh occurred due to human-to-human transmission in the period of 2001–2008 [71, 72]. Pathologically an unusual feature is systemic and CNS vasculitis with associated thrombosis and parenchymal necrosis in the CNS. This is accompanied by other usual features of encephalitis like neuronophagia, microglial nodule formation, and perivascular cuffing [72].

The incubation period varied from 4 days to 2 months in the Malaysian outbreak, while in Bangladesh this was shorter at 6–11 days [73]. Human infections may range from asymptomatic to fatal encephalitis. Patients may present with influenza-like symptoms such as fever, headache, muscle pain, vomiting, and sore throat. This may be followed by signs and symptoms of AES [71]. AES has been associated with segmental myoclonus, areflexia, hypotonia, and autonomic dysfunction [74]. Atypical pneumonia with respiratory distress can be seen in some patients. Patients from Bangladesh had high prevalence of respiratory symptoms compared to the Malaysian outbreak. Indications of poor outcome in Bangladesh were fever with temperature of >37.8 °C, altered mentation, respiratory distress, and abnormal plantar reflex [75]. Relapse of encephalitis was reported in 7.5 %, and delayed encephalitis was reported in 3.7 % patients who initially presented with non-encephalitic infection from Malaysia [76]. In contrast to this, in a study of 22 patients from Bangladesh, delayed encephalitis after Nipah fever was not observed. However, neurological sequelae and new neurological dysfunction in the form of nerve palsies and cervical dystonia were seen. There was long-term neurological and functional morbidity in survivors [77].

The definitive diagnosis of NV infection can be done by serum neutralization, ELISA tests, PCR assay, immunofluorescence assay, and viral culture [71].

Somewhat different MRI findings have been described in acute NVE from Malaysia and Bangladesh. In Malaysia, discrete T2 and FLAIR hyperintense lesions measuring 2–7 mm were seen all over the brain but with a subcortical and deep white matter predominance. These lesions showed no mass effect and did not correlate with focal neurological sign, depth of coma, or with outcome [78]. Similar findings have been reported from Singapore. Acute NVE patients showed <1 cm hyperintense lesions in the cerebral white matter including the corpus callosum and external capsules, cortex, pons, and cerebellar peduncles. On diffusion-weighted imaging, larger lesions showed restricted diffusion resembling microinfarcts. Some lesions showed contrast enhancement. On follow-up many of these lesions resolved over time with transient appearance of T1 hyperintense lesions similar to laminar cortical necrosis [79]. These lesions are thought to represent microinfarcts due to small vessel angiopathy described in postmortem studies [78]. In patients from Bangladesh, however, disseminated multifocal and confluent gray and white matter lesion has been described [77, 80]. Confluent cortical lesions have also been described in relapsed or delayed-onset NVE. The pathological correlates of these lesions were changes typical of acute encephalitis rather than vasculitis [78].

There is no vaccine or definitive treatment for NV infection. Supportive and symptomatic treatment is the main approach to the management. Preventive measures include cleaning and disinfection of pig farms and establishing animal health surveillance systems. During outbreaks, restricting animal movement and culling may be necessary. Education of people to reduce exposure to the virus should focus on cleaning and peeling of fruits and boiling raw palm juice for consumption, avoiding contact with infected people, wearing protective equipment during patient care or animal handling, and hand hygiene [71].

Rabies

Rabies is one of the oldest diseases known to mankind. It is a zoonotic encephalomyelitis with a near 100 % fatality. The virus is a single-stranded RNA virus of the genus *Lyssavirus* and family Rhabdoviridae (Fig. 6.3). Out of seven known genotypes of virus, only genotype 1 is prevalent in India and other Asian countries [81]. Though the disease is prevalent worldwide, many geographically isolated areas mainly islands and peninsulas are free of the disease. Worldwide, about 55,000 people die annually of the disease mostly in Asia and Africa [82]. More than 30 % of these deaths, estimated at about 25–30,000, occur in India alone [83]. Human infection results from bites of infected animals, dog bites being the most common mode of infection in developing countries such as India. If sufficient nerve endings are exposed through the bite, the virus may directly invade the nerves. The incubation period in this case tends to be short. Alternatively the virus replicates in the muscles and then enters the nerves supplying the muscle. This is followed by retrograde axoplasmic spread into the spinal cord and then to the brain. There is initial involvement of areas such as the hippocampus, hypothalamus, and limbic system which explains the presenting symptomatology. There is eventual involvement of the entire brain. The pathological hallmark of infection is the presence of neuronal inclusion bodies called Negri bodies (Fig. 6.3). The relative lack of pathological brain changes suggests defective neurotransmitter function or neuronal apoptosis rather than necrosis plays a role in the pathogenesis of rabies.

The progression to rabies encephalitis after exposure of an individual depends on several factors such as site and severity of the bite, host immune factors, and viral contents in the animal's saliva. Bites in the head, neck, and upper extremity carry the highest risk of disease and a have a shorter incubation period. However in India, it is more common to have bites in the legs. The incubation period is variable and may range from 7 days to 6 years. This extreme variability may be due to variable viral quantity inoculated, properties of the rabies virus strain, availability of viral receptors in the tissue, and degree of tissue innervations. In as many as 5 % of cases from India, no history of dog bite may be elicited.

Classic neurological symptoms may be preceded by a prodrome consisting of nonspecific symptoms with or without paraesthesia or itching at the site of bite. This may last for a few hours to days. This is followed by the acute neurological manifestations of rabies which is of two forms, the more classical and common encephalitic or furious form and the dumb or paralytic form. The encephalitic form starts with fever and agitation followed by classic symptoms of phobic spasms characterized by hydrophobia and aerophobia, fluctuating consciousness progressing to coma, and signs of autonomic dysfunction such as hypersalivation, papillary abnormalities, piloerection, excessive sweating, priapism, and spontaneous ejaculation. Paralytic or dumb rabies may present in approximately 20 % patients and may be more difficult to diagnose due to lack of classic phobic spasms. This presents with ascending paralysis starting from the bitten extremity and progresses to involve all limbs, face, pharyngeal, and laryngeal muscles. Features of furious rabies may at times present in the terminal phase. The cause for pathogenesis of the two clinical

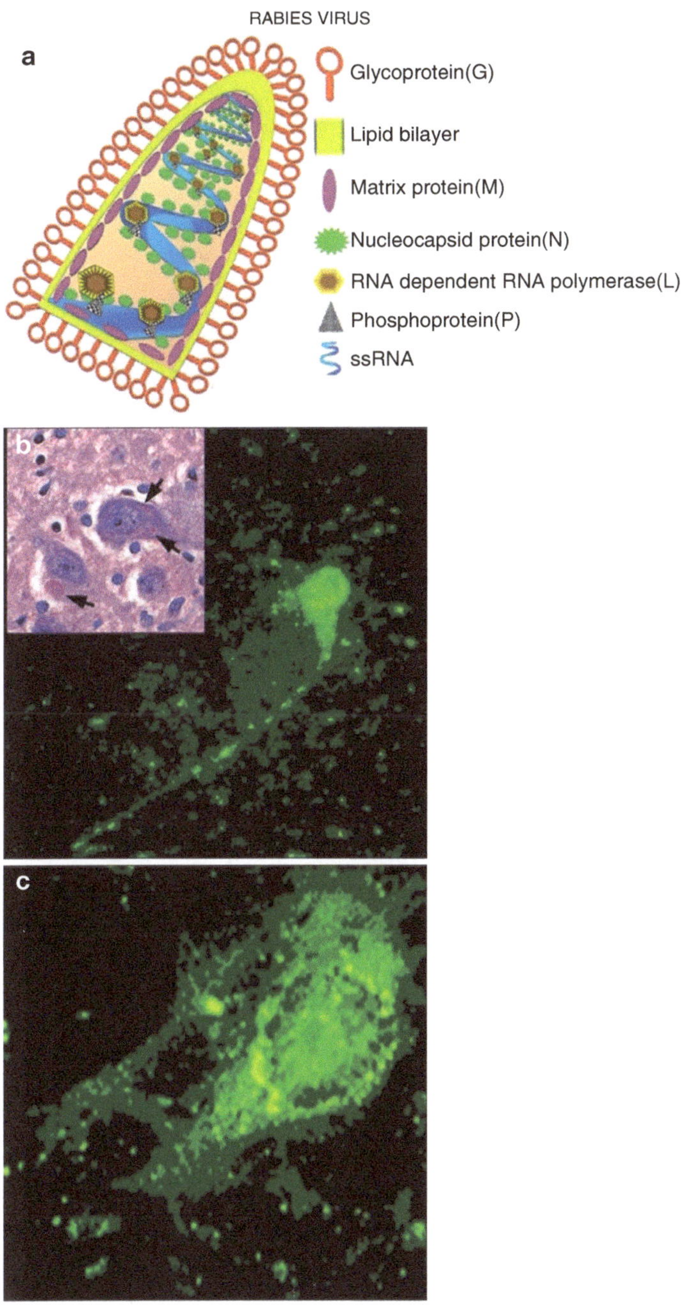

Fig. 6.3 (**a**) Schematic representation of internal structure of rabies virus and the position of various viral proteins. (**b**) Direct immunofluorescence staining on a fresh human brain smear with polyclonal antibody to nucleocapsid tagged to FITC bright greenish-yellow fluorescent rabies antigen particles inside the neuron and along the axons. ×600. *Inset*: eosinophilic intracytoplasmic Negri bodies in neuronal soma × 360. (**c**) BHK 21 cells infected with CVS strain of rabies in RFFIT. ×600 (From Ref. [81], with permission)

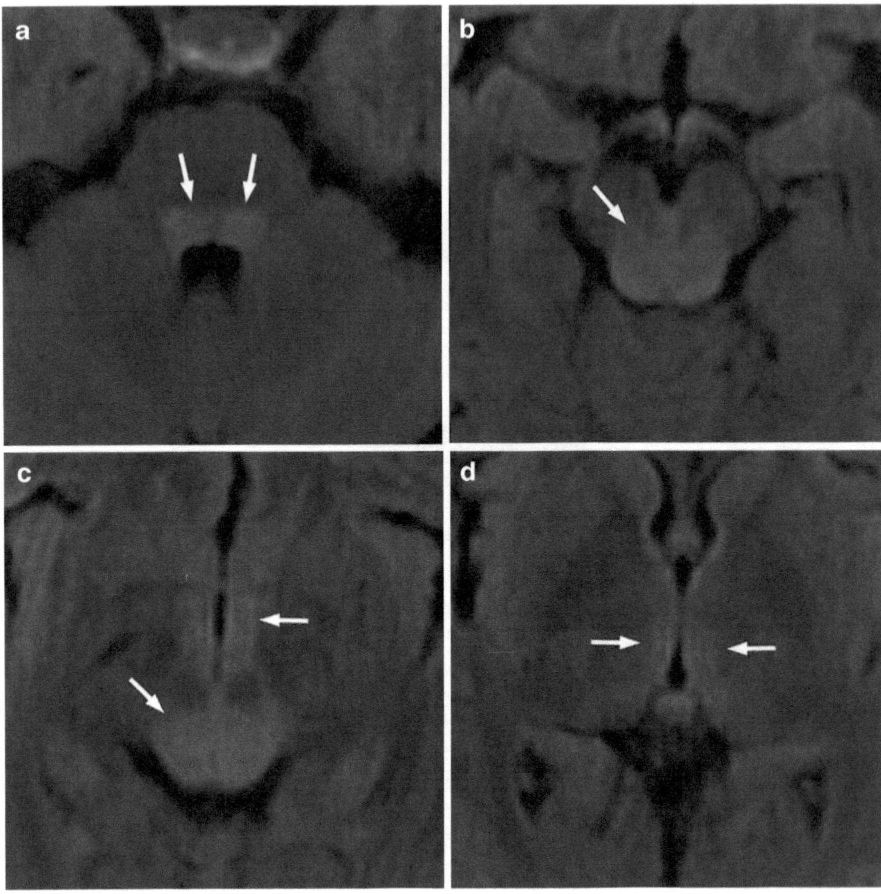

Fig. 6.4 (**a–d**) MRI in a 20-year-old woman with rabies encephalitis. Axial FLAIR MRI images of the brainstem and thalamus reveal hyperintense lesions (*arrows*) involving the pontine tegmentum (**a**), most of the midbrain (**b**, **c**), hypothalamus (**c**), and medial parts of the thalami (**d**) (With permission from Rao et al. [144])

forms of rabies is unknown. As the paralytic form is more common in partially immunized patients, a superadded immune response to virus-infected cells may be responsible for this.

There is surprisingly less imaging literature on rabies, probably because of the difficulty in imaging these patients. CT imaging may either be normal or reveal hypoattenuated lesions in the basal ganglia, hippocampi, periventricular white matter, and brainstem. No difference was found between the MRI features of paralytic and dumb rabies in a small series of five patients. T2 hyperintense ill-defined non-enhancing lesions were seen in the brainstem, hippocampi, hypothalami, deep and subcortical white matter, and deep and cortical gray matter in non-comatose patients (Fig. 6.4). Once patients became comatose, gadolinium-enhancing lesions were seen in the hypothalami, brainstem nuclei, spinal cord gray matter, and intradural

Table 6.2 Availability of antemortem diagnosis of human rabies

Tests	Specimens	Specificity %	Sensitivity %	Remarks
DFA on corneal smear (antigen)	Corneal smear	90	30	Not very sensitive
DFA on skin biopsy (antigen)	Nuchal skin	100	50–70	More sensitive than corneal test
RT-PCR on saliva for viral nucleic acid	Saliva	100	50–70	Moderate sensitivity
Real-time PCR on saliva for viral nucleic acid	Saliva	100	70–80	Higher sensitivity
Virus isolation from saliva by RTCIT	Saliva	100	70–80	Time-consuming
Antibody detection[a] in the serum/CSF by RFFIT	Serum and CSF	100	70	Time-consuming

From Ref. [81], with permission

DFA direct fluorescent antibody test, *RT-PCR* reverse transcriptase-polymerase chain reaction, *RTCIT* rabies tissue culture infection test, *RFFIT* rapid fluorescent focus inhibition test

[a]Should be interpreted based on history of prior vaccination

cervical nerve roots. Enhancement of the brachial plexus may however be seen in the prodromal phase of the disease [84].

In recent times more sensitive and specific tests for the antemortem detection of rabies have been developed (see Table 6.2). The antigen or antibody can be detected or viral isolates obtained from biological material such as serum, CSF, and saliva or from tissues such as nuchal skin or corneal swabs. The rabies virus antigen can be detected by fluorescent antibody tests in corneal smears or nuchal skin, the latter being more sensitive. Viral nucleic acid can be detected by PCR test. Both conventional reverse transcriptase-PCR or real-time PCR tests can be done and appear to be promising for antemortem diagnosis. Virus isolation can be done by mouse inoculation or rapid tissue culture infection tests. This is reliable but time-consuming. Demonstration of high titer of antibodies in nonimmunized patients or rising titer of antibodies in immunized patients in tests done 7–10 days apart provides indirect evidence of infection. Antibody detection can be done by the mouse neutralization test or the rapid tissue culture infection test, the latter being more sensitive. Antemortem diagnosis may not always be successful, and it has been seen that postmortem diagnostic tests are more sensitive and specific. Negri bodies can be demonstrated in more than 70 % of brain specimens. The viral antigen can be detected in brain smears by direct immunofluorescence tests or ELISA-based techniques.

In spite of reports of occasional survival of patients, rabies should be considered a fatal disease and treated conservatively with isolation of the patient. Antiviral agents (such as ribavarin), interferon, or intrathecal immune globulin has not been effective in treatment of rabies. In paralytic rabies when the diagnosis is not definite, more active therapy in an intensive care unit is advisable giving the benefit of doubt to the patient. Health-care personnel should take adequate precautionary measures in handling patients and take adequate preexposure prophylaxis.

Table 6.3 World Health Organization guidelines for the postexposure prophylaxis of rabies

Category of bite	Description of contact	Treatment
I	Touching, feeding of animals, or licks on intact skin	None, if history is reliable
II	Minor scratches or abrasions without bleeding and/or nibbling of uncovered skin	Immediate vaccination Stop treatment if animal remains healthy after 10 days of observation or if animal is euthanized and found to be negative for rabies by appropriate laboratory techniques
III	Single or multiple transdermal bites or scratches, licks on broken skin, contamination of mucous membrane with saliva (i.e., licks), and suspect contacts with bats	Immediate administration of rabies immunoglobulin and vaccination Stop treatment if animal remains healthy after 10 days of observation or if animal is euthanized and found to be negative for rabies by appropriate laboratory techniques

From Ref. [86]

Despite the eventual fatality of rabies, there is scope of effective disease control through postexposure prophylaxis. This consists of effective wound toilet, passive immunization with rabies immunoglobulin, and active immunization with rabies vaccine. Postexposure treatment should be started immediately for category II and III contact (see Table 6.3). Whereas no treatment other than wound toilet is necessary for category I contact, immediate vaccination along with wound toilet is recommended for category II contact. For category III contact, immediate vaccination with adequate wound toilet followed by administration of rabies immune globulin is recommended. Depending on vaccine types, the postexposure schedule recommended is intramuscular doses of 0.5 or 1 ml given as four to five doses over 4 weeks. Cell-derived vaccines recommended by the World Health Organization have been used intradermally for postexposure prophylaxis in countries like Thailand, Sri Lanka, and the Philippines, advantage being in reduced costs due to reduced dosages.

Local wound treatment should be given at the earliest. The wound should be washed in running tap water and washed with soap for at least 10 min which helps eliminate the virus. Local antiseptics should then be applied and suturing avoided as far as possible. The World Health Organization recommended dosage of rabies immunoglobulin is 40 IU/kg body weight for equine rabies immunoglobulin and 20 IU/kg body weight for human rabies immunoglobulin. This can be used for infiltrating around the wound, and the remainder can be injected intramuscularly at a site distant from the vaccine inoculation. Highly potent and safe vaccines are currently available for rabies prophylaxis. Tissue culture or duck embryo vaccines of at least 2.5 IU per single immunization dose should be used for vaccination. Intramuscular schedules involve injection of 1 dose into the deltoid region (or the anterolateral thigh in small children) on days 0, 3, 7, 14, and 30. The abbreviated multisite schedule which is a 2-1-1 regimen may be applied whereby two doses are given (one in each arm) on day 0 followed by 1 dose in the deltoid on days 7 and 21. This schedule is helpful in patients who do not receive rabies immunoglobulin, and an early immune response is necessary. The World Health Organization also recommends an intradermal regimen which may reduce costs by 60–80 %. 0.1 ml of purified Vero cell rabies vaccine or purified chick embryo cell vaccine is given intradermally in the left and right upper arm on days 0, 3, 7, and 28 [85, 86].

Preexposure vaccination is recommended for persons who have continued exposure risk like veterinarians, dog catchers, etc. Three doses of any modern vaccine are given as one standard intramuscular dose (0.5 or 1 ml) or 0.1 ml intradermally on days 0, 7, and 28. For reexposure of any person who has been previously immunized with a modern cell culture vaccine, two doses (intramuscular or intradermal) on days 0 and 3 are recommended. No immunoglobulin is applied. Use of brain tissue vaccine is no longer recommended by the World Health Organization [85, 86].

Measles

Measles is a highly infectious disease of children characterized by fever, respiratory symptoms, and a characteristic rash. The measles virus is a negative-stranded RNA paramyxovirus that is transmitted by droplet infection. Though measles is endemic to virtually all parts of the world, in recent years an appreciable reduction in deaths due to measles has been seen, principally due to effective vaccination. In the period of 2000–2011, global deaths due to measles decreased by 71 % from 5,42,000 to 1,58,000. Despite this progress, parts of South Asia, namely, India and Pakistan and parts of Africa (Ethiopia, Congo, and Nigeria), remain measles hot spots of the world due to inadequate vaccination. India remains the measles capital of the world with 29,339 cases reported in 2011 [87] and accounts for 47 % of the estimated global mortality due to measles in 2010 [88].

CNS infection by the measles virus can result in acute measles encephalitis (AME), subacute measles encephalitis (SME), or subacute sclerosing panencephalitis (SSPE). CNS complications in measles are rare. Approximately 0.5–1 in 1,000 cases of measles result in AME [89]. In North India, approximately 7–22 % of viral encephalitis in children is caused by the measles virus [67, 90]. SSPE is rarer still and occurs in a frequency of one to four cases in a million in developed countries and up to 21 cases in a million in developing countries like India [91, 92]. In recent times, however, with the introduction of mass immunization programs, the incidence of SSPE may be decreasing in India [93]. SME, also known as measles inclusion body encephalitis, is a still rarer complication of measles that occurs in the immunocompromised host and is caused by wild-type measles virus [89].

Acute measles encephalitis occurs at any time during the appearance of measles rash, usually within 8 days of onset of illness. There is controversy regarding the mechanism of AME with some studies suggesting direct viral invasion on the CNS, while others suggest autoimmune mechanisms after having failed to show viral-specific RNA in the brain of infected patients. However, an early onset may suggest direct viral invasion, while a delayed onset may suggest an autoimmune mechanism [89]. The onset is abrupt with irritability, fever, headache, vomiting, altered sensorium, seizures, and coma [94]. Mortality rate is between 10 and 20 %. The CSF may show mild pleocytosis, usually mononuclear, elevated protein, and normal sugar. Myelin basic protein in the CSF may suggest an autoimmune process, while detection of virus-specific genome in the CSF may suggest direct viral invasion [89]. MR imaging in children from Korea revealed bilateral T2 hyperintense lesions in the cerebral cortex, corpus striatum, and white matter with mild mass effect in the acute phase of the disease. These lesions showed restricted diffusion on DWI. Petechial hemorrhage, and cortical gyriform and leptomeningeal enhancement, was also seen. Encephalomalacia and atrophy was seen in the chronic phase [95]. Treatment is largely supportive, but immunomodulatory treatment with corticosteroids, immunoglobulin, and plasmapheresis has been employed with variable results [94].

SSPE is a slow virus infection of the CNS due to measles virus infection. The name is derived from the insidious nature of onset (subacute), the type of pathological lesions (sclerosis), and involvement of the entire brain (panencephalitis) [96]. The disease develops 6–8 years after the initial measles attack and is more common in males (male/female = 3:1). Risk factors of acquiring SSPE include younger age (highest risk under age 1), living in a rural area, overcrowded environments, more number of siblings, mental retardation, and lower birth order, all factors that may predispose to intensive measles exposure. A close temporal relationship of measles virus to other viruses may modify the course of measles infection and has been suggested as a risk factor for SSPE [97].

The exact pathogenesis of SSPE is not well understood. Measles virus possibly gains entry into the CNS by infection of the endothelial cells or through circulating inflammatory cells. There is evidence that an inadequate cell-mediated immune response and a resultant ineffective humoral response probably play an important role in the pathogenesis of SSPE. Once inside the neuron, the virus changes the cell machinery to bypass the immune system, and it undergoes mutations to avoid recognition. The virus remains dormant for several years before an eventual inflammatory response leading to widespread CNS destruction [96]. Despite the long latency, there is evidence that the virus gains entry into the brain soon after the acute infection with subsequent spread through the brain [97]. Early in the disease, there is variable inflammation of the meninges, cortex, deep gray matter, and white matter. This is associated with neuronophagia, gliosis, astrocytic proliferation, perivascular cuffing, lymphocytic and plasma cell infiltration, demyelination, and inclusion bodies in the neurons and glial cells. In the late stages, inflammatory changes decrease with severe loss of neurons of the cortex and deep gray matter with thinning of white matter and severe gliosis. Inclusion bodies are scanty at this time [98].

Clinically, the disease presents with minor behavioral and intellectual changes in a previously healthy child. This is followed by development of motor dysfunction and characteristic myoclonic jerks. Focal paralysis, seizures, autoimmune dysfunction, and rigidity also develop, finally leading to akinetic mutism and death [96, 97]. Four clinical stages have been described by Jabbour et al. In stage I there are personality changes and behavioral disturbances. Myoclonus, seizures, and severe intellectual decline are seen in stage II. Stage III is characterized by rigidity and progressive unresponsiveness. In stage IV there is mutism and coma; rigidity and myoclonus decreases [99]. Visual and ocular manifestations have been reported in 10–50 % patients and include cortical blindness, chorioretinitis, and optic atrophy [97].

The diagnosis of SSPE is based on clinical features associated with typical electroencephalographic (EEG) findings, presence of anti-measles antibody in the serum or CSF, MRI findings, and brain biopsy. CSF analysis may be normal or show elevated cells, total protein, gamma globulins and an oligoclonal band pattern. Elevated titers of anti-measles antibody of 1:256 in the serum and 1:4 or greater in the CSF is considered diagnostic for SSPE. There is a lowered CSF-to-serum ratio of the titer ranging from 1:4 to 1:128 compared to normal ratios of 1:200 to 1:500 [97].

The characteristic EEG findings in SSPE are periodic complexes, known as Radermecker complexes, which are found in 65–83 % of SSPE (Fig. 6.5b). Periodic complexes are 100–1,000 mv, 1–3 Hz waves, intermingled with spikes and sharp and slow waves of 1–3 s duration. The interval between complexes varies from 2 to 20 s. In early stages, they can recur every 5 min. They can occur during sleep and can be elicited by external stimuli. They are secondary to widespread neuronal excitability, pathological hypersynchronization, and rhythmic triggering by a pacemaker, potentially in the brainstem or perithalamic area [96]. Morphology of the complexes is highly stereotyped within one individual but differs between patients [97]. EEG background is normal in early stage of the disease. As the disease progresses, there is slowing, disorganization, and asymmetry with increasing diffuse slow wave activity in the background. At times there may be focal spikes coinciding with underlying pathology. In the progressive stage of disease, polymorphic delta activity or intermittent frontal dominant monorhythmic slow activity may be present. In the later stage, recurrence of periodic complexes increases and amplitude reduction of complexes occurs. Finally EEG becomes flat, or in rare instance, an alpha coma pattern may be seen.

Neuroimaging with MRI is preferred over CT, as CT underevaluates the disease [100]. MRI shows involvement of the white matter, gray matter, and deep gray matter with cerebral atrophy. MRI seems to follow a constant pattern with white matter changes appearing first followed by cerebral atrophy. Early in the disease, T2 hyperintense white matter changes are seen (Fig. 6.5). These are more common in the parieto-occipital than in the frontal regions. Gray matter changes are also noted that are hyperintense on T2- and hypointense on T1-weighted images. The brainstem, cerebral and cerebellar peduncles, and cerebellum may be involved. In advanced stages, cerebral atrophy is more pronounced with diffuse white matter changes and thinning of the corpus callosum [100–102]. Despite this set progressive pattern on conventional MRI, the changes do not correlate well with clinical stages of the disease [100] (Fig. 6.5). Newer MRI techniques such as diffusion-weighted imaging

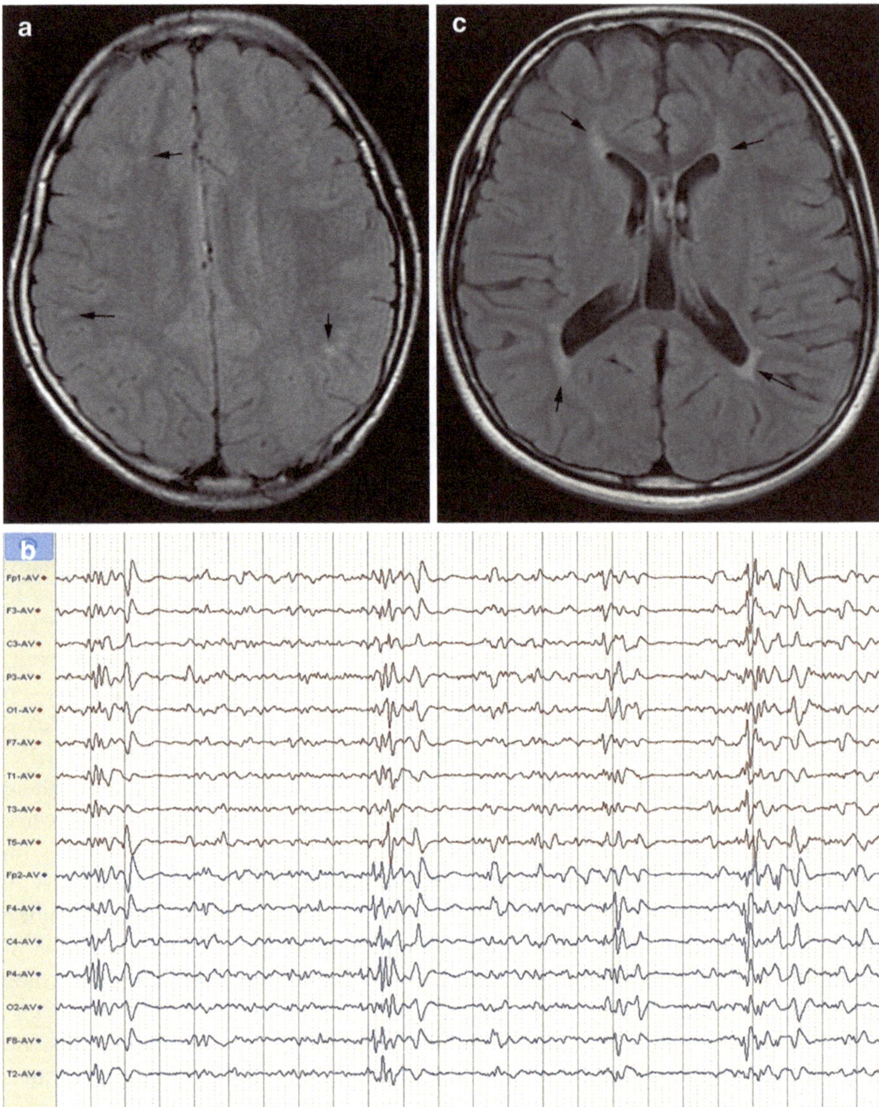

Fig. 6.5 (**a**) A 12-year-old male with subacute sclerosing panencephalitis (SSPE) in clinical stage III. Axial fluid-attenuated inversion recovery MRI image. Note subtle white matter lesions in the subcortical regions (*arrows*). There is no cerebral atrophy. MRI changes do not correlate well with the clinical stage of disease. (**b**) Electroencephalography of the same patient as (a) showing characteristic periodic complexes, appearing in 6 s and lasting for 2 s on a slow background. Focal frontal slow waves are also recorded. (**c**) Axial fluid-attenuated inversion recovery MRI in a different 13-year-old male patient with stage II SSPE. White matter lesions (*arrows*) are seen in the parieto-occipital periventricular and frontal periventricular white matter. There is cerebral atrophy. The patient had a worse looking MRI than the patient in (a) despite being clinically better

(DWI), MR spectroscopy (MRS), diffusion tensor imaging (DTI), and diffusion tensor tractography (DTT) have been reported to be of more help in early detection and staging of the disease. DWI has shown a significant difference in apparent diffusion coefficient (ADC) values between clinical stages II and III of the disease with the highest ADC values in stage III [103]. Similar ability to differentiate stage II from III has been reported with MRS. In one such study, there were differences in brain metabolites of stage II and III disease in relation to controls. Stage II disease revealed elevated myoinositol (MI) and choline levels with normal *N*-acetyl aspartate (NAA), while stage II disease revealed decreased NAA with increased choline and MI with increased lactate and lipid peaks. The findings possibly reflect the inflammation in stage II and the demyelination, gliosis, cell necrosis, and anaerobic metabolism in stage III [104]. DTI has been shown to detect abnormal mean diffusivity (MD) and fractional anisotropy (FA) values in normal-appearing white matter in stage II patients. Tract-specific FA values in some major white matter tracts have been shown to correlate inversely with clinical grades II through IV [105, 106].

No adequate therapy for SSPE exists in the current time. Three drugs, Isoprinosine, interferon-alpha (INF-α), and ribavarin have been reported as effective but not curative of the disease. Isoprinosine, an antiviral drug that acts by increasing CD4+ lymphocytes, has been shown to prolong survival and cause clinical improvement in some patients. A dose of 100 mg/kg/day is given daily, and it needs to be continued even during remissions and possibly for life [97]. INF-α did not meet with much success when used through the intravenous or intramuscular route. However, the intraventricular route has been successful in showing improvement in patients [107, 108]. Combination therapy with intraventricular INF-α and oral Isoprinosine has been found to be effective in treating SSPE. Combination of weekly intrathecal INF-α offered a benefit of 35 % compared to the 34 % benefit with Isoprinosine monotherapy in one study. This was more beneficial than the 5–10 % spontaneous remission reported in literature. Even though no statistical difference in combination therapy versus Isoprinosine monotherapy was seen in the study [109], the combination therapy is still considered the most effective treatment available for SSPE today [107]. Intraventricular administration of ribavarin, another antiviral drug, has also shown efficacy in the control of SSPE. Used in high doses it has shown doubtful results; but used in combination with INF-α, it has shown better results [110, 111]. At the current time, SSPE remains a fatal disease with a case fatality of 95 % and mean survival in children being 1 year and 9 months to 3 years [96].

Subacute measles encephalitis (SME) also known as measles inclusion body encephalitis (MIBE) or immunosuppressive measles encephalitis (IME) is an uncommon complication of measles in immunocompromised children, primarily occurring in patients of acute lymphocytic leukemia but also seen in other immunosuppressive conditions such as AIDS, organ transplantation and immunosuppressive therapy, or immunodeficiencies. Unlike SSPE which has a latency of several years, SME presents a few weeks to 7 months after the acute measles infection [112]. Recently, a cluster of eight patients of SME in HIV-positive patients have been reported during a large outbreak of measles in South Africa underscoring the importance of immunization programs in an HIV-endemic population. Unlike SSPE, the brain virus was similar to the epidemic strain, possibly due to the short time from infection to brain disease in these patients [113, 114]. CSF analysis, EEG, and measurement of measles antibody in the serum and CSF are not helpful in the diagnosis. Brain biopsy and measles polymerase chain reaction on brain tissue are required for diagnosis of SME. Brain biopsy reveals eosinophilic inclusion bodies in neurons and oligodendrocytes with non-necrotizing encephalitis with paucity of inflammation [112, 113]. Patients present with partial seizures often with epilepsia partialis continua, altered sensorium, and variable neurological deficits. It has a mortality rate of 85 %, and survivors frequently have severe psychomotor deficit. CT is not helpful in imaging these patients. On MRI, cortical T2 hyperintense lesions are seen with patchy involvement of the parieto-occipital, frontal, and temporal regions and in the deep gray matter. White matter abnormalities are infrequent [113, 115, 116]. Intravenous ribavarin therapy is effective if administered early [112].

Chandipura

Chandipura virus (CHP) is an emerging rhabdovirus that has recently been associated with a number of outbreaks of encephalitis in India. It is transmitted to humans by sandflies and mosquitoes. The sandfly may be the main vector as well as maintenance host of the virus. The virus was first isolated in 1965 during an outbreak of febrile illness in a village called Chandipura in the state of Maharashtra in India [117, 118]. Its epidemic potential was realized only during large outbreaks of acute encephalitis reported from South India in 2003 and West India in 2004 with high case fatality rates [119, 120]. Earlier believed to be prevalent only in Asia, CHP today is today known to be prevalent in India, Sri Lanka, and Western Africa [117]. There is some controversy regarding the CHP etiology of epidemic encephalopathy. One investigating group did not find any conclusive evidence of invasion by any pathogen as the cause of the outbreak. They suggested that the outbreak was not of encephalitis but because of "epidemic brain attacks" presumably due to a vascular cause [121]. Nevertheless in recent years CHP may have emerged as one of the most common agents causing acute encephalitis syndrome in India [7]. CHP encephalitis is characterized by acute-onset fever, altered sensorium, seizures, diarrhea, and vomiting. Death or recovery occurs within 2–3 days with no sequel in survivors. Most deaths occur within 24 h of illness. The symptoms have been attributed to brainstem encephalitis. CSF and blood parameters are usually normal. High-grade fever, absent oculocephalic reflex, and a Glasgow Coma Scale of less than 7 are poor prognosticators of the disease [122, 123]. The diagnosis is established by (1) virus isolation in cell culture, infant mice, and embryonated eggs; (2) antigen detection by ELISA and immunofluorescence assay; (3) genome detection by reverse transcriptase-polymerase chain reaction (RT-PCR); and (4) serological tests: IgM and IgG ELISA, hemagglutination inhibition, complement fixation, and virus neutralization test [118, 119]. As the disease has a rapid course and high fatality, RT-PCR is the diagnostic method of choice with the advantage of high sensitivity, speed, accuracy, and reproducibility [124]. Neuroimaging by CT and MRI was found to be normal in a study from South India [121]. However, there is incidental mention that one group of investigators saw lesions in the cortical regions of the frontal and temporal lobes in 11 MRI scans in patients from South India [125]. CT scans of eight patients in another study from South India showed diffuse brain swelling and dilated ventricles [126]. No specific treatment or vaccine exists. Treatment is symptomatic, aimed at symptoms and complications. Early treatment with mannitol to reduce brain edema is lifesaving [127].

Chikungunya

Chikungunya (CHIK) is an emerging virus infection that has resulted from enhanced vector competence. It is caused by a togavirus. *Aedes aegypti* mosquito was the principal vector in earlier times. Later the viral host range extended into the *Aedes albopictus* mosquito, presumably due to favorable mutation of the virus that increases infectivity of the virus for *A. albopictus*, facilitates entry into the salivary gland, and increases efficiency of transmission from mosquitoes to vertebrates [128]. It was first detected in modern-day Tanzania. Initially it was limited to sub-Saharan Africa, India, and parts of Southeast Asia. Subsequently in 2005–2006, large outbreaks have been reported from La Réunion, with subsequent spread to the Indian subcontinent and Indonesia. There were an estimated 1.5 million cases in India in 2006. A small outbreak was reported in Italy where the disease spread from an index Indian traveler through native *A. Albopictus* [72, 129].

CHIK is a dengue-like illness characterized by fever, malaise, body ache, joint pains, rash, headache, and nausea. The illness is self-limiting. Fever may last for 36 days, but arthropathy may last for 3–6 months. Neurological manifestations are rare and include meningoencephalitis, myelopathy, and neuropathy. These were seen in isolation or in combination in a large case series reported from India. Carpal tunnel syndrome and retinopathy were also seen. Neurological manifestations occur within a few days after onset of fever. Headache, altered sensorium, and focal neurological deficits were seen in patients with encephalitis. Myelopathy presented with retention of urine and paraparesis. Two types of neuropathy were seen as follows: (1) early, characterized by rapid quadriparesis and facial weakness, and (2) late, presented few weeks after onset of fever [129]. Altered sensorium, headache, seizures, sensory abnormalities, and motor dysfunction have been reported in patients with neurological disease from La Réunion [130]. In children with neurological manifestations, febrile seizures, meningitis, and acute encephalopathy have been reported [131]. Overall mortality in studies from India and La Réunion was similar at 10 % [129, 130].

MRI abnormalities in patients with encephalopathy from India were in the form of multiple punctuate white matter lesions that are more prominent on diffusion-weighted MRI than on T2- or T1-weighted images. Although these resembled those of Nipah viral encephalitis, the prominence on diffusion imaging and lack of brainstem or cortical lesions differentiated CHIK from Nipah viral encephalitis. Occasional contrast enhancement of the lesions was seen. MRI rarely showed cord changes in CHIK with myelopathy. Nerve root enhancement involving the ventral cauda equina nerve roots has been reported in patients with neuropathy [129, 132]. MRI abnormalities reported from La Réunion were somewhat different. Brain MRI was abnormal in 5 out of 14 children with neurological complications. Two out of ten patients more than 1 month of age showed abnormal MRI with increased T2 signal in the cingulate, limbic areas, and white matter. No diffusion abnormalities were seen. Three out of four patients of less than 1 month age showed abnormal MRI, with areas of restricted diffusion in the white matter and regions of increased signal in the white matter and/or cortex on T1- and T2-weighted images. Areas of hemorrhagic change were also noted. Patients with MRI abnormalities and severe clinical symptoms had more sequel or fatalities [131]. No imaging abnormalities were seen in another study of 23 patients from La Réunion [130].

While almost all patients of neurological CHIK from India showed lymphocytic pleocytosis and elevated protein [129], those from La Réunion showed variable pleocytosis [130, 131]. Electroencephalogram (EEG) was nonspecific and showed diffuse slowing [130]. In children EEG showed diffuse slowing that was anteriorly predominant in half of the cases and paroxysmal polyspikes in 40 % [131]. The diagnosis can be confirmed by the detection of IgM in the serum and CSF or by detection of the viral genome in the serum or CSF by reverse transcriptase-polymerase chain reaction [129, 131].

Treatment is nonspecific and supportive [131]. Methylprednisolone, plasmapheresis, and intravenous immunoglobulin have been tried with mixed results [129].

Viral Myelitis

Viral myelitis may involve the spinal cord gray matter, white matter, or both, extending through variable vertebral segments. If the anterior horn cells are involved, acute flaccid paralysis (AFP) can result. When both halves of the spinal cord are involved, acute transverse myelitis (ATM) can result. A chronic from of myelitis that is associated with human immunodeficiency virus 1 (HIV-1) and human T-cell lymphotropic virus 1 (HTLV-1) has also been described.

AFP is characterized by rapid-onset progressive weakness that may involve muscles of respiration and swallowing with maximum severity within days to weeks. If untreated, AFP may not only persist but lead to death. Poliomyelitis is the prototype AFP. It is of great public health importance in the context of the global polio eradication program. With poliomyelitis on the wane in endemic areas, other emerging viruses are gaining importance in the etiology of AFP. These include non-polio enteroviruses, West Nile virus, Japanese encephalitis virus, Coxsackie viruses, and tick-borne encephalitis virus [133, 134]. Out of more than 50,000 cases of AFP reported to the World Health Organization in 2013, more than 30,000 were from India, though no poliomyelitis patients were reported from the country since 2012. The annualized world non-polio AFP incidence rate is approximately 4 per 100,000 population [135]. The exact incidence of viral myelitis is unknown but is possibly more than this [134]. Viral myelitis may accompany several of the tropical CNS viral infections described above.

In AFP due to poliomyelitis, there is a prodrome consisting of headache, fever, or altered mental status. Within days, motor deficit involving one or more limbs occurs. There are no sensory abnormalities or bladder dysfunction. AFP caused by non-polio viruses may be associated with other symptoms which may provide a clue to the viral etiology of symptoms. AFP caused by enterovirus 71 may be associated with hand, foot, and mouth disease; aseptic meningitis; or acute hemorrhagic conjunctivitis. Muscle weakness and wasting associated with enterovirus 70 may be severe and permanent [133]. Acute myelitis, on the other hand, presents with sensory disturbances, urinary retention, and weakness with decreased or increased reflexes. The involvement may be asymmetric when a part of the transverse extent of the cord is involved and bilaterally uniform when both halves of the cord are involved, when it is called acute transverse myelitis. Typically viral myelitis occurs in a matter of days. Faster evolution of symptoms in the order of minutes or hours may represent a vascular event such as anterior spinal artery infarct. Clues to the viral etiology can again be provided by symptoms such as prior vesicular rash in the buccal mucosa and on the hands and feet 3–7 days before in enterovirus 71; dermatomal zoster up to 2 weeks prior in varicella-zoster virus; fever, petechiae, and rash with dengue myelitis; and fever and arthropathy with Chikungunya. Associated aseptic meningitis, meningoencephalitis, and neuritis can be seen with several types of tropical viral myelitis (see above).

Differential diagnosis of myelitis includes nonviral infective myelitis and structural, vascular, traumatic, metabolic, hereditary, and autoimmune causes. These can be distinguished by appropriate clinical evaluation and laboratory tests [133, 134].

MRI is the imaging modality of choice and should include the entire spine as the clinical level may not always be accurate. The brain should be included when clinically indicated or at least screened because this may provide important clues to the diagnosis in acute transverse myelitis (e.g., silent demyelination in multiple sclerosis and demyelination typical of acute disseminated encephalomyelitis). MRI in viral myelitis may be normal or show the level and extent of lesions and vertebral segments involved. Cord swelling and hemorrhagic changes may be seen. Gadolinium enhancement of the cord, meninges, or nerve roots may be evident. In patients with AFP due to enterovirus 71 etiology, unilateral or bilateral anterior horn cell T2 hyperintense lesions and ventral nerve root enhancement in post-gadolinium images have been reported [136]. T2 hyperintense lesions in the anterior horn cells in AFP due to poliomyelitis have also been reported [137]. Spinal cord involvement has also been seen on MRI in Japanese encephalitis [138].

The CSF may show elevated protein and lymphocytic pleocytosis. A definitive diagnosis can be arrived at by demonstration of the virus, viral genome, and antibodies in the CSF or serum. Virus culture is difficult and rarely successful. The viral genomic sequence can be demonstrated by polymerase chain reaction (PCR) for DNA viruses and reverse transcriptase-PCR (RT-PCR) for RNA viruses. The yield is highest if CSF testing is done within 5 days of onset of symptoms [139]. Intrathecal antibody detection by demonstrating virus-specific IgM is a complementary test to PCR/RT-PCR. A ratio of virus-specific serum/CSF IgG antibody titers of less than 100:1 may be suggestive of CNS antibody synthesis. More than fourfold rise of serum antibody titers against a virus may also be diagnostic of viral CNS infection [134]. The definitive diagnosis of viral myelitis is nevertheless elusive and is arrived at by the exclusion of other differential diagnosis.

Electrodiagnostic tests may provide supportive diagnostic evidence, clues to the differential diagnosis, and prognostic information in AFP and ATM. In AFP due to poliomyelitis, non-polio enteroviruses, Japanese encephalitis virus, and West Nile virus, nerve conduction tests indicate anterior horn cell disease with reduced compound muscle action potential (CMAP) amplitude with evidence of denervation on electromyography (EMG). Differentiation of AFP from Guillain-Barré syndrome (GBS) may be possible as the latter shows reduced CMAP amplitude and demyelination on nerve conduction tests but usually does not show denervation on EMG up to 3 weeks [133]. Electrodiagnostic tests may suggest peripheral nerve demyelination or less commonly a compound demyelination and axonal process in GBS [140, 141]. ATM does not show abnormalities on nerve conduction or EMG [133]. It may not be possible however to differentiate between various etiological types of ATM on the basis of electrodiagnostic tests. Prognostic information from electrodiagnostic tests in ATM has been reported. In a large series of patients of ATM, outcome was correlated to somatosensory evoked potentials, EMGs, and central motor conduction times to the tibialis anterior and abductor digiti minimi muscles.

Though the treatment of HSV myelitis is with the antiviral drug, acyclovir, administering acyclovir for all cases of viral myelitis till HSV-2 is excluded is not advisable unless there is a history of recurrent genital infection [134]. Treatment of enterovirus myelitis is mainly supportive. There are anecdotal reports of the efficacy of pleconaril, a drug that blocks enterovirus receptor interaction and viral uncoating, and intravenous immunoglobulin against acute flaccid paralysis caused by enterovirus [142]. Similarly anecdotal reports for efficacy of intravenous immunoglobulin for the treatment of West Nile virus neuroinvasive disease exist [143]. Few drugs are also under evaluation for the treatment of Japanese encephalitis virus disease (see above). Corticosteroids have a doubtful role in the treatment of neuroinvasive viral disease (see sections on JEV, measles, Chikungunya). High doses of intravenous methylprednisolone may have to be started in acute transverse myelitis as it is usually impossible to differentiate between postinfectious (immune-mediated) myelitis and viral myelitis in the acute setting. A dose of 1 g daily for 5–7 days is given [134].

In conclusion, CNS viral disease in the tropics presents a challenging task to the treating physician due to several offending endemic and epidemic viruses that are different from those seen in the western world. This is frequently compounded by inadequate health-care systems and adverse sociopolitical conditions that have posed a challenge to the control of several of these diseases. Issues such as emergence of viruses, climate, and environmental change pose fresh challenges to their control. Though commendable strides have been taken in the control of age-old problems such as poliomyelitis, much needs to be done for the control of Japanese encephalitis, rabies, and measles. Fresh challenges have been presented by the emergence of West Nile, Chandipura, Nipah, and occasional neuroinvasive viruses like dengue and Chikungunya.

Our acknowledgments are due to our colleagues N. C. Borah, B. Saharia, Diganta Dutta, Meghali Gohain, and Firdaus Ahmed for their help and support. We would also like to thank Rathin Sharma for his help in preparing the map of Japanese encephalitis prevalence.

References

1. Kumar R. Aseptic meningitis: diagnosis and management. Indian J Pediatr. 2005;72(1):57–63.
2. Sathish N, Scott JX, Shaji RV, et al. An outbreak of echoviral meningitis in children. Indian Pediatr. 2004;41(4):384–8.
3. Handique SK. Viral infections of the central nervous system. Neuroimaging Clin N Am. 2011;21:777–94.
4. Wang RJ, Wang DX, Wang JW, Feng ZJ. Analysis of 62 adult patients with viral meningitis. Zhonghua Shi Yan He Lin Chuang Bing Du Xue Za Zhi. 2009;23(3):218–20.
5. Jmor F, Emsley HC, Fischer M, Solomon T, Lewthwaite P. The incidence of acute encephalitis syndrome in Western industrialised and tropical countries. Virol J. 2008;5:134.
6. Joshi R, Mishra PK, Joshi D, et al. Clinical presentation, etiology, and survival in adult acute encephalitis syndrome in rural Central India. Clin Neurol Neurosurg. 2013. doi:http://dx.doi.org/10.1016/j.clineuro.2013.04.008.
7. Joshi R, Kalantri SP, Reingold A, et al. Changing landscape of acute encephalitis syndrome in India: a systematic review. Natl Med J India. 2012;25:212–20.
8. Booss J, Esiri MM. Pathological features of encephalitis in humans. In: Booss J, Esiri MM, editors. Viral encephalitis in humans. Washington, DC: ASM Press; 2013. p. 3–19.
9. Solomon T, Dung NM, Kneen R, et al. Japanese encephalitis. J Neurol Neurosurg Psychiatry. 2000;68:405–41.
10. Burke DS, Leake CJ. Japanese encephalitis. In: Monath TP, editor. The Arboviruses: epidemiology and ecology, vol. 3. Boca Raton: CRC Press; 1988. p. 63–92.
11. Campbell GL, Hills SL, Fischer M, et al. Estimated global incidence of Japanese encephalitis: a systematic review. Bull World Health Organ. 2011;89:766–4E. doi:10.2471/BLT.10.085233.
12. Solomon T. Recent advances in Japanese encephalitis. J Neurovirol. 2003;9:274–83.
13. Chen WR, Tesh RB, Rico-Hesse R. Genetic variation of Japanese encephalitis virus in nature. J Gen Virol. 1990;71:2915–22.
14. Chen WR, Rico-Hesse R, Tesh RB. A new genotype of Japanese encephalitis virus from Indonesia. Am J Trop Med Hyg. 1992;47(1):61–9.
15. Uchil PD, Satchidanandam V. Phylogenetic analysis of Japanese encephalitis virus: envelope gene based analysis reveals a fifth genotype, geographic clustering, and multiple introductions of the virus into the Indian subcontinent. Am J Trop Med Hyg. 2001;65:242–51.
16. Tiwari S, Singh RK, Tiwari R, et al. Japanese encephalitis: a review of the Indian perspective. Braz J Infect Dis. 2012;16:564–73.
17. Kanojia PC, Shetty PS, Geevarghese G. A long-term study on vector abundance & seasonal prevalence in relation to the occurrence of Japanese encephalitis in Gorakhpur district, Uttar Pradesh. Indian J Med Res. 2003;117:104–10.

18. Vaughn DW, Hoke Jr CH. The epidemiology of Japanese encephalitis: prospects for prevention. Epidemiol Rev. 1992;14:197–221.
19. Umenai T, Krzysko R, Bektimorov TA, et al. Japanese encephalitis: current worldwide status. Bull World Health Organ. 1985;63:625–31.
20. Huong VTQ, Ha DQ, Deubel V. Genetic study of Japanese encephalitis viruses from Vietnam. Am J Trop Med Hyg. 1993;49:538–44.
21. Misra UK, Kalita J. Overview: Japanese encephalitis. Prog Neurobiol. 2010;91:108–20.
22. Bai L, Morton LC, Liu Q. Climate change and mosquito borne diseases in China: a review. Global Health. 2013;9:10. doi:10.1186/1744-8603-0-10.
23. NVBDC P. Directorate General of Health Services. Ministry of Health and Family Welfare. New Delhi. 2010. Available from http://nvbdcp.gov.in/je-cd.html.
24. Dutta K, Rangarajan PN, Vrati S, et al. Japanese encephalitis: pathogenesis, prophylactics and therapeutics. Curr Sci. 2010;98:326–34.
25. Diamond MS. Evasion of innate and adaptive immunity by flaviviruses. Immunol Cell Biol. 2003;81:196–206.
26. Shankar SK, Vasudev Rao T, Mruthyunjayanna BP, et al. Autopsy study of brains during an epidemic of Japanese encephalitis in Karnataka. Indian J Med Res. 1983;78:431–40.
27. Zimmerman HM. The pathology of Japanese B encephalitis. Am J Pathol. 1946;22:965–91.
28. Gourie-Devi M, Ravi V, Shankar SK. Japanese encephalitis. An overview. In: Clifford Rose F, editor. Recent advances in tropical neurology. Amsterdam: Elsevier Science B.V.; 1995. p. 17–35.
29. Tiroumourougane SV, Raghava P, Srinivasan S. Japanese viral encephalitis. Postgrad Med J. 2002;78:205–15.
30. Kumar R, Mathur A, Kumar A, et al. Clinical features & prognostic indicators of Japanese encephalitis in children in Lucknow (India). Indian J Med Res. 1990;91:321–7.
31. Solomon T, Kneen R, Dung NM, et al. Poliomyelitis-like illness due to Japanese encephalitis like virus. Lancet. 1998;351:1094–7.
32. Pradhan S, Gupta RK, Singh MB, et al. Biphasic illness pattern due to early relapse in Japanese-B virus encephalitis. J Neurol Sci. 2001;183:13–8.
33. Handique SK, Barkataky N. MR imaging in biphasic Japanese encephalitis. AJNR Am J Neuroradiol. 2008;29:E3.
34. Kalita K, Misra UK. EEG in Japanese encephalitis: a clinico-radiological correlation. Electroencephalogr Clin Neurophysiol. 1998;106:238–43.
35. Kalita J, Misra UK. Comparison of CT scan and MRI findings in the diagnosis of Japanese encephalitis. J Neurol Sci. 2000;174:3–8.
36. Handique SK, Das RR, Barman K, et al. Temporal lobe involvement in Japanese encephalitis – problems in differential diagnosis. AJNR Am J Neuroradiol. 2006;27:1027–31.
37. Shoji H, Kida H, Hino H, et al. Magnetic resonance imaging findings in Japanese encephalitis. White matter lesions. J Neuroimaging. 1994;4:206–11.
38. Dung NM, Turtle L, Chong WK, et al. An evaluation of the usefulness of neuroimaging for the diagnosis of Japanese encephalitis. J Neurol. 2009;256:2052–60.
39. Basumatary LJ, Raja D, Bhuyan D, et al. Clinical and radiological spectrum of Japanese encephalitis. J Neurol Sci. 2013;325:15–21.
40. Burke DS, Nisalak A, Ussery MA. Antibody capture immunoassay detection of Japanese encephalitis virus immunoglobulin M and G antibodies in cerebrospinal fluid. J Clin Microbiol. 1982;16:1034–42.
41. Solomon T, Dung NM, Wills B, et al. Interferon alfa-2a in Japanese encephalitis: a randomised double-blind placebo-controlled trial. Lancet. 2003;361:821–6.
42. Saxena SK, Mathur A, Srivastava RC. Inhibition of Japanese encephalitis virus infection by diethyldithiocarbamate is independent of its antioxidant potential. Antivir Chem Chemother. 2003;14:91–8.
43. Hoke Jr CH, Vaughn DW, Nisalak A, et al. Effect of high dose dexamethasone on the outcome of acute encephalitis due to Japanese encephalitis virus. J Infect Dis. 1992;165:631–7.
44. Dutta K, Basu A. Use of minocycline in viral infections. Indian J Med Res. 2011; 133:467–70.

45. Sebastian L, Desai A, Shampur MN, et al. N-methylisatin-beta thiosemicarbazone derivative (Sch 16) is an inhibitor of Japanese encephalitis virus infection in vitro and in vivo. Virol J. 2008;5:64.
46. Rossi SL, Ross TM, Evans JD. West Nile virus. Clin Lab Med. 2010;30:47–65.
47. Paramasivan R, Mishra AC, Mourya DT. West Nile virus: the Indian scenario. Indian J Med Res. 2003;118:101–8.
48. Gajanana A. West Nile virus epidemics: lessons for India. ICMR Bull. 2002;32(7).
49. World Health Organisation. West Nile Virus. Media centre. Fact sheet, July 2011. [Internet] 2013 [cited 2013 June 19]. Available from http://www.who.int/mediacentre/factsheets/fs354/en/#.
50. Banker DD. Preliminary observations on antibody patterns against certain viruses among inhabitants of Bombay city. Indian J Med Sci. 1952;6:733–46.
51. Khan SA, Dutta P, Khan AM, et al. West Nile virus, Assam, India. Emerg Infect Dis. 2011;17:947–8.
52. Samuel MA, Diamond MS. Pathogenesis of West Nile Virus infection: a balance between virulence, innate and adaptive immunity, and viral evasion. J Virol. 2006;80:9349–60.
53. Sampson BA, Ambrosi C, Charlot C, et al. The pathology of human West Nile Virus infection. Hum Pathol. 2000;31:527–31.
54. Kelly TW, Prayson RA, Ruiz AI, et al. The neuropathology of West Nile virus meningoencephalitis: a report of 2 cases and review of the literature. Am J Clin Pathol. 2003;119: 749–53.
55. Zak IT, Altinok D, Merline JR, et al. West Nile virus infection. AJR Am J Roentgenol. 2005; 184:957–61.
56. Ali M, Safriel Y, Sohi J, et al. West Nile virus infection: MR imaging findings in the nervous system. AJNR Am J Neuroradiol. 2005;26:289–97.
57. Petropoulou KA, Gordon SM, Prayson RA, et al. West Nile virus meningoencephalitis: MR imaging findings. AJNR Am J Neuroradiol. 2005;26:1986–95.
58. World Health Organisation. Dengue: guidelines for diagnosis, treatment, prevention and control. Geneva: WHO; 2009.
59. World Health Organization. Dengue haemorrhagic fever; diagnosis, treatment, prevention and control. Geneva: WHO; 1997.
60. Gulati S, Maheshwari A. Atypical manifestations of dengue. Trop Med Int Health. 2007; 12:1087–95.
61. Murthy JMK. Neurological manifestations of dengue infection. Neurol India. 2010;58:581–4.
62. Varatharaj A. Encephalitis in the clinical spectrum of dengue infection. Neurol India. 2010;58:585–91.
63. World Health Organisation. Media centre. Poliomyelitis. Available at. http://www.who.int/mediacentre/factsheets/fs114/en/. Accessed 5 July 2013.
64. Tyler KL. Emerging viral infections of the central nervous system: part 1. Arch Neurol. 2009;66:939–48.
65. Sarma N. Hand, foot, and mouth disease: current scenario and Indian perspective. Indian J Dermatol Venereol Leprol. 2013;79:165–75.
66. Shen WC, Chiu HH, Chow KC, et al. MR Imaging findings of enteroviral encephalomyelitis: an outbreak in Taiwan. AJNR Am J Neuroradiol. 1999;20:1889–95.
67. Karmarkar SA, Aneja S, Khare S, et al. A study of acute febrile encephalopathy with special reference to viral etiology. Indian J Pediatr. 2008;75:801–5.
68. Lewthwaite P, Perera D, Ooi MH, Last A, Kumar R, Desai A, et al. Enterovirus 75 encephalitis in children, southern India. Emerg Infect Dis [serial on the Internet]. 2010 Nov [date cited]. http://www.cdc.gov/EID/content/16/11/1780.htm. doi: 10.3201/eid1611.100672.
69. Sapkal GN, Bondre VP, Fulmali PV, Patil P, Gopalkrishna V, Dadhania V, et al. Enteroviruses in patients with acute encephalitis, Uttar Pradesh, India. Emerg Infect Dis. 2009;15:295–8.
70. Laxmivandana R, Yergolkar P, Gopalkrishna V, et al. Characterization of the non-polio enterovirus infections associated with acute flaccid paralysis in South-Western India. PLoS ONE. 2013;8(4):e61650. doi:10.1371/journal.pone.0061650.

71. Nipah virus factsheet (revised in July 2009). Wkly Epidemiol Rec. 2010;85:64–67.
72. Tyler KL. Emerging viral infections of the central nervous system: part 2. Arch Neurol. 2009;66:1065–74.
73. Lo MK, Rota PA. The emergence of Nipah virus, a highly pathogenic paramyxovirus. J Clin Virol. 2008;43:396–400.
74. Goh KJ, Tan CT, Chew NK, et al. Clinical features of Nipah virus encephalitis among pig farmers in Malaysia. N Engl J Med. 2000;342:1229–35.
75. Hossain MJ, Gurley ES, Montgomery JM, et al. Clinical presentation of Nipah virus infection in Bangladesh. Clin Infect Dis. 2008;46:977–84.
76. Tan CT, Goh KJ, Wong KT, et al. Relapsed and late-onset Nipah encephalitis. Ann Neurol. 2002;51:703–8.
77. Sejvar JJ, Hossain J, Saha SK, et al. Long-term neurological and functional outcome in Nipah virus infection. Ann Neurol. 2007;62:235–42.
78. Sarji SA, Abdullah BJJ, Goh KJ, et al. MR imaging features of Nipah encephalitis. Am J Roentgenol. 2000;175:437–42.
79. Lim CC, Lee KE, Lee WL, et al. Nipah virus encephalitis: serial MR study of an emerging disease. Radiology. 2002;222:219–26.
80. Quddus R, Alam S, Majumdar SA, et al. A report of 4 patients with Nipah encephalitis from Rajbari district, Bangladesh in the January 2004 outbreak. Neurol Asia. 2004;9:33–7.
81. Madhusudana SN, Sukumaran SM. Antemortem diagnosis and prevention of human rabies. Ann Indian Acad Neurol. 2008;11:3–12.
82. WHO Factsheet. Rabies. Available at http://www.who.int/mediacentre/factsheets/fs099/en/. Accessed 3 Nov 2013.
83. Sudarshan MK. Assessing burden of rabies in India. WHO sponsored national multi-centric rabies survey (May 2004). Assoc Prev Control Rabies India J. 2004;6:44–5.
84. Laothamatas J, Hemachuda T, Mitrabhakdi PW, et al. MR imaging in human rabies. AJNR Am J Neuroradiol. 2003;24:1102–9.
85. World Health Organization. Rabies. Guide for post exposure prophylaxis. Available at http://www.who.int/rabies/human/postexp/en/#. Accessed 3 Nov 2013.
86. WHO guide for rabies pre and post-exposure prophylaxis in humans (revised 15 June 2010). Available at http://www.who.int/rabies/PEP_prophylaxis_guidelines_June10.pdf. Accessed 3 Nov 2013.
87. WHO: Measles deaths decline, but elimination progress stalls in some regions. Available at http://www.who.int/mediacentre/news/notes/2013/measles_20130117/en/. Accessed 3 Nov 2013.
88. Simons E, Ferrari M, Fricks J, et al. Assessment of the 2010 global measles mortality reduction goal: results from a model of surveillance data. Lancet. 2012;379(9832):2173–8. doi:10.1016/S0140-6736(12)60522-4. Epub 2012 Apr 24.
89. Hosoya M. Measles encephalitis: direct viral invasion or autoimmune-mediated inflammation? Intern Med. 2006;45:841–2.
90. Beig FK, Malik A, Rizvi M, et al. Etiology and clinic-epidemiological profile of acute viral encephalitis in children of western Uttar Pradesh, India. Int J Infect Dis. 2010;14:e141–6.
91. Saha V, John TJ, Mukundan P, et al. High incidence of subacute sclerosing panencephalitis in South India. Epidemiol Infect. 1990;104:151–6.
92. Garg RK, Karak B, Sharma AM. Subacute sclerosing panencephalitis. Indian Pediatr. 1998;35:337–44.
93. Mishra B, Kakkar N, Ratho RK, et al. Changing trend of SSPE over a period of 10 years. Indian J Public Health. 2005;49:235–7.
94. Fernandez-Muñoz R, Carabaña J, Caballero M, Ortego J, et al. Subacute sclerosing panencephalitis and other lethal encephalitis caused by measles virus infection: pathogenesis and new approaches to treatment, non-flavivirus encephalitis. Dr. Sergey Tkachev, editor. InTech; 2011. ISBN 978-953-307-720-8. Available from http://www.intechopen.com/books/non-

flavivirus-encephalitis/subacutesclerosing-panencephalitis-and-other-lethal-encephalitis-caused-by-measles-virus-infection. Accessed 5 Aug 2013.
95. Lee KY, Cho WH, Kim SH, et al. Acute encephalitis associated with measles: MRI features. Neuroradiology. 2003;45:100–6.
96. Gutierrez J, Issacson RS, Koppel BS. Subacute sclerosing panencephalitis: an update. Dev Med Child Neurol. 2010;52:901–7.
97. Garg RK. Subacute sclerosing panencephalitis. Postgrad Med J. 2002;78:63–70.
98. Esiri MM, Kennedy PG. Virus diseases. In: Adams JH, Duchen LW, editors. Greenfield's neuropathology. 5th ed. London: Edward Arnold; 1992. p. 335–99.
99. Jabbour JT, Garcia JH, Lemmi H, et al. Subacute sclerosing panencephalitis: a multidisciplinary study of eight cases. JAMA. 1969;207:2248–54.
100. Brismar J, Gascon GG, von Steyern KV, et al. Subacute sclerosing panencephalitis: evaluation with CT and MR. AJNR Am J Neuroradiol. 1996;17:761–72.
101. Tuncay R, Akman-Demir G, Gokygit A, et al. MRI in subacute sclerosing panencephalitis. Neuroradiology. 1996;38:636–40.
102. Sener RN. Subacute sclerosing panencephalitis findings at MR imaging, diffusion MR imaging, and proton MR spectroscopy. AJNR Am J Neuroradiol. 2004;25:892–4.
103. Alkan A, Korkmaz L, Sigirci A, et al. Subacute sclerosing panencephalitis: relationship between clinical stage and diffusion-weighted imaging findings. J Magn Reson Imaging. 2006;23:267–72.
104. Alkan A, Sarac K, Kutlu R, et al. Early- and late subacute sclerosing pan encephalitis: chemical shift imaging and single-voxel MR spectroscopy. AJNR Am J Neuroradiol. 2003;24: 501–6.
105. Trivedi R, Gupta RK, Agarawal A, et al. Assessment of white matter damage in subacute sclerosing panencephalitis using quantitative diffusion tensor MR imaging. AJNR Am J Neuroradiol. 2006;27:1712–6.
106. Trivedi R, Anuradha H, Agarwal A, et al. Correlation of quantitative diffusion tensor tractography with clinical grades of subacute sclerosing panencephalitis. AJNR Am J Neuroradiol. 2011;32:714–20.
107. Garg RK. Subacute sclerosing panencephalitis. J Neurol. 2008;255:1861–71.
108. Panitch HS, Gomez-Plascencia J, Noris FS, et al. Subacute sclerosing panencephalitis remission after treatment with interferon. Neurology. 1986;36:562–6.
109. Gascon GG. International Consortium on Subacute Sclerosing Panencephalitis. Randomized treatment study of inosiplex versus combined inosiplex and intraventricular interferon-alpha in subacute sclerosing panencephalitis (SSPE): international multicenter study. J Child Neurol. 2003;18:819–27.
110. Hosoya M, Shigeta S, Mori S, et al. High-dose intravenous ribavirin therapy for subacute sclerosing panencephalitis. Antimicrob Agents Chemother. 2001;45:943–5.
111. Hara S, Kimura H, Hoshino Y, et al. Combination therapy with intraventricular interferon-alpha and ribavirin for subacute sclerosing panencephalitis and monitoring measles virus RNA by quantitative PCR assay. Brain Dev. 2003;25:367–9.
112. Mustafa MM, Weitman SD, Winick NJ, et al. Subacute measles encephalitis in young immunocompromised host: a review of two cases diagnosed by polymerase chain reaction and treated with ribavirin and review of the literature. Clin Infect Dis. 1993;16:654–60.
113. Albertyn C, van der Plas H, Hardie D, et al. Silent casualties from the measles outbreak in South Africa. S Afr Med J. 2011;101(5):313–4, 316–7.
114. Hardie DR, Albertyn C, Heckmann JM, et al. Molecular characterisation of virus in the brains of patients with measles inclusion body encephalitis (MIBE). Virol J. 2013;10(1):283.
115. Poon TP, Tchertkoff V, Win H. Subacute measles encephalitis with AIDS diagnosed by fine needle aspiration biopsy. A case report. Acta Cytol. 1998;42:729–33.
116. Chong HT, Ramli N, Wong KT, et al. Subacute measles encephalitis: a case of long term survival with follow-up MR brain scans. Neurol Asia. 2007;12:121–5.

117. John TJ. Chandipura virus – what we know & do not know. Indian J Med Res. 2010; 132:125–7.
118. Chandipura encephalitis. Available at http://icmr.nic.in/pinstitute/niv/CHANDIPURA%20 ENC.pdf. Accessed 3 Nov 2013.
119. Rao BL, Basu A, Wairagkar NS, Gore MM, et al. A large outbreak of acute encephalitis with high fatality rate in children in Andhra Pradesh, India. Lancet. 2004;364:869–74.
120. Chadha MS, Arankalle VA, Jadi RS, et al. An outbreak of Chandipura virus encephalitis in the eastern districts of Gujarat state, India. Am J Trop Med Hyg. 2005;73:566–70.
121. Rao PN, Kumar PA, Rao TA, et al. Role of Chandipura virus in an "epidemic brain attack" in Andhra Pradesh, India. J Pediatr Neurol. 2004;2:131–43.
122. Rao NS, Wairagkar NS, Mohan MV, et al. Brain stem encephalitis associated with Chandipura virus in Andhra Pradesh outbreak. J Trop Pediatr. 2008;54:25–30.
123. Gurav YK, Tandale BV, Jadi RS, et al. Chandipura virus encephalitis outbreak among children in Nagpur division, Maharashtra, 2007. Indian J Med Res. 2010;132:395–9.
124. Kumar S, Jadi RS, Anakkathil SB, Tandale BV, Mishra AC, Arankalle VA. Development and evaluation of a real-time one step reverse-transcriptase PCR for quantitation of Chandipura Virus. BMC Infect Dis. 2008;8:168–74.
125. Mishra AC. Chandipura virus, encephalitis, and epidemic brain attack in India. Lancet. 2004;364(9452):2175–6.
126. Tandale BV, Tikute SS, Arankalle VA, et al. Chandipura virus: a major cause of acute encephalitis in children in North Telangana, Andhra Pradesh, India. J Med Virol. 2008;80(1): 118–24.
127. Jacob JT. Chandipura Virus, encephalitis and epidemic brain attack in India. Lancet. 2004; 364:2175.
128. Tsetsarkin KA, Vanlandingham DL, McGee CE, Higgs S. A single mutation in chikungunya virus affects vector specificity and epidemic potential. PLoS Pathog. 2007;3(12):e201. PubMed: 18069894.
129. Wadia RS. A neurotropic virus (chikungunya) and a neuropathic amino acid (homocysteine). Ann Indian Acad Neurol. 2007;10:198–213.
130. Tournebize P, Charlin C, Lagrange M. Neurological manifestations in Chikungunya: about 23 cases collected in Reunion Island [in French]. Rev Neurol (Paris). 2009;165(1):48–51. PubMed: 18835614.
131. Robin S, Ramful D, Le Seach F, Jaffar-Bandjee MC, Rigou G, Alessandri JL. Neurologic manifestations of pediatric chikungunya infection. J Child Neurol. 2008;23(9):1028–35. PubMed: 18287573.
132. Ganesan K, Diwan A, Shankar SK, et al. Chikungunya encephalomyeloradiculitis: report of 2 cases with neuroimaging and 1 case with autopsy findings. AJNR Am J Neuroradiol. 2008;29:1636–7.
133. Marx A, Glass JD, Sutter RW. Differential diagnosis of acute flaccid paralysis and its role in poliomyelitis surveillance. Epidemiol Rev. 2000;22(2):298–316.
134. Kincaid O, Lipton HL. Viral myelitis: an update. Curr Neurol Neurosci Rep. 2006;6:469–74.
135. World Health organization. Weekly epidemiological record. 2013;88:381–8.
136. Chen CY, Chang YC, Huang CC, et al. Acute flaccid paralysis in infants and young children with enterovirus 71 infection: MR imaging findings and clinical correlates. AJNR Am J Neuroradiol. 2001;22(1):200–5.
137. Malzberg MS, Rogg JM, Tate CA, et al. Poliomyelitis: hyperintensity of the anterior horn cells on MR images of the spinal cord. Am J Roentgenol. 1993;161(4):863–5.
138. Kumar S, Misra UK, Kalita J, et al. MRI in Japanese encephalitis. Neuroradiology. 1997; 39:180–4.
139. Davies NW, Brown LJ, Irish D, et al. Factors influencing PCR detection of viruses in cerebrospinal fluid of patients with suspected CNS infections. J Neurol Neurosurg Psychiatry. 2005;76:82–7.
140. Gorson K, Ropper A. Nonpoliovirus poliomyelitis simulating Guillain-Barré syndrome. Arch Neurol. 2001;58:1460–4.

141. Asbury A, Arnason B, Karp H. Criteria for diagnosis of Guillain-Barré syndrome. Ann Neurol. 1978;3:565–6.
142. Starlin R, Reed N, Leeman B. Acute flaccid paralysis syndrome associated with echovirus 19 managed with pleconaril and intravenous immunoglobulin. Clin Infect Dis. 2001; 33:730–2.
143. Shimoni Z, Niven MJ, Pitlick S, et al. Treatment of West Nile virus encephalitis with intravenous immunoglobulin. Emerg Infect Dis. 2001;7:759.
144. Rao AS, Varma DR, Chalapathi Rao MV, et al. Case report: magnetic resonance imaging in rabies encephalitis. Indian J Radiol Imaging. 2009;19:301–4.

Chapter 7
Fungal Infection of the CNS

Mansa Amul Munshi, Antonella Rella, and Maurizio Del Poeta

Abstract Fungal infections in the central nervous system have been known to lead to significant morbidity and mortality. Most of these infections are chronic and develop in patients with altered immune response. The most common predisposing factors for fungal CNS infections are HIV, organ transplant, tumors, prolonged antimicrobial therapy, chemotherapy, and long-term use of ventilators and catheters. The most common fungal pathogens are *Cryptococcus* spp., *Candida albicans*, *Aspergillus* spp., *Histoplasma capsulatum*, *Coccidioides* spp., and *Zygomycetes*. Occasionally there are serious outbreaks of rare fungal infections that affect also immunocompetent subjects, bringing to focus the enormity of unknown fungi that pose a threat to humans. The diagnosis is often difficult and the treatment options are limited. Hence, the prognosis of these infections is poor with high morbidity and high mortality. This chapter will discuss the most common fungal infections of the CNS and their challenges.

Keywords Fungal infection • Central nervous system • Meningitis • *Cryptococcus neoformans* • Cerebrospinal fluid • Amphotericin B • Fluconazole

Abbreviations

ABLC	Amphotericin B lipid complex
AIDS	Acquired immunodeficiency syndrome
AmB	Amphotericin B
AmBd	Amphotericin B deoxycholate
CNS	Central nervous system

M.A. Munshi, MS Microbiology • A. Rella, PhD Microbiology • M. Del Poeta, MD (✉)
Department of Molecular Genetics and Microbiology, Stony Brook University,
150, Life Sciences Building, Stony Brook, NY 11794, USA
e-mail: maurizio.delpoeta@stonybrook.edu

J.C. García-Moncó (ed.), *CNS Infections*,
DOI 10.1007/978-1-4471-6401-2_7, © Springer-Verlag London 2014

CSF	Cerebrospinal fluid
CT	Computerized tomography scan
GMS stain	Gomori methenamine silver stain
HIV	Human immunodeficiency virus
LF-AmB	Lipid formulations of amphotericin B
MALDI-TOF	Matrix-assisted laser desorption ionization mass spectrometry-time of flight
NMR	Nuclear magnetic resonance
PAP stain	Papanicolaou stain
PAS stain	Periodic acid schiff stain
PCR	Polymerase chain reaction

Introduction

Among the causative agents of infection of the central nervous system (CNS), fungi have the highest morbidity and mortality [1]. This is mostly due to two factors: (1) it is difficult, if not impossible, to totally eradicate the fungus once it is discovered in the brain tissue, and (2) fungal infections of the CNS occur mostly, although not exclusively, in immunocompromised hosts.

In fact, most fungal microorganisms cause a chronic instead of an acute or sub-acute meningitis [2], with a significant delay in the diagnosis. Some fungi, such as *Cryptococcus* spp., cause a self-contained cystic lesion called "cryptococcoma," which, by limiting the diffusion of antifungal drugs, allows fungal cells to replicate indefinitely. Coupled with a weak host response, these brain lesions will eventually affect key areas of the brain tissue necessary to sustain life.

Throughout the years, numerous studies have attempted (i) to improve the methodologies that allow an early diagnosis of fungal infections, (ii) to improve the formulation of antifungal drugs that would better penetrate the brain tissue and better diffuse into fungal lesions, and (iii) to treat the underlying host disease, when possible, so that the host immune response would take control of fungal replication.

A condition in which the host immunity is markedly depressed includes the acquired immunodeficiency syndrome (AIDS). To give a perspective of the fungal problem within the AIDS pandemic, recent estimates revealed that *Cryptococcus* spp. kill over 600,000 AIDS patients per year in sub-Saharan Africa [3], whereas before the advent of AIDS, only few hundred cases of cryptococcosis have been reported in the literature since the first case described in 1894 [4].

The improvement and increasing use of many surgical procedures during the last 20 years, such as organ transplants, or the use of intravenous, intratracheal, intraspinal, and intrathecal catheters, have also increased the incidence of fungal infections. In particular, in transplant recipients, the incidence of fungal infection ranges from 5 to 10 % with a mortality rate of about 83 % for aspergillosis, 40 % for candidiasis, and 42 % for cryptococcosis [5–9]. These infections are normally late-occurring infections. For cryptococcosis, the median time to onset is 16–21 months after the organ transplantation [7, 10, 11]. As expected, the time of onset is earlier when the patient is subjected to higher doses of immunosuppressive therapy, such as in liver and lung compared to kidney transplants [7].

The immunosuppressive drugs used during solid organ transplantation may influence the physiopathology of fungal infections. Compared to corticosteroids, calcineurin inhibitors are the common drugs used for immunosuppression in solid organ transplant recipients. Although these agents do not influence the incidence, they may affect the severity of the certain fungal disease [7].

Corticosteroids are associated with an increased risk of developing infections after solid organ transplantation although the risk-conferring dose remains unknown. Those solid organ transplant patients using T-cell depleting antibodies as induction therapy or as treatments of rejection have a very high risk to develop fungal infections [12].

Disseminated aspergillosis is observed in 41–72 % of liver transplant and about 3.3–14 % of heart transplant recipients [13]. Cryptococcal meningitis is observed in 20–60 % of all solid organ transplant patients: this is only in the USA and in HIV-negative subjects [14]. It is particularly frequent in heart transplant recipients as compared to other transplant groups. However, the immunosuppressive regime is not the only risk factor for cryptococcal meningitis in solid organ transplant patients, since studies have shown geographic variations in cryptococcosis rates. Since *C. neoformans* is associated with birds and areas contaminated with pigeon droppings, it is suggested that organ transplant patients avoid birds or areas contaminated with bird droppings.

Other fungal infections of the CNS in solid organ transplant recipients are relatively less frequent. *Scedosporium* infections are observed in 30–35 % of transplant patients [15]. Disseminated zygomycosis is mostly associated with liver transplant recipients [16]. Most phaeohyphomycotic infections in transplant recipients (79 %) are localized as skin and soft-tissue infections, with 21 % of known incidences of systemic invasive infections [17, 18]. Disseminated fusariosis is rare and localized [19]. *Candida* infections are common after organ transplant and they can lead to CNS infection [20].

In addition to AIDS patients and organ transplant recipients, fungal infection of the CNS also occurs in subjects with tumors, particularly in those undergoing prolonged chemotherapy, and in subjects that are under long-term treatments with immunosuppressive drugs, such as corticosteroids. Under this condition, the common fungal infections are *Cryptococcus neoformans*, *Aspergillus* spp., and *Candida albicans*.

The CNS fungal infections could occur in various forms: (1) brain meningitis, (2) hydrocephalus, (3) space occupying lesions, (4) stroke syndromes, and (5) spinal infections [21]. Due to its high mortality, a great effort has been placed in developing diagnostic methods that can detect the fungal involvement of the CNS as early as possible. Most of these methods are focused on the examination of the cerebrospinal fluid (CSF), whose analysis may directly, or indirectly, reveal the fungus responsible for the CNS involvement [2]. These methods include cell count, CSF staining, microbiological culture, polymerase chain reaction (PCR), and more sophisticated methods, such as matrix-assisted laser desorption ionization mass spectrometry-time of flight (MALDI-TOF) [22–25]. These laboratory tests are often coupled with brain imaging using computerized tomography (CT) scan or nuclear magnetic resonance (NMR) to determine the extent of the disease so that an aggressive antifungal therapy can be promptly established.

Overview of Common Fungal Pathogens Affecting the CNS

The most common fungi reported to infect the CNS are *Cryptococcus* spp., *Aspergillus* spp., *Candida albicans*, *Histoplasma capsulatum*, *Coccidioides* spp., and *Zygomycetes* with *Cryptococcus* spp. being the most frequent [26].

Cryptococcus spp.

Cryptococcosis is an infection caused by fungi that belong to the genus *Cryptococcus*. This genus has 30 different species, but two species, *Cryptococcus neoformans* and *Cryptococcus gattii*, cause nearly all cryptococcal infections in humans and animals. Although most people who develop cryptococcosis have weakened immune systems, there are also cases of infections in healthy, or apparently healthy, individuals. Every year, there are reports of over a million cases of cryptococcal meningitis [3].

Cryptococcus spp. is found in soils contaminated with bird feces and is a cosmopolitan yeastlike fungus. It generally enters the body via the respiratory tract, reaching the alveolar spaces and colonizing the lung. Eventually, it disseminates to the CNS, most often causing meningitis. Dissemination occurs after reactivation of a lung cryptococcal granuloma upon immunosuppression or during a primary infection in a subject severely immunocompromised. Although showing high tropism for the brain, the reason for this remains largely speculative. Perhaps the high concentration of catecholamines in the brain, which can be used by the fungus to make melanin, and the high concentration of inositol, which is necessary for the fungus to survive in the CNS, are interesting possibilities that may explain its brain tropism [27]. Additional fungal properties that allows colonization and growth of *Cryptococcus* in the brain are its ability to grow at 37 °C and 5 % of CO_2 and to survive a very low hypoxic environment (such as brain parenchyma), to produce a thick polysaccharide capsule that protects it from the host immunity, and to synthesize different fungal molecules, such as specific lipids, that enables it to quickly adapt to a variety of host environments.

As discussed above, cryptococcal meningoencephalitis is particularly common in human immunodeficiency virus (HIV) patients and organ transplant recipients [28, 29]. Reports show that the mortality of patients with organ transplant with cryptococcal infection is 20–100 % [30, 31]. A recent study of *Cryptococcus* infection revealed that HIV-positive patients were more likely than those without HIV infection to have CNS involvement (91.9 % versus 21.7 %). Particularly interesting in this study was the significant similarity of mortality rates of the two groups (22.2 % in HIV versus 34.5 % without HIV) [32].

Clinical Manifestation and Diagnosis

Cryptococcal meningitis usually presents as severe, chronic, or subacute headache with or without fever. Headache could be accompanied with vomiting and vision obscurations. Patients can also present papilledema, hydrocephalus, focal deficits, and seizures. These symptoms and signs should prompt consideration for a lumbar puncture for evidence of meningeal inflammation. On occasion, the diagnosis is made when an imaging study (CT or NMR) show contrast enhancement of the meninges. Once chronic meningitis is confirmed by CSF examination, effort is focused on identifying the cause by (1) further analysis of the CSF, (2) diagnosis of an underlying systemic infection or noninfectious conditions, and (3) pathological examination of meningeal biopsy samples. The presentation of CNS cryptococcoma, although rare in immunocompetent patients, is similar to CNS tumors and can be difficult to differentiate [33]. Ring-shaped mass lesions with or without cystic changes in the NMR imaging may indicate cryptococcoma, but confirmatory diagnosis depends on detection of cryptococcal antigen and/or by visualization under the microscope of cryptococcal cells in the CSF using India ink stain. Using this relatively simple method, the diagnosis can be made in >90 % of patients with AIDS and in >50 % of the cases of cryptococcal meningitis in HIV-negative subjects [26, 34, 35].

Therapeutic Treatment

Cryptococcosis can be managed successfully in the vast majority of patients if the diagnosis is made early and the treatment is instituted promptly (Table 7.1). The primary therapy for the treatment of cryptococcal meningoencephalitis in HIV-infected individuals is amphotericin B (AmB) deoxycholate (0.7–1.0 mg/kg per day intravenously [IV]) and flucytosine 100 mg/ kg per day orally in four divided doses. For severe cases, IV formulations are recommended for at least 2 weeks, followed by consolidation with fluconazole (400 mg [6 mg/kg] per day orally) for a minimum of 8 weeks. Lipid formulations of AmB (LFAmB), including liposomal AmB (3–4 mg/kg per day IV) and AmB lipid complex (ABLC; 5 mg/kg per day IV) for at least 2 weeks, could be substituted to AmBd among patients with or predisposed to renal dysfunction. Suppressive and prophylactic therapy is fluconazole (200 mg per day orally) or itraconazole (200 mg twice per day orally; along with drug-level monitoring). The therapy for non-HIV, non-transplant hosts is AmBd (0.7–1.0 mg/kg per day IV) and flucytosine (100 mg/kg per day orally in four divided doses) for 6 weeks followed by consolidation with fluconazole (400 mg per day) for 8 weeks [28].

Table 7.1 Overview of common fungal pathogens of CNS

Etiology	Epidemiology	Clinical features	Diagnosis	Treatment
Cryptococcus neoformans	Sporadic, endemic exposure to bird, bird droppings or eucalyptus trees	Chronic meningitis ± lung involvement	Microscopic observation of cryptococcal cell by India ink, fungal culture, cryptococcal antigen	Amphotericin B Oral flucytosine Fluconazole
Aspergillus spp.	Diffuse worldwide	Chronic meningitis ± lung involvement	Galactomannan antigen, observation of hyphae in biopsy, PCR, culture	Voriconazole Amphotericin B
Candida albicans	Commensal	Meningitis, most likely disseminated candidiasis, micro-abscess, high WBC count	Culture, antigen, fungal stain, imaging	Amphotericin B Oral flucytosine Fluconazole
Histoplasma capsulatum	Endemic in Ohio and Mississippi river valleys in US and other microfoci	Chronic meningitis	Fungal stain, antigen in urine or blood, antibody detection in serum or CSF	Amphotericin B Itraconazole
Coccidioides spp.	Endemic in the Southwest USA, Mexico, and South America	Subacute or chronic meningitis	Antibodies, skin testing, complement fixation test, wet smear, culture of serum sputum, urine, or CSF	Amphotericin B Fluconazole
Zygomycetes	Inhabit acidic and carbohydrate rich environment	Headache, fever, vision loss, altered mental status, retro orbital headache, visual changes	CSF culture, CT, endoscopy, biopsy, PCR, antibody detection in serum or CSF	Amphotericin B Posaconazole

Aspergillus spp.

Aspergillus spp. are ubiquitous filamentous fungi, also called molds. A normal subject inhales many *Aspergillus* conidia every day, but in contrast to cryptococcosis, aspergillosis manifests mainly, although not exclusively, in condition of immunosuppression. Thus, cases of infection of the CNS by *Aspergillus* in healthy individuals are very rare [36, 37]. Unfortunately, despite treatment, aspergillosis of the CNS is associated with a very high mortality rate (88 %) [38]. In addition, there has been a significant increase of *Aspergillus* infections caused by resistant conidia to common antifungal drugs [39].

Aspergillus fumigatus is the most common isolate [40], followed by *Aspergillus flavus*, *Aspergillus terreus*, *Aspergillus oryzae*, and *Aspergillus niger*. The most common risk factor for aspergillosis of the CNS is solid organ transplantation. Hematologic malignancies and chemotherapy are also predisposing conditions for *Aspergillus* brain abscess [41]. These are also associated with very poor prognosis. Since *Aspergillus* conidia are present everywhere, including normal operating rooms, it is very difficult to limit the exposure of subjects at risk from contracting this disease (e.g., solid organ transplant recipients).

Clinical Manifestation and Diagnosis

CNS aspergillosis usually presents with altered mental status, meningitis, or seizures. The clinical symptoms observed in patients with aspergillosis are focal neurological deficits and focal seizures [42]. The pathobiological lesions observed in *Aspergillus* infection are basilar meningitis, dural abscess, and mycotic aneurysm [43, 44]. Aspergilloma in the brain (fungus ball) is observed rarely [45].

Diagnosis of *Aspergillus* infection is difficult. Culture methods of the CSF or blood are often negative. Detection of galactomannan or/and β-glucan antigen in CSF or/and serum suggests the diagnosis but sensitivity is low and false positive results occur [46]. Histological examination can reveal *Aspergillus* hyphae, but culture is required for the identification of the precise species. For instance, only culture can reliably distinguish aspergillosis from pseudallescheriasis: therapy for these two diseases differs.

Therapeutic Treatment

For invasive disease involving the brain parenchyma, a surgical approach may be useful, if technically feasible, with some debunking of the infectious mass. Antifungal treatment for *Aspergillus* infection has in the past been hampered by the lack of antifungal activity of some azoles and the toxicity of amphotericin B. However, primary treatment would begin with voriconazole 6 mg/kg IV twice a day followed by 4 mg/kg IV every 12 h and by oral administration of 200 mg dose every 12 h (Table 7.1).

Alternatively, liposomal-AMB (3–5 mg/kg/day IV), amphotericin B lipid complex (5 mg/ kg/day IV), caspofungin (70 mg day 1 IV and 50 mg/day IV thereafter), or micafungin (IV 100–150 mg/day, dose not established), posaconazole (200 mg 4 times a day initially, then 400 mg orally twice a day after stabilization of disease), and itraconazole (dosage depends upon formulation) can be also used [42].

Candida albicans

Candida spp. is a commensal yeast, usually found in the oral cavity, skin, gastrointestinal tract, and genitourinary tract. Although it is part of the normal human flora, it can cause systemic infection in immunocompromised hosts. *Candida* spp. and in particular *Candida albicans*, *Candida glabrata*, *Candida tropicalis*, *Candida parapsilosis*, and *Candida krusei* cause more than 90 % of invasive infections, although the relative prevalence of the species depends on the geographical location, patient population, and clinical settings [47].

Out of the 80 known *Candida* species, *C. albicans* is the species most commonly known to lead to neurocandidiasis [48]. *C. albicans* initially infects the oral cavity and esophagus, eventually progressing to submucosal blood vessels and finally disseminating hematogenously to the CNS [1]. About 50 % infections of candidemia have CNS involvement, and the mortality of these patients is 80–97 % [49, 50]. Candidal meningitis can be a result of complications of infected wounds, ventriculostomy, or direct introduction of the fungus during surgery [1].

The disease may have different symptomatology depending on the underlying immunosuppressive diseases, antibiotic or corticosteroid treatment, abdominal surgery, premature birth, intravenous drug use, neurosurgery, intravascular catheter carriers, or prolonged use of ventriculoperitoneal shunt [48]. In fact, in addition to CNS involvement due to bloodstream dissemination, CNS infection by *Candida* can also occur exogenously (e.g., postoperative infection, craniofacial trauma, lumbar puncture, or shunt placement) [51].

Clinical Manifestation and Diagnosis

Initial symptoms of *Candida* infection include fever, headache, stiff neck, and mental instability along with reduced consciousness with or without vomiting, altered vision, paralysis, and confusion. *Candida* meningitis has no unique symptoms and usually presents signs similar to those of *Cryptococcus* meningitis [52].

In the absence of *Candida* isolation in CSF, the laboratory tests may show mild pleocytosis and hypoglycorrhachia, also present in other mycoses like cryptococcal meningitis [52, 53]. The main clinical manifestations of *Candida* infection in the CNS are cerebral micro- and macroabscesses, meningitis, and vascular complications.

Diagnosis of *C. albicans* infection primarily relies on CSF analysis and culture. The CSF shows increased WBC counts, low glucose, high adenosine deaminase levels, and high protein levels. Also mannan detection in the CSF is a promising test for detecting *Candida* infection in CNS [54, 55]. CT and NMR can assist in the confirmation of this infection by visualization of lesions.

Therapeutic Treatment

One of the primary steps for treatment and control of *Candida* infection is the removal and sterilization of catheters that could be a source harboring the pathogen. The treatment strategy includes administration of lipid formulation of amphotericin B 3–5 mg/kg with or without 5-flucytosine 25 mg/kg for several weeks, followed by fluconazole 400–800 mg (6–12 mg/kg) daily. Alternatively, fluconazole 400–800 mg (6–12 mg/kg) daily can be administered in patients unable to tolerate lipid formulation of amphotericin B (Table 7.1). These treatments are applied until all symptoms (CSF abnormalities and radiologic abnormalities) are resolved [56].

Dimorphic Fungi

Histoplasma capsulatum

Histoplasma capsulatum is found between tropics of Cancer and Capricorn and is endemic in Ohio and Mississippi River Valley [57]. It has been known to inhabit bird droppings, commonly known to affect people exploring caves and bridge workers [58, 59]. Twenty percent of patients with disseminated infection of *H. capsulatum* develop CNS infection. *H. capsulatum* causes meningitis in 5–25 % of patients with disseminated disease [60]. In addition to AIDS, predisposing factors are age and organ transplant. Farmers, roofers, landscapers, and geologists are at higher risk of contracting the infection for their exposure to the pathogen [58, 59]. This infection can occur in immunocompetent subjects in which case it is mostly limited to the lung.

Clinical Presentation and Diagnosis

Histoplasmosis of the CNS usually takes the form of a chronic meningitis often complicated with communicating hydrocephalus [61]. Acute meningitis, encephalitis, small ring-enhancing lesions throughout the brain and spinal cord (with and without meningeal involvement), larger brain abscesses, and stroke (due to infected emboli) are infrequent manifestations of this disease.

Signs and symptoms of CNS involvement in histoplasmosis, such as headache, fever, lethargy, or altered mental status, are similar to those of other chronic fungal meningitis. Thus, histoplasmosis should be suspected in patients with chronic meningitis or parenchymal lesions, which have negative reports for other causes, particularly if they have traveled to areas where *H. capsulatum* is endemic [62].

Diagnosis of suspected *Histoplasma* meningitis requires any of the following: (i) fungal culture; (ii) *Histoplasma* antigen testing and anti-*Histoplasma* antibody testing for CSF and blood; (iii) *Histoplasma* antigen testing in urine; (iv) in situations of inconclusive results from the above, cisternal and ventricular fluid is tested for fungal culture, *Histoplasma* antigen, and anti-*Histoplasma* antibody; and (v) final histopathologic testing of the brain and meninges. Bone marrow biopsy is recommended in cases of suspected disseminated histoplasmosis [63]. Detection of *Histoplasma* DNA by PCR may also suggest the diagnosis [62, 64].

Therapeutic Treatment

Although there is no optimal treatment for this pathogen, CNS histoplasmosis requires prolonged and aggressive therapy [62]. CNS histoplasmosis is generally treated with liposomal amphotericin B (5.0 mg/kg daily for a total of 175 mg/kg given over 4–6 weeks) followed by itraconazole (200 mg 2 or 3 times daily) for at least 1 year and until CSF abnormalities and *Histoplasma* antigen levels are cleared (Table 7.1) [60].

***Coccidioides* spp.**

Coccidioides spp. infection has a high rate of CNS involvement. The fungus is saprophytic, and it is mostly found in hot and dry regions like the Southwest USA [65, 66]. Inhalation of only a few arthroconidia by an immunocompetent subject is sufficient to cause a lung infection, but CNS involvement is rare. The risk of blood stream dissemination after inhalation is 30 % in AIDS patients, and one-third of these show CNS involvement [67, 68]. Coccidioidal meningitis has a high morbidity and mortality. However, there are also known cases in which the infection has been successfully treated [69]. Among the *Coccidioides* spp., *C. immitis* is reported to be the most frequent infecting agent of the CNS. Similar to other fungi, lowered immunity is a major risk factor. However, prolonged soil exposure increases the risk of acquiring this infection also in immunocompetent subjects. This is generally applicable to archeologists, construction workers, and agricultural workers. Interestingly, the incidence of coccidioidomycosis is rapidly increasing. There are reports of 100,000 cases of *C. immitis* in the USA every year. And a major cause of mortality of these patients is due to CNS infection [70, 71].

Clinical Presentation and Diagnosis

The most common clinical manifestation of *Coccidioides* spp. is a subacute or chronic granulomatous meningitis. The majority of the patients show no signs of respiratory trouble, the rest display "flulike" symptoms or pneumonia and therefore it is difficult to make a prompt diagnosis [66]. Fever, cough, chest discomfort, malaise, and fatigue are most commonly observed in symptomatic patients, and coccidioidal meningitis is a more severe complication of coccidioidomycosis. Once the meninges are affected, the following symptoms/signs may develop: (i) hydrocephalus with increased intracranial pressure causing stupor, nausea and vomiting, dizziness, diplopia, and papilledema; (ii) diplopia, facial numbness or weakness, dysarthria, dysphagia, and hearing loss caused by cranial nerves trapped by the basilar meningitis; and (iii) cerebral infarctions from meningeal vessel thrombosis producing hemiparesis, aphasia, visual loss, and cerebellar ataxia [68].

Diagnosis of *C. immitis* requires taking into consideration the geographic location of the individual. This should be followed by physical examination to detect any signs of infection by this pathogen, like cough, rales, pleural effusion, wartlike nodules, erythema nodosa, papules, and draining ulcers in the sinus tract. Other signs include arthritic pains, joint swelling, and painful bony areas. Radiological and laboratory tests include CT, NMR, lumbar puncture for CSF, further confirmation by fungal culture, and brain or meningeal biopsy [68]. Detection of anticoccidioidal antibodies from CSF is a more confirmatory mode of diagnosis compared to culture of *Coccidioides* spp. from the CSF [72]. IgG levels in serum are generally not indicatory of meningeal disease and should be accompanied with CT or NMR [73].

Therapeutic Treatment

Treatment begins with the induction phase using liposomal amphotericin B 3–5 mg/kg/day intravenously for 6–10 weeks with a total dose of 100–150 mg/kg or, alternatively, fluconazole 400–600 mg/day. This phase is followed by the consolidation phase in which oral fluconazole (400–600 mg/day for 9–18 months) can be administered. The last phase or maintenance phase consists of a life-long administration of fluconazole 200–400 mg/day given orally [68] (Table 7.1).

For nonresponsive patients to azoles, intrathecal amphotericin B is used, with normal dosage ranging from 0.1 mg to 1.5 mg per dose, administered at intervals ranging from daily to weekly, beginning at a low dosage and increasing the dosage until the appearance of patient intolerance (severe vomiting, prostration, or transient dose-related mental status) [67, 74].

Normalization of CSF cell count, protein and glucose level, neuroimaging, and serum IgG titer can help follow the progress of treatment.

Zygomycetes

Zygomycosis are common fungal infections and represent approximately 5–12 % of all opportunistic fungal infections [75]. Clinical cases of zygomycosis have dramatically increased in recent years, with unexpected high morbidity and mortality [76]. There are two orders of *Zygomycetes*, the Mucorales and the Entomophthorales. The majority of human diseases are generally associated with the Mucorales, and in particular, the most clinically relevant microorganisms are *Rhizopus*, *Mucor*, and *Cunninghamella* spp. They are ubiquitous fungi, mostly found in the environment and associated with soil, decomposing plants and animal material. These fungi require acidic and carbohydrate rich environment to grow.

Zygomycosis generally affect immunocompromised hosts with neutropenia or neutrophil dysfunction, with very poor prognosis. The infections are uncommon in immunocompetent individuals [77]. However, there are reports of cases of zygomycosis in immunocompetent subject due to antibiotic abuse or damage of mucocutaneous barrier [75]. This opportunistic pathogen is also known to affect intravenous drug addicts [78].

The sporangiospores are largely present in the environment; therefore, the common port of entry of the pathogen is through inhalation. Studies in rabbits showed that upon nasal infection with sporangiospores, the rabbits developed a lung disease with subsequent spreading of the pathogen to CNS [79]. CNS infection is generally correlated with high mortality [54]. Sporangiospores can also infect the gastrointestinal tract or can directly pass through skin damage or contaminated catheters. In addition to immunosuppression, a variety of risk factors are known to be associated with zygomycosis including diabetes mellitus, ketoacidosis, neutropenia, iron overload, transplantation, malnutrition, and breakdown in the cutaneous barrier (trauma, burn, wounds). Zygomycosis can appear as a wide spectrum of diseases depending on the port of entry and the risk factors of the patients. For example, an overload of iron (diabetic ketoacidosis) facilitates fungal growth and their rapid progression to CNS. Moreover, it appears that deferoxamine treatment (agent that chelates iron and aluminum) increases iron uptake by the fungus, promoting fungal growth and dissemination. In this case the disseminated zygomycosis is fatal with a mortality rate of 90 % [75].

Clinical Presentation and Diagnosis

The major clinical manifestations of this disease are sinusitis-rhinocerebral, pulmonary, cutaneous-subcutaneous, gastrointestinal, and eventually disseminated zygomycosis. Zygomycosis of the CNS is often associated with three different clinical presentations: (i) rhinocerebral zygomycosis characterized by hyphal invasion of CNS via the nasal cavity or sinus, (ii) disseminated zygomycosis with brain involvement characterized by a hyphal invasion of the whole body via blood, and (iii) isolated cerebral zygomycosis [80]. The most frequent symptoms of cerebral zygomycosis are headache, nausea, fever, lethargy, impaired vision, bulging eyes, blurred vision, seizures, convulsions, and altered mental status.

For the diagnosis of cerebral zygomycosis, CSF analysis and biopsy obtained from rhinofacial and cerebral areas (rich in necrotic and infarcted tissue) are needed. Isolation and identification of *Zygomycetes* from human specimens is difficult. The identification is made through direct microscopic examination of the clinical specimens looking for hyaline hyphal elements. The stain techniques usually used are calcofluor-white stain, Gomori methenamine silver stain (GMS), periodic acid schiff (PAS), Gram's stain, and Papanicolaou stain (PAP stain). However, the hyphae could be present only in some parts of the specimens. Serologic tests and molecular techniques are not diagnostically useful or used only for epidemiologic studies [75]. CT and NMR are reported to be sensitive for the detection of *Zygomycetes* in CNS infection [81].

Therapeutic Treatment

There are two treatments for zygomycosis: (i) surgical intervention (dead and infected tissue needs to be removed surgically) and (ii) antifungal drugs. If untreated, mortality rate is 100 %. Zygomycosis is treated with amphotericin B lipid complex (ABLC) ≥ 5 mg/kg once per day or liposomal amphotericin B ≥ 3–5 mg/kg once per day with possible escalation to 10 mg/kg/d in patients with CNS infection administered intravenously. Reduction of immunosuppressants could be helpful to control this infection. Echinocandins have been reported to be unsuccessful for infection by this pathogen. When toxicity develops or patients do not respond anymore to amphotericin B, 200 mg of posaconazole four times a day can be administered orally [82] (Table 7.1).

Rare Fungi Affecting CNS

There is an increasing number of rare fungal infections observed, some causing serious outbreaks among the population [83–91]. Unusual and emerging fungal pathogens causing meningitis include *Sporothrix schenckii* [92], *Rhodotorula glutinis* [91], *Sporobolomyces roseus* [93], *Scedosporium apiospermum* (*Pseudallescheria boydii*) [94], *Blastomyces dermatitidis* [95], *Geotrichum capitatum* (*Blastoschizomyces capitatus*) [96], and others. A rare case of meningitis by *Pseudallescheria boydii* was recently observed [97]. Another unusual case of meningitis due to *Rhodotorula glutinis* was seen in a 35-year-old HIV-positive male [98].

The most recent case of fungal infection outbreak was reported in September 2012 and arose from glucocorticoid injections for the treatment of chronic musculoskeletal pain [99]. Such infections are extremely rare in medical history [100–107]. This particular outbreak was due to the contamination of three lots of methylprednisolone acetate injections by the black mold *Exserohilum rostratum. Aspergillus fumigatus* was also detected in some cases. This contamination affected almost 14,000 people, with 741 confirmed drug-related infections and 55 deaths [108, 109]. Antifungal treatment should be maintained for a minimum of 3 months up to 1 year [110]. It is interesting, though, that the majority of the subjects did not actually developed any infection even if they received an injection of fungal-contaminated steroid directly into their spine.

Differential Diagnosis of CNS Fungal Infection

CNS fungal infections may be difficult to diagnose. This is because of the enormous number of pathogens, common symptoms, and underlying disease. When a fungal infection of the CNS is suspected, the key diagnostic procedures are lumbar puncture to obtain CSF followed by microscopic observation and other laboratory tests of the CSF. Fungal meningitis is usually chronic and persistent, in contrast to the common relapsing course of viral meningitis. Bacterial CNS involvement mostly causes acute or subacute meningitis.

The epidemiological history is of considerable importance and may provide the choice of the laboratory test to be performed: travel history to areas endemic for fungal infections (e.g., *Histoplasma* and *Blastomyces*), exposure of an immunocompromised host to birds and their droppings (e.g., *Cryptococcus*), or gardening (*Sporothrix*). Once the clinical syndrome is recognized, proper diagnosis of the CSF is essential. It is important that if the possibility exists for raised intracranial pressure, a brain imaging study should be performed *before* lumbar puncture. Unfortunately, certain fungal infection (e.g., cryptococcosis) can be associated with a drastic increase of the intracranial pressure without visible hydrocephalous.

Often, it is necessary to broaden the number of diagnostic tests if the initial laboratory results of the CSF or brain imaging are inconclusive. If a fungal organism is suspected, the identification of the species may require the withdrawal of a large quantity of CSF, which can be obtained by a cervical cisternal tap.

CSF analysis in fungal meningitis will show lymphocytic pleocytosis with increased proteins. Specific tests can be done to detect fungi by direct examination under the microscope, to detect specific fungal antigens or antibodies, and to detect fungal DNA by PCR [23]. Novel molecular techniques are emerging as highly useful tools of successful and quick diagnosis. Among them, MALDI-TOF is proven to be one of the most effective modes of detection of fungal pathogen. It is a quick and inexpensive method of direct identification of the pathogen to the subspecies and strain level (reviewed in [111]). As discussed, neuroimaging may be helpful in the diagnostic process to visualize specific areas affected. CT is highly recommended in cases of diminishing consciousness [112]. Neuroimaging is also important as a follow-up exam to monitor the efficacy of the antifungal therapy. In up to 30 % of chronic meningitis, the diagnosis is not known. If fungal meningitis is suspected, the drug of choice for empirical therapy is amphotericin B.

Conclusion

CNS infections by fungal pathogens have increased rapidly over the last two decades. The developments in modern medicine, the increase in procedures like solid organ transplantation, predisposing conditions such as AIDS, and immunosuppressive therapy are the major reasons for this rise. New diagnostic methods and more efficient therapies are needed to better control these life-threatening diseases and improve the prognosis. Till date, fungal infections of the central nervous system remain a life-threatening condition that needs to be carefully evaluated in order to administer a prompt and effective antifungal therapy.

Acknowledgments This work was supported by National Institute of Health (NIH) awards AI56168, AI71142, AI87541, and AI100631 to MDP. Maurizio Del Poeta is a Burroughs Welcome New Investigator in the Pathogenesis of Infectious Diseases. The authors have no conflicts of interest that are directly relevant to the content of this review.

References

1. Raman Sharma R. Fungal infections of the nervous system: current perspective and controversies in management. Int J Surg. 2010;8(8):591–601.
2. Sundaram C, et al. Pathology and diagnosis of central nervous system infections. Patholog Res Int. 2011;878263.
3. Park BJ, et al. Estimation of the current global burden of cryptococcal meningitis among persons living with HIV/AIDS. AIDS. 2009;23(4):525–30.
4. Knoke M, Schwesinger G. One hundred years ago: the history of cryptococcosis in Greifswald. Medical mycology in the nineteenth century. Mycoses. 1994;37(7–8):229–33.
5. Minari RHA, Avery RK, Longworth DL, DeCamp M, Bertin M, Schilz R, Smedira N, Haug MT, Mehta A, Gordon SM. The incidence of invasive aspergillosis among solid organ transplant recipients and implications for prophylaxis in lung transplants. Transpl Infect Dis. 2002;4:195–202.
6. Schaenman JM, Austin JM, Baron EJ, Gamberg P, Miller J, Oyer PE, Robbins RC, Montoya JG. Trends in invasive disease due to Candida species following heart and lung transplantation. Transpl Infect Dis. 2009;11(2):112–21.
7. Husain S, Wagener MM, Singh N. Cryptococcus neoformans infection in organ transplant recipients: variables influencing clinical characteristics and outcome. Emerg Infect Dis. 2001;7(3):375–81.
8. Silveira FP, Husain S. Fungal infections in solid organ transplantation. Med Mycol. 2007;45(4):305–20.
9. Pappas PG, et al. Invasive fungal infections among organ transplant recipients: results of the Transplant-Associated Infection Surveillance Network (TRANSNET). Clin Infect Dis. 2010;50(8):1101–11.
10. Pappas PG, Alexander B, Andes D, Hadley S, Patterson T, Walker R, Morrison V, Perl T, Wannemuehler K, Chiller T. Prospective surveillance of invasive fungal infections (IfIs) among organ transplant recipients (OTRs) in the U.S. 2001–2006. 47th interscience conference on Antimicrobial Agents and Chemotherapy; Chicago; 17–20 Sept 2007.
11. Singh N, et al. Cryptococcus neoformans in organ transplant recipients: impact of calcineurin-inhibitor agents on mortality. J Infect Dis. 2007;195(5):756–64.
12. Silveira FP, et al. Cryptococcosis in liver and kidney transplant recipients receiving anti-thymocyte globulin or alemtuzumab. Transpl Infect Dis. 2007;9(1):22–7.
13. Singh N, Paterson DL. Aspergillus infections in transplant recipients. Clin Microbiol Rev. 2005;18(1):44–69.
14. Vilchez RA, Fung J, Kusne S. Cryptococcosis in organ transplant recipients: an overview. Am J Transplant. 2002;2(7):575–80.
15. Husain S, et al. Infections due to Scedosporium apiospermum and Scedosporium prolificans in transplant recipients: clinical characteristics and impact of antifungal agent therapy on outcome. Clin Infect Dis. 2005;40(1):89–99.
16. Singh N, et al. Zygomycosis in solid organ transplant recipients: a prospective, matched case–control study to assess risks for disease and outcome. J Infect Dis. 2009;200(6):1002–11.
17. Nina Singh FYC, Gayowski T, Marino IR. Infections due to dematiaceous fungi in organ transplant recipients: case report and review. Clin Infect Dis. 1997;24(3):369–74.
18. Husain S, et al. Opportunistic mycelial fungal infections in organ transplant recipients: emerging importance of non-Aspergillus mycelial fungi. Clin Infect Dis. 2003;37(2):221–9.
19. Sampathkumar P, Paya CV. Fusarium infection after solid-organ transplantation. Clin Infect Dis. 2001;32(8):1237–40.
20. Kulberg B-J. Fungal infections of the central nervous system. Advanced studies in medicine 2003;(1A):S1–S11.
21. Murthy JM. Fungal infections of the central nervous system: the clinical syndromes. Neurol India. 2007;55(3):221–5.
22. Posteraro B, et al. MALDI-TOF mass spectrometry in the clinical mycology laboratory: identification of fungi and beyond. Expert Rev Proteomics. 2013;10(2):151–64.

23. Davis JA, Costello DJ, Venna N. Laboratory investigation of fungal infections of the central nervous system. Neurol India. 2007;55(3):233–40.
24. Thomson Jr RB, Bertram H. Laboratory diagnosis of central nervous system infections. Infect Dis Clin North Am. 2001;15(4):1047–71.
25. Bader O. MALDI-TOF-MS-based species identification and typing approaches in medical mycology. Proteomics. 2013;13(5):788–99.
26. Khanna N, et al. Cryptococcal infections of the central nervous system: an analysis of predisposing factors, laboratory findings and outcome in patients from South India with special reference to HIV infection. J Med Microbiol. 1996;45(5):376–9.
27. Liu TB, et al. Brain inositol is a novel stimulator for promoting cryptococcus penetration of the blood–brain barrier. PLoS Pathog. 2013;9(4):e1003247.
28. Perfect JR, et al. Clinical practice guidelines for the management of cryptococcal disease: 2010 update by the infectious diseases society of america. Clin Infect Dis. 2010;50(3):291–322.
29. Eghwrudjakpor PO, Allison AB. Neurocryptococcosis in a 10-year-old immunocompetent girl. Acta Neurochir (Wien). 2009;151(6):711–2; discussion 712.
30. Voelz K, May RC. Cryptococcal interactions with the host immune system. Eukaryot Cell. 2010;9(6):835–46.
31. Mitchell TG, Perfect JR. Cryptococcosis in the era of AIDS – 100 years after the discovery of Cryptococcus neoformans. Clin Microbiol Rev. 1995;8(4):515–48.
32. Davis JA, et al. Central nervous system involvement in cryptococcal infection in individuals after solid organ transplantation or with AIDS. Transpl Infect Dis. 2009;11(5):432–7.
33. Li Q, et al. Central nervous system cryptococcoma in immunocompetent patients: a short review illustrated by a new case. Acta Neurochir (Wien). 2010;152(1):129–36.
34. Chuck SL, Sande MA. Infections with Cryptococcus neoformans in the acquired immunodeficiency syndrome. N Engl J Med. 1989;321(12):794–9.
35. Satishchandra P, et al. Cryptococcal meningitis: clinical, diagnostic and therapeutic overviews. Neurol India. 2007;55(3):226–32.
36. Lee GJ, et al. Cerebral aspergillosis with multiple enhancing nodules in the right cerebral hemisphere in the immune-competent patient. J Korean Neurosurg Soc. 2013;53(5):312–5.
37. Kose S, et al. Central nervous system aspergillosis in an immunocompetent patient. J Infect Dev Ctries. 2011;5(4):313–5.
38. Lin SJ, Schranz J, Teutsch SM. Aspergillosis case-fatality rate: systematic review of the literature. Clin Infect Dis. 2001;32(3):358–66.
39. Marr KA, et al. Epidemiology and outcome of mould infections in hematopoietic stem cell transplant recipients. Clin Infect Dis. 2002;34(7):909–17.
40. Xess I, et al. Prevalence of Aspergillus species in clinical samples isolated in an Indian tertiary care hospital. Indian J Med Sci. 2004;58(12):513–9.
41. Bodey G, et al. Fungal infections in cancer patients: an international autopsy survey. Eur J Clin Microbiol Infect Dis. 1992;11(2):99–109.
42. Walsh TJ, et al. Treatment of aspergillosis: clinical practice guidelines of the Infectious Diseases Society of America. Clin Infect Dis. 2008;46(3):327–60.
43. Kleinschmidt-DeMasters BK. Central nervous system aspergillosis: a 20-year retrospective series. Hum Pathol. 2002;33(1):116–24.
44. Shamim MS, et al. Craniocerebral aspergillosis: a review of advances in diagnosis and management. J Pak Med Assoc. 2010;60(7):573–9.
45. Figueiredo EG, et al. Tumoral form of aspergillosis in central nervous system (cerebral aspergilloma): case report. Sao Paulo Med J. 2003;121(6):251–3.
46. Verweij PE, et al. Aspergillus meningitis: diagnosis by non-culture-based microbiological methods and management. J Clin Microbiol. 1999;37(4):1186–9.
47. Spampinato C, Leonardi D. Candida infections, causes, targets, and resistance mechanisms: traditional and alternative antifungal agents. Biomed Res Int. 2013;2013:204237.
48. Sanchez-Portocarrero J, et al. The central nervous system and infection by Candida species. Diagn Microbiol Infect Dis. 2000;37(3):169–79.

49. Parker Jr JC, McCloskey JJ, Lee RS. Human cerebral candidosis – a postmortem evaluation of 19 patients. Hum Pathol. 1981;12(1):23–8.
50. Nakayama H, et al. Histopathological study of candidal infection in the central nervous system. Nippon Ishinkin Gakkai Zasshi. 2010;51(1):31–45.
51. Pfaller MA. Nosocomial candidiasis: emerging species, reservoirs, and modes of transmission. Clin Infect Dis. 1996;22 Suppl 2:S89–94.
52. Casado JL, et al. Candidal meningitis in HIV-infected patients: analysis of 14 cases. Clin Infect Dis. 1997;25(3):673–6.
53. Voice RA, et al. Chronic candidal meningitis: an uncommon manifestation of candidiasis. Clin Infect Dis. 1994;19(1):60–6.
54. Black KE, Baden LR. Fungal infections of the CNS: treatment strategies for the immunocompromised patient. CNS Drugs. 2007;21(4):293–318.
55. Verduyn Lunel FM, et al. Detection of the Candida antigen mannan in cerebrospinal fluid specimens from patients suspected of having Candida meningitis. J Clin Microbiol. 2004;42(2):867–70.
56. Pappas PG, et al. Clinical practice guidelines for the management of candidiasis: 2009 update by the Infectious Diseases Society of America. Clin Infect Dis. 2009;48(5):503–35.
57. Edwards JA, Rappleye CA. Histoplasma mechanisms of pathogenesis – one portfolio doesn't fit all. FEMS Microbiol Lett. 2011;324(1):1–9.
58. Ashford DA, et al. Outbreak of histoplasmosis among cavers attending the National Speleological Society Annual Convention, Texas, 1994. Am J Trop Med Hyg. 1999;60(6):899–903.
59. Jones TF, et al. Acute pulmonary histoplasmosis in bridge workers: a persistent problem. Am J Med. 1999;106(4):480–2.
60. Wheat LJ, et al. Clinical practice guidelines for the management of patients with histoplasmosis: 2007 update by the Infectious Diseases Society of America. Clin Infect Dis. 2007;45(7):807–25.
61. Kauffman CA. Histoplasmosis: a clinical and laboratory update. Clin Microbiol Rev. 2007;20(1):115–32.
62. Wheat LJ, Musial CE, Jenny-Avital E. Diagnosis and management of central nervous system histoplasmosis. Clin Infect Dis. 2005;40(6):844–52.
63. Bajwa S, Kulshrestha A. Fungal infections in intensive care unit: challenges in diagnosis and management. Ann Med Health Sci Res. 2013;3(2):238–44.
64. Klein CJ, et al. Central nervous system histoplasmosis mimicking a brain tumor: difficulties in diagnosis and treatment. Mayo Clin Proc. 1999;74(8):803–7.
65. Kirkland TN, Fierer J. Coccidioidomycosis: a reemerging infectious disease. Emerg Infect Dis. 1996;2(3):192–9.
66. Saubolle MA, McKellar PP, Sussland D. Epidemiologic, clinical, and diagnostic aspects of coccidioidomycosis. J Clin Microbiol. 2007;45(1):26–30.
67. Galgiani JN, et al. Coccidioidomycosis. Clin Infect Dis. 2005;41(9):1217–23.
68. Davis LE, Porter BS. Central nervous system Coccidioides immitis infections. Curr Treat Options Neurol. 2005;7(2):157–65.
69. Kokseng SL, Blair JE. Successful kidney transplantation after coccidioidal meningitis. Transpl Infect Dis. 2011;13(3):285–9.
70. Mischel PS, Vinters HV. Coccidioidomycosis of the central nervous system: neuropathological and vasculopathic manifestations and clinical correlates. Clin Infect Dis. 1995;20(2):400–5.
71. Lee CH, et al. Coccidioides immitis: two cases of misidentified mycosis. Can Respir J. 2008;15(7):377–9.
72. Trible R, et al. Antiretroviral therapy-associated coccidioidal meningitis. Emerg Infect Dis. 2013;19(1):163–5.
73. Arsura EL, et al. Neuroimaging as a guide to predict outcomes for patients with coccidioidal meningitis. Clin Infect Dis. 2005;40(4):624–7.
74. Stevens DA, Shatsky SA. Intrathecal amphotericin in the management of coccidioidal meningitis. Semin Respir Infect. 2001;16(4):263–9.

75. Ribes JA, Vanover-Sams CL, Baker DJ. Zygomycetes in human disease. Clin Microbiol Rev. 2000;13(2):236–301.
76. Waness A, Dawsari GA, Al Jahdali H. The rise of an opportunistic infection called "Invasive Zygomycosis". J Glob Infect Dis. 2009;1(2):131–8.
77. Rahman A, et al. Rhino-orbital mucourmycosis in a non-immunocompromised patient. BMJ Case Rep. ;2013. pii:bcr2012007863.
78. Hopkins RJ, et al. Cerebral mucormycosis associated with intravenous drug use: three case reports and review. Clin Infect Dis. 1994;19(6):1133–7.
79. Reinhardt DJ, et al. Experimental cerebral zygomycosis in alloxan-diabetic rabbits: variation in virulence among zygomycetes. Sabouraudia. 1981;19(4):245–56.
80. Skiada A, et al. Disseminated zygomycosis with involvement of the central nervous system. Clin Microbiol Infect. 2009;15 Suppl 5:46–9.
81. Reed C, et al. Combination polyene-caspofungin treatment of rhino-orbital-cerebral mucormycosis. Clin Infect Dis. 2008;47(3):364–71.
82. Cornely OA, Vehreschild JJ, Ruping MJ. Current experience in treating invasive zygomycosis with posaconazole. Clin Microbiol Infect. 2009;15 Suppl 5:77–81.
83. To CA, et al. Cryptococcal osteomyelitis and meningitis in a patient with non-hodgkin's lymphoma treated with PEP-C. BMJ Case Rep. ;2012. pii: bcr0820114578.
84. Nguyen FN, et al. Isolated central nervous system histoplasmosis presenting with ischemic pontine stroke and meningitis in an immune-competent patient. JAMA Neurol. 2013;70(5): 638–41.
85. Louro R, et al. Fungal meningitis in an immunocompetent patient. Clin Drug Investig. 2013;33 Suppl 1:S47–50.
86. Simsek H, et al. Concomitant tubercular and fungal cerebellar abscess in an immunocompromised girl. Turk Neurosurg. 2013;23(1):88–94.
87. Dusart A, et al. Fatal rhinocerebral mucormycosis with intracavernous carotid aneurysm and thrombosis: a late complication of transsphenoidal surgery? Acta Neurol Belg. 2013;113(2):179–84.
88. Igusa R, et al. Escherichia coli pneumonia in combination with fungal sinusitis and meningitis in a tsunami survivor after the Great East Japan Earthquake. Tohoku J Exp Med. 2012;227(3):179–84.
89. Kawakami Y, et al. Disseminated aspergillosis associated with tsunami lung. Respir Care. 2012;57(10):1674–8.
90. Lokuhetty MD, et al. Iatrogenic Aspergillus infection of the central nervous system in a pregnant woman. Indian J Pathol Microbiol. 2009;52(3):427–9.
91. Lanzafame M, et al. Rhodotorula glutinis-related meningitis. J Clin Microbiol. 2001;39(1):410.
92. Galhardo MC, et al. Sporothrix schenckii meningitis in AIDS during immune reconstitution syndrome. J Neurol Neurosurg Psychiatry. 2010;81(6):696–9.
93. McNicholas S, et al. Sporobolomyces roseus in the cerebrospinal fluid of an immunocompetent patient – to treat or not to treat? J Med Microbiol. 2012;61(Pt 2):295–6.
94. Gopinath M, et al. An elusive diagnosis: Scedosporium apiospermum infection after near-drowning. Ann Indian Acad Neurol. 2010;13(3):213–5.
95. Dobre MC, Smoker WR, Kirby P. A case of solitary Blastomyces dermatitidis meningitis. Clin Neurol Neurosurg. 2011;113(8):665–7.
96. Romano A, et al. Pulmonary infection caused by Blastoschizomyces capitatus. Infez Med. 2005;13(3):187–91.
97. Poza G, et al. Meningitis caused by Pseudallescheria boydii treated with voriconazole. Clin Infect Dis. 2000;30(6):981–2.
98. Shinde RS, Mantur BG, Patil G, Parande MV, Parande AM. Meningitis due to Rhodotorula glutinis in an HIV infected patient. Indian J Med Microbiol. 2008;26(4):375–7.
99. Smith RM, et al. Fungal infections associated with contaminated methylprednisolone injections – preliminary report. N Engl J Med. 2013;369:1598–1609.
100. Staal JB, et al. Injection therapy for subacute and chronic low back pain: an updated Cochrane review. Spine (Phila Pa 1976). 2009;34(1):49–59.

101. Hooten WM, Kinney MO, Huntoon MA. Epidural abscess and meningitis after epidural corticosteroid injection. Mayo Clin Proc. 2004;79(5):682–6.
102. Cooper AB, Sharpe MD. Bacterial meningitis and cauda equina syndrome after epidural steroid injections. Can J Anaesth. 1996;43(5 Pt 1):471–4.
103. Park MS, et al. Paraspinal abscess communicated with epidural abscess after extra-articular facet joint injection. Yonsei Med J. 2007;48(4):711–4.
104. Michal W, Olena W, Wojciech O. Bilateral endogenous fungal endophthalmitis. Int Ophthalmol. 2014;34:321–25.
105. Kim EC, Kim MS, Kang NY. Fungal corneal ulcer and bacterial orbital cellulitis occur as complications of bacterial endophthalmitis after cataract surgery in an immunocompetent patient. Semin Ophthalmol. 2013;28(2):75–8.
106. Ostensson A, Geborek P. Septic arthritis as a non-surgical complication in rheumatoid arthritis: relation to disease severity and therapy. Br J Rheumatol. 1991;30(1):35–8.
107. Centers for Disease, C. and Prevention. Exophiala infection from contaminated injectable steroids prepared by a compounding pharmacy – United States, July-November 2002. MMWR Morb Mortal Wkly Rep. ;51(49):1109–12.
108. Smith RM, et al. Relapse of fungal meningitis associated with contaminated methylprednisolone. N Engl J Med. 2013;368(26):2535–6.
109. Centers for Disease, C. and Prevention. Multistate outbreak of fungal infection associated with injection of methylprednisolone acetate solution from a single compounding pharmacy – United States, 2012. MMWR Morb Mortal Wkly Rep. ;61(41):839–42.
110. Centers for Disease, C. and Prevention. Multistate fungal meningitis outbreak – interim guidance for treatment. MMWR Morb Mortal Wkly Rep. ;61(41):842.
111. Croxatto A, Prod'hom G, Greub G. Applications of MALDI-TOF mass spectrometry in clinical diagnostic microbiology. FEMS Microbiol Rev. 2012;36(2):380–407.
112. Kastrup O, Wanke I, Maschke M. Neuroimaging of infections. NeuroRx. 2005;2(2):324–32.

Chapter 8
CNS Tuberculosis and Other Mycobacterial Infections

Juan Carlos García-Moncó and Aida Rodriguez-Sainz

Abstract Tuberculous meningitis is the most severe form of tuberculous infection (*Mycobacterium tuberculosis*) and presents as a subacute syndrome with lymphocytic pleocytosis and low glucose in the cerebrospinal fluid (CSF) and meningeal enhancement of the basal cisterns and hydrocephalus on neuroimaging.

Diagnosis is challenging, since CSF cultures take long and are positive in less than two-thirds of patients. Empirical therapy is thus often employed. Mortality rate of this infection remains at approximately 25 % of the patients.

Parenchymal involvement (tuberculomas and spinal cord damage) may also appear.

Nontuberculous mycobacteria affect AIDS patients. *M. avium* complex is most frequently implicated. CNS infection is rare and occurs with disseminated disease. Diagnosis is made by culture of involved tissues, and therapy requires a prolonged, multidrug regimen.

Keywords Tuberculosis • *Mycobacterium tuberculosis* • Tuberculoma • Tuberculous abscess • Tuberculous meningitis

Tuberculosis (TB) remains a major public health problem with approximately 9.2 million new cases and 1.7 million deaths throughout the world in 1 year (data from 2006). Thirty percent of the global population is infected with *M. tuberculosis*, 15 million people around the globe are coinfected with HIV and *M. tuberculosis*, and 50 million are infected with multidrug-resistant tuberculosis [1]. Every untreated individual with active TB will infect 10–15 persons every year.

J.C. García-Moncó, MD (✉) • A. Rodriguez-Sainz, MD
Department of Neurology, Hospital de Galdakao-Usansolo,
Barrio Labeaga S/N, Galdakao, Vizcaya, 48960, Spain
e-mail: hospit05@sarenet.es

J.C. García-Moncó (ed.), *CNS Infections*,
DOI 10.1007/978-1-4471-6401-2_8, © Springer-Verlag London 2014

The HIV epidemic together with rising immigration, homelessness, and urban crowding and the increase in drug-resistant *M. tuberculosis* strains have contributed significantly to this burden. Tuberculosis is currently the leading infectious cause of death and undoubtedly represents a global public health priority.

Central nervous system (CNS) involvement occurs in 5–10 % of extrapulmonary tuberculosis cases [2].

M. tuberculosis: The Etiologic Agent

Human tuberculosis is caused by mycobacteria belonging to the *Mycobacterium tuberculosis* complex, which consists of *M. tuberculosis*, *M. bovis*, and *M. africanum*.

M. tuberculosis is the main agent in humans and the term *tuberculosis* should be reserved exclusively for infection caused by this organism. The other two species belonging to the *Mycobacterium tuberculosis* complex, *M. bovis* and *M. africanum*, are implicated in very few human cases.

M. tuberculosis is an obligate aerobic, slowly growing, acid-fast bacillus with a cell wall abundant in lipids and glycolipids that conform an external hydrophobic layer that interferes with antibiotic penetration, thus explaining its difficult and lengthy therapy.

Pathogenesis of CNS Tuberculosis

Human tuberculosis is acquired by inhalation of aerosolized droplet nuclei containing a few bacilli (1–10 are needed) that reach the alveoli where they multiply and interact with macrophages, resulting in cytokine and chemokine release with activation of T-helper immunity and granuloma formation.

Within 2–4 weeks a silent hematogenous spread to extrapulmonary sites occurs, including the brain, where tubercles of mononuclear cells surrounding a caseous center are formed. Neuroimaging at this stage may reveal the presence of CNS granulomas in neurologically asymptomatic patients with miliary tuberculosis [3].

These tubercles, also known as Rich focus, remain latent for months or years until they reactivate for unclear reasons. Tubercles rupturing into the subarachnoid space cause meningitis. Those tubercles deeper in the brain or spinal cord parenchyma may expand resulting in tuberculomas or, more rarely, tuberculous abscesses.

Neurological Manifestations

Tuberculous meningitis (TBM) is the most frequent and severe manifestation of CNS involvement in tuberculosis [4]. Tuberculoma and abscess formation as well as spinal cord involvement can also occur.

Table 8.1 Tuberculous meningitis: associated features

	Adults	Children
Mean duration of illness prior to admission (range)	2 weeks (1 day–9 months)	2 weeks (3 days–3 months)
Mean frequency of close contact with tuberculosis (range)	28 % (2–50 %)	56 % (45–70 %)
Prior history of tuberculosis	23 % (5–45)	NA
Abnormal chest X-ray (range)	45 % (25–55 %)	61 % (35–75 %)
Positive tuberculin skin test (range)	51 % (40–70 %)	72 % (50–95 %)
Patients with hyponatremia (plasma sodium level <135 mEq/dl) (range)	46 % (25–75 %)	44 % (25–65 %)
Mortality	27 % (7–45 %)	19 % (3–40 %)

Modified from Ref. [4]
NA not available or incomplete data

Table 8.2 Signs and symptoms in patients with tuberculous meningitis

	Adults		Children	
	Mean (%)	Range (%)	Mean (%)	Range (%)
Fever	72	55–85	76	45–95
Headache	67	45–85	34	20–40
Meningismus	67	55–90	62	25–75
Abnormal mental status	59	30–80	42	25–75
Hydrocephalus (CT scan)	52	40–65	85	75–100
Vomiting	43	30–70	58	30–70
Malaise-anorexia	41	45–65	52	30–70
Cranial nerve palsies	24	20–40	29	10–45
Papilledema	15	5–30	9	9
Hemiparesis/hemiplegia	12	5–20	24	5–40
Seizures	11	7–10	25	10–55

Modified from Ref. [4]

Tuberculous Meningitis

The clinical characteristics of patients with TBM in adults and children have been pooled on Tables 8.1 and 8.2.

There is a consistent prodromal period of 2–4 weeks before presentation of nonspecific symptoms, including fatigue, malaise, myalgia, and fever. Chest X-ray abnormalities, a history of close contact with tuberculosis patients, and tuberculin test positivity are present more frequently in children, reflecting the shorter period between contagion and development of meningitis. Hyponatremia is present in half of the patients, often due to inappropriate secretion of antidiuretic hormone (SIADH).

The most prominent clinical features of tuberculous meningitis in adults are fever, headache, vomiting, mental status abnormalities, and meningismus. Cranial nerve palsies occur in one-fourth of patients, involving mainly the sixth and, less frequently, the third, fourth, seventh, and eighth cranial nerves. Hemiparesis,

Table 8.3 CSF profile in patients with tuberculous meningitis

	Adults	Children
Mean cell count (range)	223 cells/μl (0–4,000)	200 cells/μl (5–950)
Mean percentage of patients with neutrophilic pleocytosis (>50 % neutrophils) (range)	27 % (15–55)	21 % (15–30)
Percentage of CSFs with normal cell count	6 % (5–15)	3 % (1–5)
Mean protein level in mg/dl (range)	224 mg/dl (20–1,000)	219 mg/dl (50–1,300)
Percentage of CSFs with normal protein content	6 % (0–15)	16 % (10–30)
Percentage of patients with depressed glucose levels (<45 mg/dl or 40 % of serum glucose)	72 % (50–85)	77 % (65–85)
Positive smear	25 % (5–85)	3 % (0–6)
Positive culture	61 % (40–85)	58 % (35–85)

Modified from Ref. [4]

papilledema, and seizures occur in 10–15 % of the patients. Funduscopic evidence of choroidal tubercles is pathognomonic but is present in <10 % of patients, most frequently in association with miliary tuberculosis [5].

Children presentation is similar except for a lower percentage of headache complaints and a higher frequency of hydrocephalus.

The severity of TBM is assessed by the British Medical Research Council into three stages [6]: from conscious patients with no neurological signs (stage 1) to confused patients with focal findings (stage 2) to patients in coma or with hemiplegia or paraplegia (stage 3).

CSF Findings

The CSF shows a lymphocytic pleocytosis with an average of 200 cell/μl, increased protein contents (around 200 mg/dl), and low glucose levels (Table 8.3). In 20–25 % of non-HIV-infected patients, neutrophilic predominance is present; it shifts to lymphocytic predominance over the next 24–48 h [7]. Occasionally neutrophils persist, resulting in the so-called persistent neutrophilic meningitis, a syndrome of varied etiology in which tuberculosis has to be carefully excluded [8]. This syndrome seems more frequent in HIV-infected patients, particularly when meningitis is caused by multidrug-resistant mycobacteria [9].

On the other hand, an initial mononuclear pleocytosis may briefly change in the direction of polynuclear predominance when therapy is initiated, and this may be associated with clinical deterioration. This "therapeutic paradox" has been regarded by some authors as virtually pathognomonic of tuberculous meningitis [10] and manifests a few days after the start of antituberculous therapy by rapid deterioration. It likely represents an uncommon hypersensitivity reaction to the massive release of tuberculoproteins into the subarachnoid space.

Normal protein contents are seen in 5–15 % of patients and normal glucose levels in less than one-third, and cells are absent in up to 16 % of HIV patients as compared to 3–6 % in non-HIV-infected patients. Acellular CSF samples may show pleocytosis if a spinal tap is repeated 24–48 h later [11].

Over time, CSF sugar levels seem to normalize first, followed by the cell count and the protein contents [7, 12]. In a series, the most rapid return to normal of CSF glucose was 19 days and the slowest 11 weeks [7].

Diagnosis

The diagnosis of TBM remains an important challenge, since clinical presentation is nonspecific and microbiological confirmation is often difficult and late. From a clinical standpoint, the best predictors of TBM are as follows: (a) duration of symptoms >6 days; (b) CSF total cell count <1,000/μl with lymphocytic predominance; and (c) peripheral blood white cell count <15,000 × 10^3/ml [13, 14].

Acid-fast stains (Ziehl-Neelsen, Kinyoun, and auramine-rhodamine): These methods are fast to detect acid-fast bacilli with a conventional smear microscopy but have a low sensitivity (up to 20 %). The reasons are that acid-fast dyes cannot stain *M. tuberculosis* once it enters into the cell and that high volumes (5–10 mL) of CSF are needed, since approximately 10^4 organisms are required for their reliable detection [15]. The sensitivity of Ziehl-Neelsen stain increases with large CSF volumes, but sensitivity rarely exceeds 60 % [16].

Recently, a highly efficient Ziehl-Neelsen stain has been developed. It requires low CSF volumes (0.5 mL) that are first cytospinned to compactly collect the bacilli and cells in the CSF with permeabilization of the cells by a detergent, Triton X100, allowing the staining of the intracellular bacilli. This modified stain managed a 93.8 % of intracellular detection rate and a 100 % extracellular detection rate, results that need to be replicated [15].

Interferon-gamma release assays (IGRAs): This technique measures the interferon-gamma release in response to stimulation with specific *M. tuberculosis* antigens. In whole blood, it is useful for the diagnosis of active pulmonary tuberculosis or to distinguish between active and latent tuberculosis [17]. IGRA determination in the CSF requires high CSF volume samples, the results are commonly indeterminate, and its sensitivity (58–84 %) and specificity (73–94 %) vary among studies depending on the cutoff of the number of spots (interferon-gamma producing lymphocytes) [16].

CSF culture: When productive, it takes 4–8 weeks for unequivocal identification. Their sensitivity in TBM ranges from 25 to 85 % with an average of 50 %. Newer culture media, either radiometric – such as BACTEC – or nonradiometric systems, may give positive results in 7–10 days [18]. The WHO has endorsed the microscopic observation drug susceptibility (MODS) assay, a liquid culture with a sensitivity of 65 % and specificity of 100 %, and a median detection time of 6 days. It can be used for diagnosis and for drug resistance [19].

Adenosine deaminase (ADA) determination in CSF: Increased ADA values are useful for the diagnosis of tuberculous meningitis [20–23], although false positives and negatives do occur in other infectious and neoplastic CNS disorders [22, 24].

ADA values may increase during the first 1–2 weeks of therapy and then progressively decrease [23]. A recent systematic search on the value of ADA in the CSF of TBM patients found that values >8 U/l provided a sensitivity <59 % and specificity >96 % in TBM diagnosis [25].

Nucleic acid amplification test: The paucity of organisms in TBM and the availability of a completely sequenced genome of *M. tuberculosis* [26] made the polymerase chain reaction (PCR) an important diagnostic tool, but its sensitivity seems too low (56 %, 95 % CI 46–66) and perhaps not better than bacteriology [27]. Furthermore, performance of PCR assays is heterogeneous, which makes difficult the comparisons between different studies. PCR assays remain positive up to 1 month after antituberculous therapy [19]. The detection of mycobacterial proteins (GlcB, HspX, MPT51) in CSF by ELISA and qPCR in children with tuberculous meningitis has shown a 98–100 % sensitivity and 96–98 % specificity [28] and gives new perspectives in fast methods for TBM diagnosis. Metabolomics or gene-expression profiles in preliminary studies suggest a future role but are not in routine use at present [16].

Neuroimaging

The predilection of TBM for the basal cisterns is revealed on neuroimaging by intense meningeal enhancement (Fig. 8.1), corresponding to the thick exudate that is observed pathologically [29]. The interpeduncular fossa, the ambiens cistern, and the chiasmatic region are the sites of predilection. Meningeal enhancement is more common in HIV-infected patients. In one study, meningeal enhancement was present in 23 % of HIV-positive patients but only in 6 % of HIV-negative individuals [30]. Hydrocephalus is observed on CT scan and MRI, usually of the communicating type, although obstructive hydrocephalus may result from a focal parenchymal lesion and the associated mass effect. As mentioned before, hydrocephalus is more common in children.

Complications

Ischemic brain infarctions occur in about 25–40 % of patients during the course of tuberculous meningitis [31], as a consequence of the inflammatory arterial occlusion. When there is basal ganglia involvement, abnormal movements result, including unilateral choreoathetoid movements, myoclonus, and dystonia [32, 33]. Hyponatremia or true SIADH frequently develops in TBM.

Syringomyelia can occur several years after the initial infection, although a few acute cases have been reported [34]. Inflammatory edema and spinal cord ischemia appear to be the mechanisms implicated in early cases, whereas chronic arachnoiditis underlies late cases.

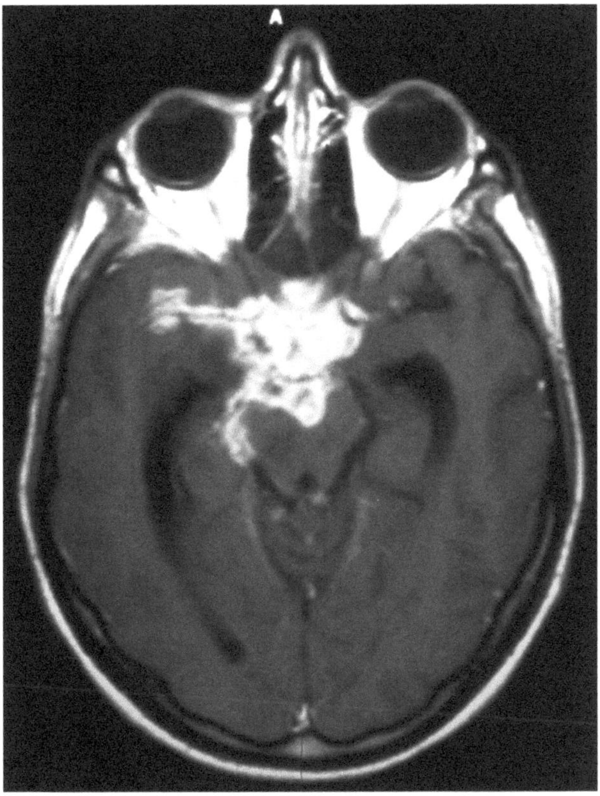

Fig. 8.1 Magnetic resonance imaging (T1-weighted sequence after gadolinium administration) of a patient with tuberculous meningitis showing a prominent exudate involving the basal meninges and extending toward the middle cerebral artery

Management

Guidelines for therapy of tuberculosis have been established by the American Thoracic Society, the Centers for Disease Control and Prevention [35], the Infectious Disease Society of America [36], and the British Infection Society [37].

Unlike its pulmonary counterpart, from where it has often been extrapolated, the optimal therapy for TBM is not the result of controlled studies and therefore is not so well established. Many patients will be empirically treated due to the diagnostic difficulties of TBM. Not infrequently, the response to therapy constitutes a key to the diagnosis. Identification and early empiric treatment of patients at risk is critical to their outcome. TBM should be suspected in patients with subacute meningitis and moderate (<1,000 cells/μl) lymphocytic pleocytosis in the CSF.

An initial four-drug course of 2 months is generally accepted, particularly in areas of multiple-drug resistance, with isoniazid, rifampin, pyrazinamide, and ethambutol (particularly appropriate in patients over 50 years of age or with renal disease), followed by 10 additional months with two drugs (isoniazid and rifampin) to a total duration of 12 months. Drug dosages and specific comments are described on Table 8.4. Isoniazid and rifampin as well as several second-line agents

Table 8.4 Drug therapy for tuberculous meningitis

Drug	Penetration into the CSF with normal meninges[a]	Penetration into the CSF with inflamed meninges	Daily dose (route)	Special remarks	Duration
First-line drugs					
Isoniazid	+ (20 % of plasma levels)	+++ (90 % of plasma levels)	A: 300 mg/day (PO, IM) Ch: 10 mg/kg	Monitor for liver toxicity Add pyridoxine to avoid peripheral neuropathy	9–12 months
Rifampin	No	+ (up to 10 % of plasma levels)	A: 600 mg/day (PO, IV) Ch: 10–20 mg/kg	Monitor for liver toxicity Interacts with protease inhibitors for HIV infection	9–12 months
Ethambutol	No	++ (10–50 % of plasma levels)	15–25 mg/kg/day (PO)	Monitor for optic neuritis	2 months
Pyrazinamide	+++ (similar to plasma levels)	+++ (similar to plasma levels)	A: 20–35 mg/kg(PO) Ch: 20–30 mg/kg	Monitor for liver toxicity	2 months
Second-line drugs					
Streptomycin	No	++ (25 % of plasma levels)	A: 15 mg/kg (IM) Ch: 20–30 mg/kg Maximum daily dose 1 g	Monitor for vestibular and auditory toxicity	2 months
Cycloserine	+++ (similar to plasma levels)	+++ (similar to plasma levels)	A: 10–15 mg/kg (1 g/day, PO) Ch: same dosage	Neurologic side effects; avoid in epileptic patients	18–24 months
Ethionamide	+++ (similar to plasma levels)	+++ (similar to plasma levels)	A: 15–20 mg/kg (1 g/day, PO) Ch: same dosage	Gastrointestinal adverse effects	18–24 months

Capreomycin Kanamycin	NO	++	A: 15 mg/kg (10 mg/kg if older than 50, IM or IV) Ch: 15–30 mg/kg (1 g/d, IM or IV)	Auditory (high-frequency hearing loss), vestibular, and renal dysfunction	6 months
p-Aminosalicylic acid (PAS)	NO	+	A: 8–12 g/day in 2–3 doses (PO) Ch: 200–300 mg/kg/day in 2–4 doses	Gastrointestinal adverse effects	18–24
Levofloxacin	+	+	A: 500–1,000 mg/day Ch: unknown	Gastrointestinal and neurologic side effects	18–24
Moxifloxacin Gatifloxacin	+	+	A. 400 mg Ch: unknown	Gastrointestinal and neurologic side effects	18–24

A adult, *Ch* children, *PO* oral route, *IM* intramuscular, *IV* intravenous

[a]Penetration arbitrarily graded as low (+), intermediate (++), or high (+++)

(aminoglycosides, capreomycin, and fluoroquinolones) are available in parenteral form if an altered mental status precludes oral intake. Isoniazid, the cornerstone of TBM therapy, and pyrazinamide readily cross the blood-brain barrier, while rifampin and ethambutol have significantly less penetration into the CNS. Isoniazid and rifampin are bactericidal against intra- and extracellular organisms, and pyrazinamide against intracellular organisms at high concentrations, whereas all the other first- and second-line drugs are bacteriostatic (streptomycin is bactericidal in vitro, but it is bacteriostatic in vivo, acting only against intracellular bacteria).

In areas where the incidence of drug resistance to *M. tuberculosis* is lower than 4 % (it is higher in Africa, Asia, and parts of South America), an initial regimen with three drugs (isoniazid, rifampin, and pyrazinamide, all daily) for 2 months and two drugs (isoniazid and rifampin, daily or twice a week) for 7–10 additional months is acceptable [38]

Liver enzymes should be monitored throughout the therapy; in the event of significant elevations of alanine aminotransferase (>5 times normal), isoniazid and rifampin are usually stopped, and ethambutol and streptomycin started and continued until enzymes return to normal, at which time isoniazid may be resumed with biweekly determinations. In most cases a combination of isoniazid, ethambutol, pyrazinamide, and streptomycin will be well tolerated. During pregnancy, streptomycin (can cause congenital deafness) and pyrazinamide (not enough experience) should be avoided, and the preferred regimen is isoniazid, ethambutol, and rifampin.

Shorter regimens may suffice, although there have been few controlled trials of treatment in patients with extrapulmonary disease. Two studies reported that the 6-month therapeutic regimen resulted in a morbidity/mortality ratio similar to that found in the longer-course therapies [39]. Chemotherapy with isoniazid and rifampin for 9 months has also proven successful in 95 % of patients, equivalent to conventional therapy with two to three drugs for 18–24 months [40]. The authors claimed that their twice-weekly regimen has the additional advantages of reduced cost, fewer doses, and ease of supervision when needed. A prospective study concluded that young children with TBM can be safely treated for 6 months with high doses of antituberculous agents (isoniazid, rifampin, ethionamide, and pyrazinamide) without overt hepatotoxicity and with a low risk of relapse [41].

Intensification of treatment in an attempt to reduce mortality has been recently evaluated. High dose of intravenous rifampicin (600 mg or 13 mg/kg) for the first 14 days resulted in significant mortality reduction (65 % vs. 35 %) [42]. A trial will be ended in the next few years comparing the use of high dose of intravenous rifampicin and oral levofloxacin as the fourth drug compared to conventional treatment [43].

Surgery in TBM patients is considered in patients with hydrocephalus in whom an external drainage is required. The most effective management of communicating hydrocephalus in these patients is unclear but requires neurosurgical consultation to alleviate hydrocephalus not responsive to medical therapy and intracranial pressure monitoring.

Corticosteroid therapy was suggested to improve neurologic outcomes of TBM of moderate severity [44]. Another study showed that corticosteroids significantly improved the survival rate and intellectual outcome of children with TBM, although they did not affect the intracranial pressure or the incidence of basal ganglia infarction [45]. A recent controlled trial in Vietnamese adults with TBM has shown that steroid therapy was strongly associated with a reduced risk of death (relative risk 0.69; 95 % CI, 0.52–0.92), although it did not prevent disability in survivors [46]. Steroids were beneficial regardless of the severity grades of disease, but did not affect those patients with HIV coinfection; this aspect requires further study.

Therefore, dexamethasone use is warranted in TBM patients not infected with HIV, regardless of age and disease severity. The regimen employed in the most recent trial was 0.4 mg/kg of intravenous dexamethasone for the first week, tapering 0.1 mg/kg per week over the 3 ensuing weeks until a dose of 0.1 mg/kg was reached, and then 4 mg daily PO, thereafter reducing 1 mg/kg per week to drug stop [46].

Drug Resistance in TBM

Although drug resistance does not seem to represent a serious threat for TBM at present since only occasional single cases of multidrug-resistant (MDR) meningitis (as defined by resistance to both isoniazid and rifampin) have been reported [47–49], this aspect requires utmost vigilance because it is associated with a decreased probability of cure. MDR meningitis should be considered in patients with prior antituberculous treatment, contact with a patient with MDR tuberculosis, or with a poor clinical response to first-line drugs within 2 weeks of therapy.

Therapy in MDR cases includes a combination of first- and second-line drugs (Table 8.4) and should be individualized and based on susceptibility studies. Second-line drugs include capreomycin, ethionamide, para-aminosalicylic acid (PAS), cycloserine, streptomycin (SM), some fluoroquinolones (levofloxacin and moxifloxacin mainly), and aminoglycosides (kanamycin and amikacin). Among these agents, ethionamide and cycloserine have a good CNS penetration and may be the only agents for extensively resistant TBM (XDR, resistance to isoniazid, rifampin, fluoroquinolones, and either capreomycin, kanamycin, or amikacin), although they are not commonly used in pulmonary tuberculosis because of their high side-effect profile. Amikacin, kanamycin, and capreomycin are injectable agents with moderate antituberculosis activity. Moxifloxacin and levofloxacin are the preferred fluoroquinolones and are commonly used as second-line agents. Intrathecal therapy with amikacin and levofloxacin was successful in an HIV patient with multidrug-resistant TBM [50]. Drug monitoring, if feasible, is useful in the management of these patients.

Regimens should consist of at least four drugs with proven effectiveness and are based on the history of drugs taken by the patient. Occasionally, 5–6 drugs are needed simultaneously. The minimum length of treatment is usually 18 months. The WHO has published guidelines with recommendations on the management of these patients [51].

Prognosis

The level of consciousness at hospital admission and the timing of therapy initiation are two important prognostic markers in TBM. Patients initially classified as having stage 3 at admission and those in whom therapy is delayed show a poor prognosis [52]. Also, patients under the age of 3 or over 65, as well as those with associated miliary tuberculosis, may have a poorer outcome.

Verdon et al. carried out a study on adults admitted to the intensive care unit with tuberculous meningitis and found three variables that correlated with outcome: time to onset of treatment ≥3 days, coma, and a simplified acute physiology score of >11 [7]. Another study observed important neurological sequelae one year after disease onset in 78.5 % of patients that included cognitive impairment in 55 %, motor deficit in 40 %, optic atrophy in 37 %, and other cranial nerve palsy in 23 %. Focal motor deficit at admission was the most important predictor of neurologic deficits at 1 year, whereas GCS score predicted the cognitive and motor sequelae [53].

Parenchymal CNS Disease: Tuberculomas and Tuberculous Abscesses

Tuberculous granulomas (*tuberculomas*) are composed of a central zone of caseation necrosis with few bacilli surrounded by a capsule of collagenous tissue and mononuclear inflammatory cells [54]. They are most commonly supratentorial in adults (infratentorial in children) and are multiple in one-third of patients [55]. The clinical course is subacute or chronic, and the commonest presentation includes headache, intracranial hypertension, seizures, and papilledema [56]. The tuberculin skin test is positive in 85 % of patients, and chest X-rays show tuberculous changes in 30–80 % of patients. CSF findings are unremarkable, and microbiology is usually negative [57]. A retrospective review of 23 tuberculoma patients from high-risk countries found a laboratory-proven meningitis in 43.5 % [56].

The diagnosis is made on the basis of neuroimaging findings, skin test, and response to empirical therapy. On CT scan, tuberculomas appear as solid-enhancing, ring-enhancing, or mixed lesions; on occasions, there is a central calcification surrounded by a hypodense area with peripheral ring enhancement (target sign) [58], a pattern highly suggestive of tuberculosis, although occasionally present in metastatic adenocarcinoma [59]. Lesions are most often located at the corticomedullary junction and periventricular regions, consistent with hematogenous spread.

Magnetic resonance imaging (MRI) shows tuberculomas as isointense to gray matter on T1-weighted images, sometimes with a hyperintense rim [60] (Fig. 8.2). Noncaseating lesions are bright on T2-weighted images with nodular enhancement. Caseating tuberculomas vary from isointense to hypointense on T2-weighted images and also exhibit rim enhancement [60]. There is a variable degree of perilesional edema and mass effect [60]. Normal diffusion-weighted MRI with normal apparent diffusion coefficient (ADC) values has been described in tuberculomas [61].

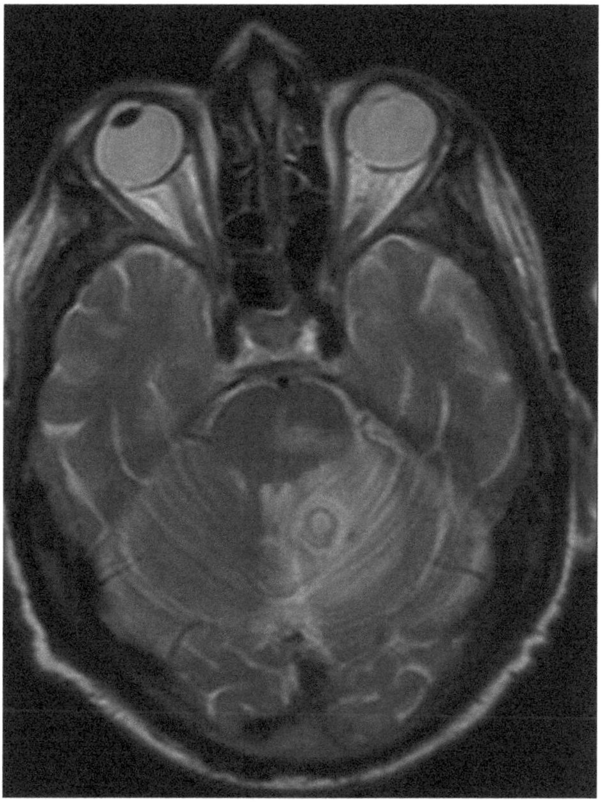

Fig. 8.2 Magnetic resonance imaging (T2-weighted sequence) showing a ring-shaped cerebellar tuberculoma surrounded by edema. Another smaller tuberculoma was present in the pons (observe the presence of pons edema). Both disappeared with a four-drug antituberculous therapy for 1 year

The differential diagnosis includes neoplasms and other granulomatous processes like sarcoidosis and parasitic diseases such as cysticercosis and toxoplasmosis. Magnetization transfer imaging analysis has proved helpful in differentiating tuberculomas and pyogenic abscess from brain tumors [62]. With therapy, tuberculomas usually decrease in size to complete resolution within 3 months although it may take longer (even years), sometimes leaving a residual calcification [63, 64]. Medical therapy alone is indicated initially, and surgery is required in the presence of intolerably increased intracranial pressure or of medical failures. Mortality with current chemotherapeutic regimens is <10 %, while prior to the availability of antituberculous drugs, mortality after decompression and excision was 35–85 % [65]. Some patients, however, develop intracranial tuberculomas or present a paradoxical enlargement of preexisting ones, during the first weeks or months of treatment for TBM [66]. Paradoxical deterioration in HIV-negative patients is frequently accompanied by an increase in peripheral blood lymphocyte count and an exaggerated tuberculin skin reaction [67]. Steroids seem to improve the general outcome, and dexamethasone is recommended for 4–8 weeks [68]. The review of the literature shows that surgery has been employed in approximately 60 % of these patients [67].

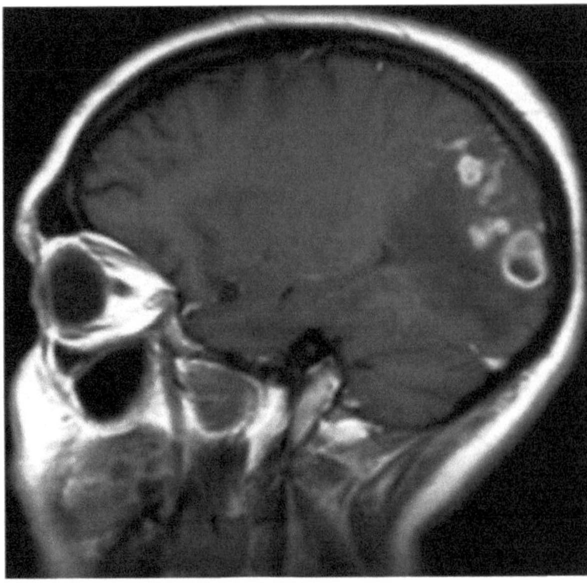

Fig. 8.3 Magnetic resonance imaging (T1-weighted sequences after gadolinium administration) showing an occipital tuberculous abscess in an HIV patient with disseminated tuberculosis and seizures. The lesion disappeared with antituberculous therapy

When the caseous core of a tuberculoma liquefies, a *tuberculous abscess* will result. They are larger and much less frequent than tuberculomas, may be multiloculated, and often have greater mass effect and edema. In contrast to the solid caseation and few organisms seen in tuberculomas, the abscess is formed by pus, where many bacilli can be found [69]. Its wall is devoid of the granulomatous reaction that surrounds the tuberculoma, with its appearance resembling that of a typical pyogenic abscess (Fig. 8.3). They have a more accelerated clinical course than tuberculomas, usually presenting acutely with fever, headache, and neurological focal signs, and are most commonly supratentorial [70]. On CT, abscesses are hypodense, with surrounding edema and mass effect, and peripheral enhancement, usually thin and uniform. On MRI, there is a central area of hyperintensity on T2-weighted images [58]. This pattern is not specific, and thus, they are difficult to differentiate from toxoplasmic, fungal, or pyogenic abscesses or even from lymphoma in AIDS patients. Localized areas of cerebritis with gyriform enhancement are less frequently observed. Appropriate therapy includes antituberculous chemotherapy and surgical excision or aspiration where needed. Ofloxacin proved successful in a patient with intracranial tuberculomas in whom first-line therapy failed [71].

Spinal Cord Involvement

Tuberculous myelitis or radiculomyelitis usually presents as an acute or subacute transverse myelitis with variable degree of radicular pain. Ischemic spinal cord infarction secondary to vasculitis may also occur [72]. CSF analysis reveals an

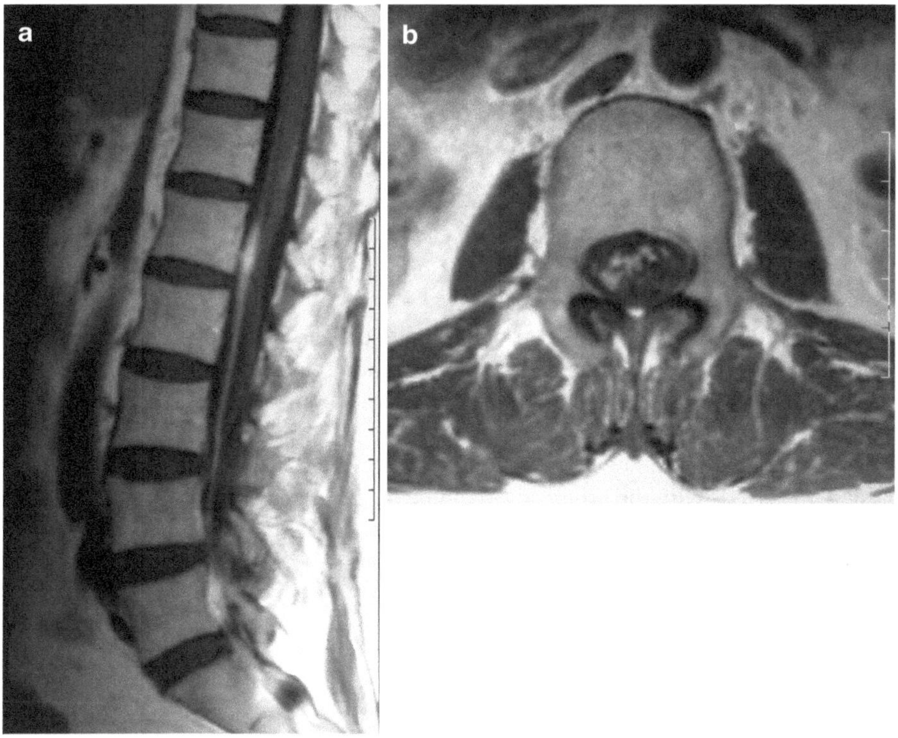

Fig. 8.4 Magnetic resonance imaging showing nodular thickening of the cauda equina roots in a patient with tuberculous meningitis and lumbosacral root involvement. Sagittal (**a**) and axial (**b**) T1-weighted sequences after gadolinium administration

increased protein content with lymphocytic pleocytosis; low glucose levels are observed in up to one-third of patients [73]. The thoracic cord is most commonly affected, followed by the lumbar and the cervical regions. MRI shows contrast-enhancing tissue that surrounds the spinal cord and the roots and obliterates the subarachnoid space with focal or diffuse increased intramedullary signal on T2-weighted images and variable degrees of edema and mass effect. Postcontrast T1-weighted images reveal leptomeningeal enhancement (Fig. 8.4). The nerve roots may be clumped and show contrast enhancement depending on the degree of involvement [74]. Corticosteroids seem to improve the prognosis [75]. Rarely, tuberculomas occur in the spinal cord, either as intramedullary lesions or located in the dural space [76], often requiring microsurgical resection and antituberculous chemotherapy. Infrequent cases of intramedullary tuberculous abscesses have been reported [77].

Tuberculous spondylitis most often involves the thoracolumbar region, with L1 being the most affected level and the cervical and sacral spine being only rarely involved [58]. The infection initially predominates in the anterior part of the vertebral body, usually involving more than one vertebral level, and disseminates to affect the disk and eventually extends along the anterior or posterior longitudinal ligaments or through the end plate. Vertebral collapse may occur, resulting in kyphosis. In the lumbar region, tuberculous spondylitis may result in a calcified psoas abscess, a finding very suggestive of tuberculosis. Neuroimaging discloses bone destruction and fragmentation with involvement of the disk space and calcified paravertebral mass. MRI seems the method of choice, with an accuracy of 94 % in vertebral osteomyelitis [78]. It reveals hypointense T1-weighted areas in the vertebral bodies alternating with areas of hyperintense T2-weighted signal in the disk space and paravertebral soft tissue. Postgadolinium images show enhancement of infected bone and disk.

Spondylitis can also complicate with an epidural abscess, resulting in different combinations of local and radicular pain, limb motor and sensory loss, and sphincter disturbances. Eventually, complete spinal cord compression with paraplegia, the most dreaded complication, may supervene.

Spinal cord disease is best treated with prolonged antituberculosis therapy and systemic steroids with the prognosis being better in those patients with recent onset disease and in whom prompt treatment is established. Surgery should be considered on an individualized basis depending on the extent and nature of the lesion and on the degree of neurologic deficit.

CNS Tuberculosis in the HIV Patient

Coinfection with HIV and tuberculosis has important implications, since the prognosis of tuberculosis is poorer due to the immunosuppression of these individuals and there is mounting evidence that the host immune response to *M. tuberculosis* enhances HIV replication and might accelerate the natural progression of HIV infection. HIV testing is recommended for all patients with tuberculosis [36].

The clinical features and CSF profiles of tuberculous meningitis are not modified by HIV infection [30, 79]. HIV-infected patients show a lower percentage of tuberculin test positivity (30 % with initial infection as compared with 50 % in the immunocompetent adult), reflecting their cell-mediated immune deficiency. Anergy develops with advanced stages of immunosuppression.

Parenchymal disease seems more common in HIV patients [30] and has been reported in 15–44 % of patients with CNS tuberculosis [80].

When treating HIV-infected individuals, several facts should be considered. First, they usually have difficulty in controlling the infection due to the associated immune deficiencies. Second, rifamycins (rifampin, rifabutin, and rifapentine) reduce the activity of protease inhibitors due to induction of cytochrome CYP450 (all protease inhibitors are metabolized by CYP450). For this reason, rifabutin – which has substantially less activity as an inducer of cytochrome enzymes – is used instead of rifampin in these individuals, at a dose of 150 mg/day. Conversely, if protease inhibitors, particularly ritonavir or saquinavir, which are potent CYP450 inhibitors, are administered with rifabutin, blood concentrations of the latter increase markedly, and most likely rifabutin toxicity increases as well. Rifabutin is efficacious in nonresistant tuberculosis; its role in multiresistant cases is less clear [81]. Finally, HIV-infected patients can have malabsorption of antituberculous drugs [82] and are particularly prone to adverse drug reactions [83], which makes drug monitoring particularly important. Ideally, the management of tuberculosis among HIV-infected patients taking antiretroviral drugs should include directly observed therapy. It has to be taken into account that paradoxical reactions might occur during the course of tuberculosis treatment when antiretroviral therapy restores immune function [84].

Aside from classical regimens of long duration (see above), 6-month (isoniazid, rifabutin, and pyrazinamide for 2 months and isoniazid and rifabutin for 4 additional moths) and 9-month schedules (isoniazid, streptomycin, and pyrazinamide daily for 2 months and then 2–3 times/week for 7 months) are accepted regimens for HIV-infected patients [85].

Paradoxical tuberculosis-associated immune reconstitution inflammatory syndrome (TB-IRIS) is an important complication in HIV-infected tuberculosis patients who start combination antiretroviral treatment (ART). Neurological manifestations occur in more than 10 % of TB-IRIS cases, mainly meningitis and tuberculomas [86].

CNS Infection by Nontuberculous Mycobacteria

Nontuberculous mycobacteria (NTM) are categorized into different groups based on characteristic colony morphology, growth rate, and pigmentation (the Runyon system of classification), although this system is being progressively replaced by more efficient and rapid systems of molecular diagnosis. Growth rates in culture remain a practical means for grouping species and classify NTM into slow (>7 days), rapid (<7 days), and intermediate (7–10 days) growing mycobacteria. The slow group includes the "*M. avium* complex" (MAC), constituted by *M. avium* and *M. intracellulare* (also known as MAI), *M. kansasii*, *M. scrofulaceum*, *M. xenopi*, and *M. genavense*, among others. Mycobacteria that grow at the intermediate rate include *M. gordonae* and *M. marinum*. Rapidly growing organisms include the *M. fortuitum* complex (*M. fortuitum group* and the *M. chelonei/abscessus* group). *M. avium* complex is responsible for most of the infections caused by NTM [87].

Currently, approximately 50 species of NTM are considered to be potential sources of disease. NTM are ubiquitous in the environment, including soil, water, and animals [87]. Most infections, including those that are hospital acquired, result from inhalation or direct inoculation from environmental sources. Ingestion may be the source of infection for children with NTM cervical adenopathy and for patients with the acquired immunodeficiency syndrome (AIDS) whose disseminated infection may begin in the gastrointestinal tract. Because person-to-person transmission is extremely rare, isolation of infected patients is not required.

NTM usually infect immunosuppressed individuals, primarily patients with AIDS and very low CD4 counts (<50 cells/ul) in whom prophylaxis with clarithromycin (500 mg twice daily) or azithromycin (1,200 mg once weekly) is recommended. NTM produce a broad spectrum of disease, including chronic pulmonary disease in adults, lymphadenitis (mainly cervical) in children, skin and soft tissue disease, skeletal infection, catheter-related infections, and disseminated infection [87]. CNS infection is rare and occurs in the setting of disseminated disease.

The definite diagnosis is made by culture of the different samples depending on the organ involved and in cases of systemic infection by blood cultures, since they may be accompanied by high mycobacteremia. The diagnosis is also established if transbronchial, percutaneous, or open-lung biopsy tissue reveals mycobacterial histopathologic changes and yields the organism. Radiometric culture systems, DNA probes, and polymerase chain reaction assays have increased the speed and accuracy of laboratory diagnosis of pulmonary and extrapulmonary infections [88, 89]. Specific skin test antigens for NTM are not available.

Since NTMs are ubiquitous bacteria, their isolation from a clinical sample may represent a contamination. Thus, it is very important to consider the clinical features when evaluating a positive culture. In contrast, isolation from a sterile fluid such as CSF usually represents a genuine infection of the nervous system.

CNS infection by NTM is infrequent and usually consists of meningitis or meningoencephalitis [90]. *M. avium* is the most common etiologic agent of this group, especially in AIDS patients. Most of the patients had evidence of extensive disseminated disease. *M. kansasii* meningitis is similar to that of tuberculous meningitis but with a somber prognosis. *M. fortuitum* meningitis is related to prior CNS surgery and trauma, frequently associated with abscess and foreign bodies; prognosis in these cases can be more favorable if the concomitant abscess can be successfully drained or the foreign body removed. Overall prognosis for NTM meningitis is poor, with a mortality rate close to 70 % [90–92]. CSF examination in NTM meningitis shows mild lymphocytic pleocytosis, with glucose and protein levels close to normal [90].

Less frequently, these infections result in brain masses [93] or rhombencephalitis [94]. A case of chronic meningitis with a brain abscess in immunocompetent patients has also been described [95]. In a patient with Hodgkin's disease, the histopathological examination of the brain showed a perivascular infiltrate of lymphocytes and macrophages containing acid-fast resistant bacilli [96].

In a series of CSF cultures from 2,083 AIDS patients with concomitant neurological manifestations, *M. tuberculosis* was the most commonly isolated microorganism (4.2 %), followed by NTM (0.7 %). Of 130 positive cultures, 89 (68.5 %) corresponded to *M. tuberculosis* and 15 (11 %) a NTM [97]. In another series, from Brazil, *Mycobacterium avium* was isolated in 11 of a total of 1,273 (0.63 %) AIDS patients [98].

A potential role has been suggested for bacteria of the *Mycobacterium avium* complex infection in contributing to AIDS peripheral neuropathy as a consequence of macrophage activation resulting in an increased macrophage-derived toxin production [99].

NTM have been implicated also in neurosarcoidosis after a positive hybridization with MAC by polymerase chain reaction assay on CSF from a patient with this disorder [100].

Therapy for disseminated NTM infections requires consultation with an expert and has been revised by the American Thoracic Society [101], although approaches to neurological infection are unclear due to their rarity. Decisions must weigh all potential drug toxicities and interactions as well as the results of susceptibility testing. Regimens usually include a macrolide (clarithromycin 500 mg twice daily or azithromycin 600 mg daily), ethambutol (15 mg/kg daily), and an additional third drug (rifampin 600 mg daily or rifabutin 150–300 mg daily, or ciprofloxacin). Optimal duration of therapy is unclear; immunocompetent patients should probably be treated for 18–24 months, and AIDS patients for life.

References

1. Kaufmann SH. Robert Koch, the Nobel Prize, and the ongoing threat of tuberculosis. N Engl J Med. 2005;353(23):2423–6.
2. Rieder HL, Snider Jr DE, Cauthen GM. Extrapulmonary tuberculosis in the United States. Am Rev Respir Dis. 1990;141(2):347–51.
3. Gupta RK, Kohli A, Gaur V, et al. MRI of the brain in patients with miliary pulmonary tuberculosis without symptoms or signs of central nervous system involvement. Neuroradiology. 1997;39(10):699–704.
4. Garcia-Monco JC. Central nervous system tuberculosis. Neurol Clin. 1999;17(4):737–59.
5. Illingworth RS. The early diagnosis of tuberculous meningitis. Br Med J. 1950;1:479–81.
6. Council BMR. Streptomycin treatment of tuberculous meningitis. Lancet. 1948;1:582–96.
7. Verdon R, Chevret S, Laissy JP, Wolff M. Tuberculous meningitis in adults: review of 48 cases [see comments]. Clin Infect Dis. 1996;22(6):982–8.
8. Pinto Jr VL, Lima MA, Boia MN. Persistent neutrophilic meningitis. J Neurol Neurosurg Psychiatry. 2009;80(6):697–8.
9. Sanchez-Portocarrero J, Perez-Cecilia E, Jimenez-Escrig A, et al. Tuberculous meningitis. Clinical characteristics and comparison with cryptococcal meningitis in patients with human immunodeficiency virus infection. Arch Neurol. 1996;53(7):671–6.
10. Garcia-Monco JC, Ferreira E, Gomez-Beldarrain M. The therapeutic paradox in the diagnosis of tuberculous meningitis. Neurology. 2005;65(12):1991–2.
11. Ogawa SK, Smith MA, Brennessel DJ, Lowy FD. Tuberculous meningitis in an urban medical center. Medicine (Baltimore). 1987;66(4):317–26.
12. Barret-Connor E. Tuberculous meningitis in adults. South Med J. 1967;60:1060–7.
13. Thwaites GE, Chau TT, Stepniewska K, et al. Diagnosis of adult tuberculous meningitis by use of clinical and laboratory features. Lancet. 2002;360(9342):1287–92.
14. Moghtaderi A, Alavi-Naini R, Izadi S, Cuevas LE. Diagnostic risk factors to differentiate tuberculous and acute bacterial meningitis. Scand J Infect Dis. 2009;41(3):188–94.
15. Chen P, Shi M, Feng GD, et al. A highly efficient Ziehl-Neelsen stain: identifying de novo intracellular Mycobacterium tuberculosis and improving detection of extracellular M. tuberculosis in cerebrospinal fluid. J Clin Microbiol. 2012;50(4):1166–70.
16. Thwaites GE. Advances in the diagnosis and treatment of tuberculous meningitis. Curr Opin Neurol. 2013;26(3):295–300.
17. Metcalfe JZ, Everett CK, Steingart KR, et al. Interferon-gamma release assays for active pulmonary tuberculosis diagnosis in adults in low- and middle-income countries: systematic review and meta-analysis. J Infect Dis. 2011;204 Suppl 4:S1120–9.

18. Watterson SA, Drobniewski FA. Modern laboratory diagnosis of mycobacterial infections. J Clin Pathol. 2000;53(10):727–32.
19. Ho J, Marais BJ, Gilbert GL, Ralph AP. Diagnosing tuberculous meningitis – have we made any progress? Trop Med Int Health. 2013;18(6):783–93.
20. Malan C, Donald PR, Golden M, Taljaard JJ. Adenosine deaminase levels in cerebrospinal fluid in the diagnosis of tuberculous meningitis. J Trop Med Hyg. 1984;87(1):33–40.
21. Mishra OP, Loiwal V, Ali Z, et al. Cerebrospinal fluid adenosine deaminase activity for the diagnosis of tuberculous meningitis in children. J Trop Pediatr. 1996;42(3):129–32.
22. Pettersson T, Klockars M, Weber TH, Somer H. Diagnostic value of cerebrospinal fluid adenosine deaminase determination [see comments]. Scand J Infect Dis. 1991;23(1):97–100.
23. Ribera E, Martinez-Vazquez JM, Ocana I, et al. Activity of adenosine deaminase in cerebrospinal fluid for the diagnosis and follow-up of tuberculous meningitis in adults. J Infect Dis. 1987;155(4):603–7.
24. Garcia-Monco C, Berciano J. Sarcoid meningitis, high adenosine deaminase levels in CSF and results of cranial irradiation [letter]. J Neurol Neurosurg Psychiatry. 1988;51(12): 1594–6.
25. Tuon FF, Higashino HR, Lopes MI, et al. Adenosine deaminase and tuberculous meningitis – a systematic review with meta-analysis. Scand J Infect Dis. 2010;42(3):198–207.
26. Cole ST, Brosch R, Parkhill J, et al. Deciphering the biology of Mycobacterium tuberculosis from the complete genome sequence [see comments]. Nature. 1998;393(6685):537–44.
27. Pai M, Flores LL, Pai N, et al. Diagnostic accuracy of nucleic acid amplification tests for tuberculous meningitis: a systematic review and meta-analysis. Lancet Infect Dis. 2003; 3(10):633–43.
28. Haldar S, Sankhyan N, Sharma N, et al. Detection of Mycobacterium tuberculosis GlcB or HspX Antigens or devR DNA impacts the rapid diagnosis of tuberculous meningitis in children. PLoS One. 2012;7(9):e44630.
29. Ozates M, Kemaloglu S, Gurkan F, et al. CT of the brain in tuberculous meningitis. A review of 289 patients. Acta Radiol. 2000;41(1):13–7.
30. Berenguer J, Moreno S, Laguna F, et al. Tuberculous meningitis in patients infected with the human immunodeficiency virus [see comments]. N Engl J Med. 1992;326(10):668–72.
31. Belorgey L, Lalani I, Zakaria A. Ischemic stroke in the setting of tuberculous meningitis. J Neuroimaging. 2006;16(4):364–6.
32. Alarcon F, Escalante L, Perez Y, et al. Tuberculous meningitis. Short course of chemotherapy [published erratum appears in Arch Neurol 1991 Sep;48(9):920]. Arch Neurol. 1990;47(12): 1313–7.
33. Leiguarda R, Berthier M, Starkstein S, et al. Ischemic infarction in 25 children with tuberculous meningitis. Stroke. 1988;19(2):200–4.
34. Daif AK, al Rajeh S, Ogunniyi A, et al. Syringomyelia developing as an acute complication of tuberculous meningitis. Can J Neurol Sci. 1997;24(1):73–6.
35. Bass Jr JB, Farer LS, Hopewell PC, et al. Treatment of tuberculosis and tuberculosis infection in adults and children. American Thoracic Society and The Centers for Disease Control and Prevention [see comments]. Am J Respir Crit Care Med. 1994;149(5):1359–74.
36. Horsburgh Jr CR, Feldman S, Ridzon R. Practice guidelines for the treatment of tuberculosis. Clin Infect Dis. 2000;31(3):633–9.
37. Thwaites G, Fisher M, Hemingway C, et al. British Infection Society guidelines for the diagnosis and treatment of tuberculosis of the central nervous system in adults and children. J Infect. 2009;59(3):167–87.
38. Small PM, Fujiwara PI. Management of tuberculosis in the United States. N Engl J Med. 2001;345(3):189–200.
39. van Loenhout-Rooyackers JH, Keyser A, Laheij RJ, et al. Tuberculous meningitis: is a 6-month treatment regimen sufficient? Int J Tuberc Lung Dis. 2001;5(11):1028–35.
40. Dutt AK, Moers D, Stead WW. Short-course chemotherapy for extrapulmonary tuberculosis. Nine years' experience. Ann Intern Med. 1986;104(1):7–12.

41. Donald PR, Schoeman JF, Van Zyl LE, et al. Intensive short course chemotherapy in the management of tuberculous meningitis. Int J Tuberc Lung Dis. 1998;2(9):704–11.
42. Ruslami R, Ganiem AR, Dian S, et al. Intensified regimen containing rifampicin and moxifloxacin for tuberculous meningitis: an open-label, randomised controlled phase 2 trial. Lancet Infect Dis. 2013;13(1):27–35.
43. Heemskerk D, Day J, Chau TT, et al. Intensified treatment with high dose rifampicin and levofloxacin compared to standard treatment for adult patients with tuberculous meningitis (TBM-IT): protocol for a randomized controlled trial. Trials. 2011;12:25.
44. Dooley DP, Carpenter JL, Rademacher S. Adjunctive corticosteroid therapy for tuberculosis: a critical reappraisal of the literature. Clin Infect Dis. 1997;25(4):872–87.
45. Schoeman JF, Van Zyl LE, Laubscher JA, Donald PR. Effect of corticosteroids on intracranial pressure, computed tomographic findings, and clinical outcome in young children with tuberculous meningitis. Pediatrics. 1997;99(2):226–31.
46. Thwaites GE, Nguyen DB, Nguyen HD, et al. Dexamethasone for the treatment of tuberculous meningitis in adolescents and adults. N Engl J Med. 2004;351(17):1741–51.
47. Fortun J, Gomez-Mampaso E, Navas E, et al. Tuberculous meningitis caused by resistant microorganisms. Therapeutic failure in 2 patients with HIV infection and disseminated tuberculosis (see comments). Enferm Infecc Microbiol Clin. 1994;12(3):150–3.
48. Horn DL, Hewlett Jr D, Peterson S, et al. RISE-resistant tuberculous meningitis in AIDS patient [letter]. Lancet. 1993;341(8838):177–8.
49. Steiner P, Rao M, Victoria MS, et al. A continuing study of primary drug-resistant tuberculosis among children observed at the Kings County Hospital Medical Center between the years 1961 and 1980. Am Rev Respir Dis. 1983;128(3):425–8.
50. Berning SE, Cherry TA, Iseman MD. Novel treatment of meningitis caused by multidrug-resistant Mycobacterium tuberculosis with intrathecal levofloxacin and amikacin: case report. Clin Infect Dis. 2001;32(4):643–6.
51. WHO. WHO guidelines for the programmatic management of drug-resistant tuberculosis. Geneva: World Health Organization (WHO); 2008.
52. Sheu JJ, Yuan RY, Yang CC. Predictors for outcome and treatment delay in patients with tuberculous meningitis. Am J Med Sci. 2009;338(2):134–9.
53. Kalita J, Misra UK, Ranjan P. Predictors of long-term neurological sequelae of tuberculous meningitis: a multivariate analysis. Eur J Neurol. 2007;14(1):33–7.
54. Dastur DK, Lalitha VS, Prabhakar V. Pathological analysis of intracranial space-occupying lesions in 1000 cases including children. 1. Age, sex and pattern; and the tuberculomas. J Neurol Sci. 1968;6(3):575–92.
55. Jinkins JR. Computed tomography of intracranial tuberculosis. Neuroradiology. 1991;33(2):126–35.
56. Man H, Sellier P, Boukobza M, et al. Central nervous system tuberculomas in 23 patients. Scand J Infect Dis. 2010;42(6–7):450–4.
57. Mayers MM, Kaufman DM, Miller MH. Recent cases of intracranial tuberculomas. Neurology. 1978;28(3):256–60.
58. Whiteman ML. Neuroimaging of central nervous system tuberculosis in HIV-infected patients. Neuroimaging Clin N Am. 1997;7(2):199–214.
59. Kong A, Koukourou A, Boyd M, Crowe G. Metastatic adenocarcinoma mimicking 'target sign' of cerebral tuberculosis. J Clin Neurosci. 2006;13(9):955–8.
60. Gupta RK, Jena A, Singh AK, et al. Role of magnetic resonance (MR) in the diagnosis and management of intracranial tuberculomas. Clin Radiol. 1990;41(2):120–7.
61. Basoglu OK, Savas R, Kitis O. Conventional and diffusion-weighted MR imaging of intracranial tuberculomas. A case report. Acta Radiol. 2002;43(6):560–2.
62. Pui MH, Ahmad MN. Magnetization transfer imaging diagnosis of intracranial tuberculomas. Neuroradiology. 2002;44(3):210–5.
63. DeAngelis LM. Intracranial tuberculoma: case report and review of the literature. Neurology. 1981;31(9):1133–6.

64. Garcia-Monco JC, Gomez Beldarrain M, Fernandez Canton G, et al. Resolution of a brainstem abscess through antituberculous therapy [see comments]. Neurology. 1997;49(1):265–7.
65. Arseni C. Two hundred and one cases of intracranial tuberculoma treated surgically. J Neurol Neurosurg Psychiatry. 1958;21:308–11.
66. Afghani B, Lieberman JM. Paradoxical enlargement or development of intracranial tuberculomas during therapy: case report and review. Clin Infect Dis. 1994;19(6):1092–9.
67. Cheng VC, Ho PL, Lee RA, et al. Clinical spectrum of paradoxical deterioration during antituberculosis therapy in non-HIV-infected patients. Eur J Clin Microbiol Infect Dis. 2002;21(11):803–9.
68. Hejazi N, Hassler W. Multiple intracranial tuberculomas with atypical response to tuberculostatic chemotherapy: literature review and a case report. Acta Neurochir (Wien). 1997;139(3):194–202.
69. Tyson G, Newman P, Strachan WE. Tuberculous brain abscess. Surg Neurol. 1978; 10(5):323–5.
70. Kumar R, Pandey CK, Bose N, Sahay S. Tuberculous brain abscess: clinical presentation, pathophysiology and treatment (in children). Childs Nerv Syst. 2002;18(3–4):118–23.
71. Sermet-Gaudelus I, Stambouli F, Abadie V, et al. Rapid improvement of intracranial tuberculomas after addition of ofloxacin to first-line antituberculosis treatment. Eur J Clin Microbiol Infect Dis. 1999;18(10):726–8.
72. Kocen RS, Parsons M. Neurological complications of tuberculosis: some unusual manifestations. Q J Med. 1970;39(153):17–30.
73. Dastur D, Wadia NH. Spinal meningitides with radiculo-myelopathy. 2. Pathology and pathogenesis. J Neurol Sci. 1969;8(2):261–97.
74. Gupta RK, Gupta S, Kumar S, et al. MRI in intraspinal tuberculosis. Neuroradiology. 1994;36(1):39–43.
75. de La Blanchardiere A, Stern JB, Molina JM, et al. Spinal tuberculous arachnoiditis. Presse Med. 1996;25(29):1333–5.
76. Lu M. Imaging diagnosis of spinal intramedullary tuberculoma: case reports and literature review. J Spinal Cord Med. 2010;33(2):159–62.
77. Hanci M, Sarioglu AC, Uzan M, et al. Intramedullary tuberculous abscess: a case report. Spine. 1996;21(6):766–9.
78. Modic MT, Feiglin DH, Piraino DW, et al. Vertebral osteomyelitis: assessment using MR. Radiology. 1985;157(1):157–66.
79. Thwaites GE, Duc Bang N, Huy Dung N, et al. The influence of HIV infection on clinical presentation, response to treatment, and outcome in adults with Tuberculous meningitis. J Infect Dis. 2005;192(12):2134–41.
80. Whiteman M, Espinoza L, Post MJ, et al. Central nervous system tuberculosis in HIV-infected patients: clinical and radiographic findings. AJNR Am J Neuroradiol. 1995;16(6): 1319–27.
81. Wallace RJ. Antimycobacterial agents. In: Mandell GI, Bennet JE, Dolin R, editors. Principles and practice of infectious diseases. Philadelphia: Churchill-Livingstone; 2000. p. 436–48.
82. Gordon SM, Horsburgh Jr CR, Peloquin CA, et al. Low serum levels of oral antimycobacterial agents in patients with disseminated Mycobacterium avium complex disease. J Infect Dis. 1993;168(6):1559–62.
83. Pozniak AL, MacLeod GA, Mahari M, et al. The influence of HIV status on single and multiple drug reactions to antituberculous therapy in Africa. Aids. 1992;6(8):809–14.
84. Rao GP, Nadh BR, Hemaratnan A, et al. Paradoxical progression of tuberculous lesions during chemotherapy of central nervous system tuberculosis. J Neurosurg. 1995;83:359–62.
85. Anonymous. Prevention and treatment of tuberculosis among patients infected with human immunodeficiency virus: principles of therapy and revised recommendations. Centers for Disease Control and Prevention. MMWR Morb Mortal Wkly Rep. 1998;47(RR-20):1–58.
86. Marais S, Scholtz P, Pepper DJ, et al. Neuroradiological features of the tuberculosis-associated immune reconstitution inflammatory syndrome. Int J Tuberc Lung Dis. 2010;14(2):188–96.

87. Brown BA, Wallace Jr RJ. Infections due to nontuberculous mycobacteria. In: Mandell GI, Bennet JE, Dolin R, editors. Principles and practice of infectious disease. Philadelphia: Churchill-Livingstone; 2000. p. 2630–6.
88. Cook VJ, Turenne CY, Wolfe J, et al. Conventional methods versus 16S ribosomal DNA sequencing for identification of nontuberculous mycobacteria: cost analysis. J Clin Microbiol. 2003;41(3):1010–5.
89. Brown-Elliott BA, Griffith DE, Wallace Jr RJ. Diagnosis of nontuberculous mycobacterial infections. Clin Lab Med. 2002;22(4):911–25, vi.
90. Flor A, Capdevila JA, Martin N, et al. Nontuberculous mycobacterial meningitis: report of two cases and review [see comments]. Clin Infect Dis. 1996;23(6):1266–73.
91. Jacob CN, Henein SS, Heurich AE, Kamholz S. Nontuberculous mycobacterial infection of the central nervous system in patients with AIDS. South Med J. 1993;86(6):638–40.
92. Weiss IK, Krogstad PA, Botero C, et al. Fatal Mycobacterium avium meningitis after misidentification of M tuberculosis. Lancet. 1995;345(8955):991–2.
93. Berman SM, Kim RC, Haghighat D, et al. Mycobacterium genavense infection presenting as a solitary brain mass in a patient with AIDS: case report and review. Clin Infect Dis. 1994;19(6):1152–4.
94. Duong M, Piroth L, Chavanet P, et al. A case of rhombencephalitis with isolation of cytomegalovirus and Mycobacterium avium complex in a woman with AIDS [letter]. Aids. 1994;8(9):1356–7.
95. Uldry PA, Bogousslavsky J, Regli F, et al. Chronic Mycobacterium avium complex infection of the central nervous system in a nonimmunosuppressed woman. Eur Neurol. 1992;32(5):285–8.
96. Gyure KA, Prayson RA, Estes ML, Hall GS. Symptomatic Mycobacterium avium complex infection of the central nervous system. A case report and review of the literature [see comments]. Arch Pathol Lab Med. 1995;119(9):836–9.
97. Landgraf IM, Palaci M, Vieira MF, et al. Bacterial agents isolated from cerebrospinal fluid of patients with acquired immunodeficiency syndrome (AIDS) and neurological complications. Rev Inst Med Trop Sao Paulo. 1994;36(6):491–6.
98. Hadad DJ, Petry TC, Maresca AF, et al. Mycobacterium avium complex (MAC): an unusual potential pathogen in cerebrospinal fluid of AIDS patients. Rev Inst Med Trop Sao Paulo. 1995;37(2):93–8.
99. Norton GR, Sweeney J, Marriott D, et al. Association between HIV distal symmetric polyneuropathy and Mycobacterium avium complex infection [see comments]. J Neurol Neurosurg Psychiatry. 1996;61(6):606–9.
100. el-Zaatari FA, Graham DY, Samuelsson K, Engstrand L. Detection of Mycobacterium avium complex in cerebrospinal fluid of a sarcoid patient by specific polymerase chain reaction assays. Scand J Infect Dis. 1997;29(2):202–4.
101. Diagnosis and treatment of disease caused by nontuberculous mycobacteria. American Thoracic Society Statement. Am J Respir Crit Care Med. 1997;156(2 Pt 2):S1–25.

Chapter 9
Parasitic Infections of the Central Nervous System

Oscar H. Del Brutto

Abstract Parasitic infections of the CNS are a public health challenge to the developing world. During the past few decades, increased tourism, migratory movements, and the AIDS epidemic have facilitated the spread of formerly geographically restricted parasitic infections that now affect thousands of people living in developed countries. Parasites are classified into protozoa and helminths, and the latter are further divided into cestodes (tapeworms), nematodes (roundworms), and trematodes (flukes). Parasitic infections are highly pleomorphic due to the unpredictable nature of the immunological reaction of the host against parasites as well as the many pathological lesions that these organisms may cause. Parasitic infections of the CNS may cause subacute or chronic meningitis, encephalitis, space-occupying brain lesions, stroke, and myelopathy. Diagnosis may be difficult due to nonspecificity of clinical manifestations and neuroimaging findings and the poor reliability of some of the most commonly used serologic tests. While the introduction of potent antiparasitic drugs has improved the prognosis in many patients, therapy still remains anecdotal for most of these conditions.

Keywords Angiostrongyliasis • Baylisascariasis • Cerebral amebiasis • Cerebral malaria • Chagas' disease • Coenurosis • Cysticercosis • Echinococcosis • Eosinophilic meningitis • Gnathostomiasis • Hydatid disease • Neurocysticercosis • Paragonimiasis • Schistosomiasis • Sleeping sickness • Trypanosomiasis • Sparganosis • Strongyloidiasis • Toxocariasis • Toxoplasmosis • Trichinellosis

O.H. Del Brutto, MD
School of Medicine, Universidad Espiritu Santo – Ecuador,
Km 3 Via Puntilla – Samborondon, Guayaquil, Ecuador
e-mail: oscardelbrutto@hotmail.com

J.C. García-Moncó (ed.), *CNS Infections*,
DOI 10.1007/978-1-4471-6401-2_9,

Protozoan Infections

Cerebral Amebiasis

Three genuses of free-living amoeba, *Naegleria*, *Acanthamoeba*, and *Balamuthia*, may invade the human CNS and cause disease. While *Naegleria fowleri* infections occur in healthy individuals, *Acanthamoeba* spp. and *Balamuthia mandrillaris* are opportunistic pathogens, typically affecting immunocompromised hosts. *N. fowleri* infection is most often acquired during swimming in warm freshwater; this parasite enters the nasal cavity and migrates through olfactory nerves to the CNS [8]. In contrast, *Acanthamoeba* spp. and *B. mandrillaris* enter the human body through the skin or the upper respiratory tract and secondarily invade the CNS by the hematogenous route [5].

N. fowleri causes a condition called "primary amoebic meningoencephalitis." This is a fulminant disease associated with hemorrhagic necrosis of the brain parenchyma that is more prominent around the olfactory bulbs and frontal lobes (as a reflection of the portal of entry of the microorganisms). Neuroimaging studies of nonspecific brain swelling and the diagnosis must be confirmed by the demonstration of mobile trophozoites in fresh cerebrospinal fluid (CSF) examination [27].

CNS infection with *Acanthamoeba* spp. and *B. mandrillaris* causes "granulomatous amoebic encephalitis," a subacute disease characterized by fever, focal neurological signs, seizures, increased intracranial pressure, and behavioral changes. These manifestations are related to the formation of hemorrhagic parenchymal brain abscesses that are seen on neuroimaging studies as multiple ring-enhancing lesions surrounded by edema. Invasion of the walls of intracranial arteries by trophozoites causes a necrotizing angiitis that may lead to ischemic strokes. As neuroimaging findings are nonspecific, diagnosis of this condition requires the demonstration of parasites in biopsy specimens [2]. Both *Acanthamoeba* spp. and *B. mandrillaris* may also cause disseminated disease with involvement of the lungs, skin, and kidneys.

Infections by free-living amoeba are highly fatal [38]. Amphotericin B, rifampin, and fluconazole may be used in *N. fowleri* infections, while surgery, pentamidine, and metronidazole are advised for *Acanthamoeba* spp. and *B. mandrillaris* brain abscesses.

Cerebral Malaria

It has traditionally been known that *Plasmodium falciparum* is the only one of the five species of human malaria parasites that invades the CNS and may cause cerebral malaria. However, there is some recent evidence suggesting that *P. vivax* infection may also be associated with this condition [4]. Human infection occurs when the sporozoite form of the parasite is inoculated through the skin during a blood meal by a female *Anopheles* mosquito. Then, sporozoites are carried into the liver where they mature to schizonts that liberate merozoites which, in turn, enter the bloodstream, parasitize red blood cells, and transform in gametocytes. The life cycle of the *Plasmodium* is completed when the mosquito ingests infected human red blood cells and gametocytes transform into sporozoites [33].

The first clinical manifestation of cerebral malaria is fever. Then, seizures, dysconjugate gaze, cloudiness of consciousness, and extensor posturing occur. Some patients (particularly children) present with focal neurological signs related to the occurrence of a cerebral infarction or intracranial hemorrhage. Neuroimaging studies are often normal or may show brain swelling or small hemorrhages in severe cases. Cytochemical analysis of CSF is normal, but a spinal tap is mandatory to rule out other causes of encephalopathy. Diagnosis is confirmed by the finding of *P. falciparum* by examining thin and thick blood smears with Giemsa stain; repeated examinations may be needed since parasitemia is cyclical. The occurrence of the so-called malarial retinopathy, which is characterized by retinal whitening, flame hemorrhages, and papilledema, is highly reliable for confirming the diagnosis of cerebral malaria in children with parasitemia and coma [3].

In fatal cases, autopsy often reveals diffuse brain swelling and subcortical ring hemorrhages, which are the result of extravasation of erythrocytes due to endothelial damage. Of interest, erythrocytes that form the ring hemorrhages are not parasitized, suggesting that blood vessel damage may be related to the liberation of vasoactive substances (immune hypothesis). On the other hand, capillaries and venules are plugged by clumped, parasitized erythrocytes, suggesting that brain damage is caused by obstruction of the cerebral microvasculature (mechanical hypothesis). The brain of patients who survived the acute phase of the disease often develops granulomatous lesions, called Dürck nodules, at the site of ring hemorrhages.

Quinine is still considered as the drug of choice for cerebral malaria in most of the developing world. It has been shown that artemether (an artemisinin derivative) is as effective as quinine. However, its effect is short lasting and artemether must be associated with mefloquine or amodiaquine [16]. Corticosteroids may be deleterious and must not be used. Due to chloroquine-resistant strains of *P. falciparum*, this drug should not be used in this setting. Hypoglycemia, pulmonary edema, renal failure, bleeding diathesis, and hepatic dysfunction may complicate the course of the disease, and up to 25 % of patients die despite medical care. Permanent sequelae are more common in children and include mental retardation, recurrent seizures, blindness, and focal motor deficits.

Toxoplasmosis

Toxoplasmosis is the most common opportunistic infection of the CNS in AIDS patients and most often occurs as the result of the reactivation of a dormant infection that had been acquired several years ago [31]. The causal agent, *Toxoplasma gondii*, is acquired by eating undercooked meat or by accidental ingestion of contaminated cat feces. While CNS invasion almost always occurs as an opportunistic infection, immunocompetent hosts may also suffer from CNS toxoplasmosis during acute infections, and the brain of fetuses may be affected due to placental transmission of tachyzoites from women who acquire the disease during pregnancy [21].

CNS invasion with *T. gondii* is associated with the development of necrotizing encephalitis related to perivascular inflammation. Focal lesions in the brain parenchyma consist of a necrotic center surrounded by tachyzoites and cysts, together with patchy areas of necrosis and perivascular cuffing of lymphocytes. The surrounding parenchyma usually shows glial nodules.

Cerebral toxoplasmosis in immunocompromised patients may present in the form of acute encephalitis or, more often, as a subacute disease characterized by fever, focal signs associated with seizures, increased intracranial pressure, and decreased level of consciousness. Those individuals may have absent or low serum antibody titers despite severe disease [1]. Neuroimaging studies usually show multiple ring-enhancing lesions surrounded by edema; lesions are most often located in the subcortical white matter, the basal ganglia, or the brainstem (Fig. 9.1). Abnormal enhancement of granulomas may be poor in severely immunosuppressed patients. These are not pathognomonic lesions, and definitive diagnosis theoretically requires histological demonstration of the parasite. However, initiation of empiric therapy followed by repeated neuroimaging studies 2 weeks later is an alternative to biopsy in these cases [34].

Combination therapy with pyrimethamine and sulfadiazine is the best option for CNS toxoplasmosis. Clindamycin, atovaquone, and trimethoprim/sulfamethoxazole are alternative drugs in patients allergic to sulfadiazine. CNS toxoplasmosis tends to recur after discontinuation of therapy; therefore, permanent maintenance therapy with pyrimethamine and sulfadiazine is advised to decrease the risk of relapses in immunosuppressed patients [21].

Trypanosomiasis

American Trypanosomiasis (Chagas' Disease)

Chagas' disease is caused by the protozoa *Trypanosoma cruzi*. Infection occurs when parasites enter the human body by direct inoculation through a bite of bugs of the genus *Triatoma* (the insect vector). Blood transfusions represent a common cause of *T. cruzi* infection in non-endemic areas [18]. Chagas' disease is a major public health problem in Latin America, where more than ten million people are infected with this parasite. The acute phase of the disease is often characterized by unilateral orbital edema (Romaña's sign) and mild constitutional symptoms. In some cases (particularly in infants and AIDS patients), early invasion of the CNS by trypanosomes may cause diffuse encephalitis [29]. In these cases, the brain shows multiple areas of hemorrhagic necrosis, glial proliferation, and perivascular infiltrates of inflammatory cells. During the chronic phase of the disease, neurological

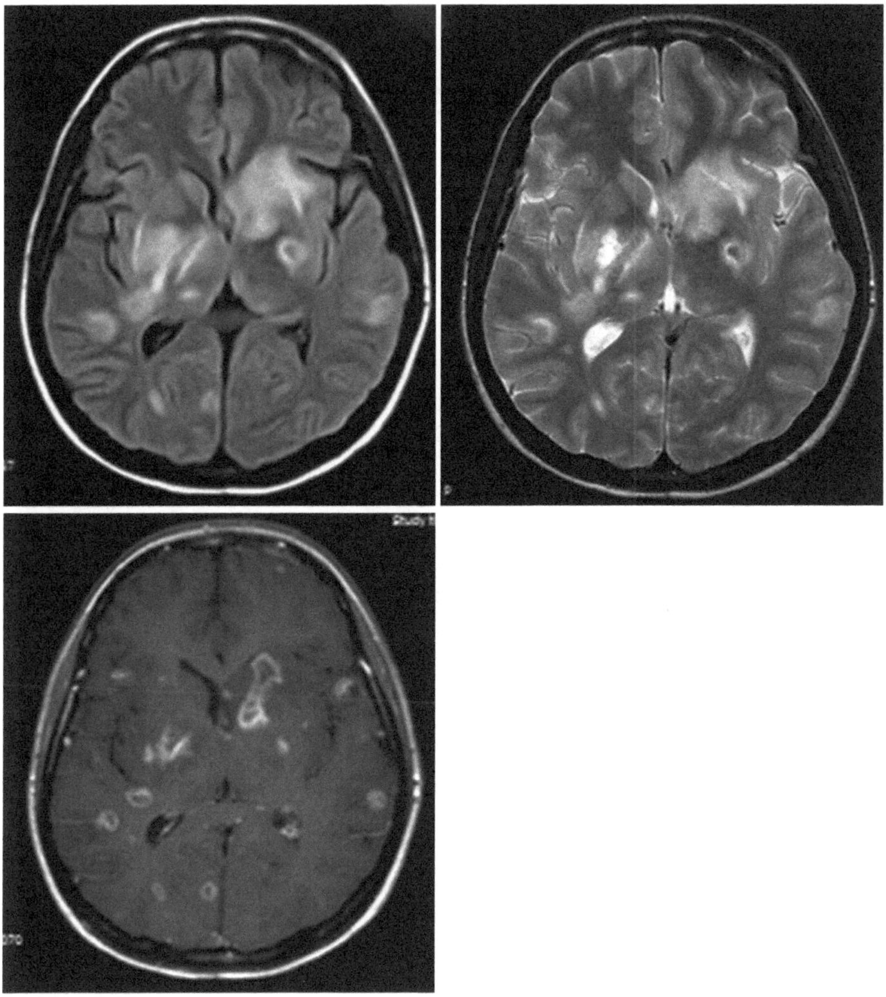

Fig. 9.1 FLAIR, T2-weighted, and contrast-enhanced T1-weighted MRIs of patient with AIDS and cerebral toxoplasmosis. Note multiplicity of lesions, predominance of involvement of the basal ganglia, and ring-enhancement of most of them

complications are most often related to the occurrence of cardiogenic brain embolisms as the result of a chagasic dilated cardiomyopathy [11]. As expected, such strokes may be multiple and most often involving the territory of cortical branches of major intracranial arteries. However, some patients develop primary neurological complications due to direct damage of cerebral blood vessels.

Immunocompromised individuals may experience reactivation of chronic infections, resulting in a fatal meningoencephalitic syndrome similar to that observed in acute infections. During the acute phase of the disease (up to 12 weeks after infection), diagnosis is possible by demonstration of *T. cruzi* in blood smears or CSF samples. Chronic disease must be confirmed by serologic testing since parasites are no longer detectable in blood smears. Nifurtimox and benznidazole may be used for patients during the acute phase of the disease, for those with acute reactivations of chronic disease, and for congenital infections. Chronic Chagas' disease has no specific treatment [10].

African Trypanosomiasis (Sleeping Sickness)

This condition may be caused by two subspecies of *Trypanosoma brucei*: *T. brucei gambiense* as the agent of West African trypanosomiasis and *T. brucei rhodesiense* as that of East African trypanosomiasis [25]. These protozoa enter the human body by direct inoculation through a bite of tsetse fly, the insect vector. In both forms of the disease, trypanosomes invade the CNS soon after inoculation and remain latent for long periods. Thereafter, the disease enters in a stage in which clinical manifestations ensue. These include fever, cervical lymphadenopathy (Winterbottom's sign), and hepatosplenomegaly, suggesting activation of the reticuloendothelial system. Then, somnolence, apathy, involuntary movements, and generalized rigidity appear. Neurological manifestations progress to severe cognitive impairment, coma, and death. The brain of fatal cases often shows diffuse gliosis, demyelination, and infiltrates of hypertrophied lymphocytes (Mott cells) involving the meninges, perivascular spaces, and brain parenchyma. Soon after infection, parasites may be isolated from the blood, CSF, and lymph nodes, and CSF examination may reveal moderate pleocytosis and the typical Mott cells. In contrast, chronic disease may only be diagnosed by immune tests performed in serum or CSF. Therapy of sleeping sickness depends on the subspecies involved and on the stage of the disease. For West African trypanosomiasis, pentamidine is recommended for early phases and eflornithine for late stages. For East African trypanosomiasis, suramin is the drug of choice for early stages and melarsoprol for late stages [25].

Nematode Infections

Eosinophilic Meningitis

While the term eosinophilic meningitis comprises all conditions causing meningitis associated with eosinophils in the CSF, it is commonly used to refer to the neurological complications related to infection with *Angiostrongylus cantonensis*, *Gnathostoma spinigerum*, and *Baylisascaris procyonis* [39]. Humans become accidental hosts of these tissue nematodes after eating raw snails (*A. cantonensis*), undercooked fish or poultry (*G. spinigerum*), or raccoon feces (*B. procyonis*). Once ingested, larvae of these parasites migrate to the tissues of the host, including the CNS.

CNS damage induced by tissue nematodes may be caused by mechanical injury or related to the immunological response of the host. The former mechanism explains the occurrence of hemorrhagic tracts in the brain parenchyma in cases of *G. spinigerum* infection. In contrast, most neuropathologic findings in *A. cantonensis* infections are related to congestion and inflammation of leptomeninges [19].

Patients with angiostrongyliasis often present with a self-limited meningitis characterized by headache, neck stiffness, and cranial nerve palsies. Seizures, intracranial hypertension, somnolence, or coma may also occur. Neurological manifestations of gnathostomiasis include radicular pain, transverse myelitis, meningitis, encephalitis, and intracranial hemorrhages. Sudden blindness due to retinal detachment may occur as the result of migration of the parasite through the eye. Only a few cases of human baylisascariasis have been reported (particularly children). Some patients have developed a severe eosinophilic meningoencephalitis, while others have presented with spinal cord involvement or with neuroretinitis without major evidence of cerebral involvement [22].

As implicit in its name, the CSF of patients with eosinophilic meningitis usually reveals moderate pleocytosis with up to 70 % eosinophils; protein contents may be increased, but glucose levels are normal. Neuroimaging studies may show abnormal meningeal enhancement, periventricular hyperintensities suggestive of demyelination, hydrocephalus, or, in patients with gnathostomiasis, hemorrhagic tracts in the brain parenchyma. While serologic tests may support the diagnosis in some cases, confirmation usually rests on identification of the larvae in tissues.

Since the course of angiostrongyliasis is usually benign, most patients improve in less than 1 month with symptomatic drugs. CSF drainage is effective for headache relief in patients who do not respond to common analgesics. A short course with corticosteroids may reduce the need of repeated spinal taps in these cases [37]. The management of *G. spinigerum*- and *B. procyonis*-related eosinophilic meningitis requires the use of intravenous dexamethasone to reduce the inflammation-mediated damage of intracranial blood vessels. Thiabendazole, mebendazole, albendazole, and ivermectin may be active against the tissue nematodes causing eosinophilic meningitis. However, the actual role of specific therapy for eosinophilic meningitis has not been settled.

Other Nematode Infections

Strongyloidiasis

Under normal conditions, *Strongyloides stercoralis* is confined to the human intestinal tract and does not invade the CNS. Disseminated disease may occur when the host's immune mechanisms fail to control the normal cycle of autoinfection (hyperinfection syndrome). Common predisposing factors include HTLV-1 infection, chronic corticosteroid therapy, transplant recipients, and chemotherapy administration [23]. Cerebral infarcts and brain abscesses may occur in such cases. Definitive diagnosis requires identification of the larvae in the CSF or tissue specimens. However, the disease should be suspected in immunosuppressed patients who

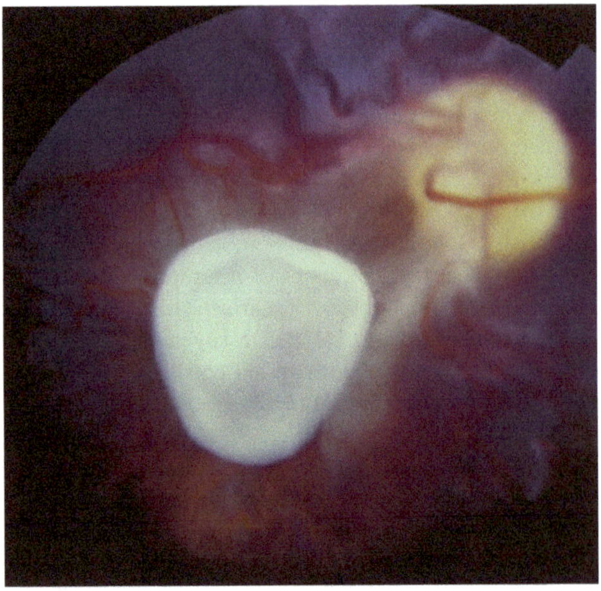

Fig. 9.2 Fundoscopic examination of a patient with ocular larva migrans (Courtesy of Dr. Nelson Matamoros, Guayaquil, Ecuador)

develop meningitis, focal neurological signs, or acute encephalopathy. Mortality of disseminated strongyloidiasis is high, although ivermectin or thiabendazole may be of value in some patients.

Toxocariasis

This disease is caused by nematodes of the genus *Toxocara*. The infection is acquired when humans ingest soil contaminated with dog or cat feces containing *Toxocara* eggs. Eggs mature into larvae which migrate to the tissues of the host producing a disease called visceral larva migrans. Migration to the eye produces ocular larva migrans, in which the parasite is easily identified by fundoscopic examination (Fig. 9.2). CNS damage is related to migration of larvae through the brain parenchyma leaving necrotic tracks or to the inflammatory response that develops around inert larvae. Clinical manifestations include subacute encephalitis, parenchymal brain granulomas, or cerebral infarcts due to angiitis [35]. Diagnosis may be suspected in patients with positive serology, particularly if intrathecal synthesis of anti-*Toxocara* antibodies is documented. Neuroimaging studies may show multiple enhancing lesions in the brain parenchyma. Albendazole and diethylcarbamazine have been useful in some cases [30].

Trichinellosis

This disease occurs after ingestion of undercooked pork contaminated with larva of *Trichinella spiralis*. Larvae enter the bloodstream and encyst in the skeletal muscle. Trichinellosis is often asymptomatic; however, CNS involvement, characterized by meningoencephalitis or stroke, may occur. Stroke subtypes associated with trichinellosis include hemorrhagic infarcts related to venous thrombosis and subcortical infarcts caused by small-artery disease. It has been suggested that migrating larval emboli are responsible for occlusion of cerebral vessels. However, other studies suggest that hypereosinophilia is responsible for these vascular lesions. Eosinophils may directly induce vascular occlusion through a prothrombotic effect or may damage the vascular endothelium after being stimulated by cytokines produced in response to *T. spiralis* infection. Neurotrichinellosis should be suspected in patients who, besides a cerebral infarct, have fever, myalgia, periorbital edema, and peripheral eosinophilia. Cytochemical analysis of the CSF is most often normal, and neuroimaging may show nonspecific patchy hyperintensities in the subcortical white matter. Support for the diagnosis is provided by the presence of anti-*Trichinella* antibodies or by the identification of the parasite in the muscle tissue. Corticosteroids suppress the eosinophilic-induced vascular damage and reduce mortality in severe cases [7].

Trematode Infections

Paragonimiasis

Paragonimiasis is caused by trematodes of the genus *Paragonimus* (lung flukes). Humans acquire the disease by ingesting undercooked crustaceans infected with larvae of these parasites. Then, larvae cross the intestinal wall, enter the peritoneal cavity, and migrate to the lungs. Further migration of the worms through the foramina of the skull base to the CNS may occur. Neurological syndromes occurring in the course of cerebral paragonimiasis include meningitis, granulomatous or calcified parenchymal brain lesions, and intracranial hemorrhages. Paragonimus meningitis may be associated with cerebral infarctions due to endarteritis. Parenchymal brain lesions may be associated with seizures, focal signs, and intracranial hypertension. Cerebral hemorrhages may occur along tracts of larva's migration or as the result of the necrotizing vasculitis that develops during early granuloma formation [12]. Diagnosis is suggested by the presence of specific antibodies in the CSF or by neuroimaging findings of confluent calcifications located in the temporal and occipital lobes that resemble "soap bubbles." Lesions may also be located at the spinal intradural space [24]. Support for the diagnosis is provided by demonstration of *Paragonimus* eggs in sputum. Therapy includes praziquantel and corticosteroids.

Schistosomiasis

Schistosomiasis occurs when humans become definitive hosts in the life cycle of trematodes of the species *Schistosoma* (*S. japonicum*, *S. mansoni*, *S. haematobium*) [17]. These parasites enter the body through the skin following aquatic exposure with their larval forms. Larvae migrate, transform into adult worms, and settle in the mesenteric veins. Larvae may also migrate to the spinal cord or the cerebral vasculature. The spectrum of neurological manifestations is related to the *Schistosoma* species and the location of parasites; *S. japonicum* almost always affect the brain. In contrast, the other two species most often affect the spinal cord and only eventually the brain [9].

Acute infection with *S. japonicum* produces meningoencephalitis – a disease called "Katayama fever" – associated with fever, seizures, visual loss, neck stiffness, disorientation and stupor, and focal neurological deficits. The chronic phase of the disease is characterized by seizures, focal signs, and intracranial hypertension related to the development of single or multiple parenchymal brain granulomas. Intracranial hemorrhages may occur; they are related to segmental damage of small leptomeningeal or parenchymal blood vessels induced by the parasites [28].

Infections with *S. mansoni* and *S. haematobium* are often associated with transverse myelitis related to inflammatory necrosis of the spinal cord. Myelitis usually affects the lower segments of the spinal cord and is characterized by flaccid paraplegia associated with sphincter dysfunction and sensory loss. In addition, granulomatous masses may involve the conus medullaris and cauda equina, causing low back pain, saddle anesthesia, sphincter dysfunction, and weakness in the lower limbs. Acute paraplegia has resulted from occlusion of the anterior spinal artery by the parasite.

Cytochemical analysis of the CSF may be normal or may show a nonspecific mononuclear pleocytosis and increased protein contents. Neuroimaging studies may show discrete hemorrhagic or enhancing lesions in patients with *S. japonicum* schistosomiasis and enlargement of the lower spinal cord in some patients with spinal schistosomiasis (Fig. 9.3). Most patients with spinal cord involvement have specific antibodies detected by ELISA. The absence of schistosomal eggs in stool and urine does not exclude the diagnosis. Praziquantel associated with corticosteroids is effective for some patients with brain or spinal cord involvement. Surgical decompression of the spinal canal is still an option in some cases [9].

Cestode Infections

Cysticercosis

Cysticercosis is the most common helminthic infection of the CNS. It is caused by the larval stage of *Taenia solium*, a cestode with a complex life cycle involving humans as definitive hosts and either pigs or humans as intermediate hosts. Cysticercosis in humans occurs after the ingestion of *Taenia* eggs through direct or indirect contact with feces of a *T. solium* carrier. Cysticerci may invade almost every organ; however, relevant clinical manifestations are almost always related to CNS involvement [13].

Cysticerci are liquid-filled vesicles including an invaginated scolex that has a similar appearance than the adult *T. solium*. These cysts may be located anywhere within the CNS. Parenchymal brain cysticerci are mainly located in the cerebral cortex or the basal ganglia. In contrast, subarachnoid and ventricular cysticerci may

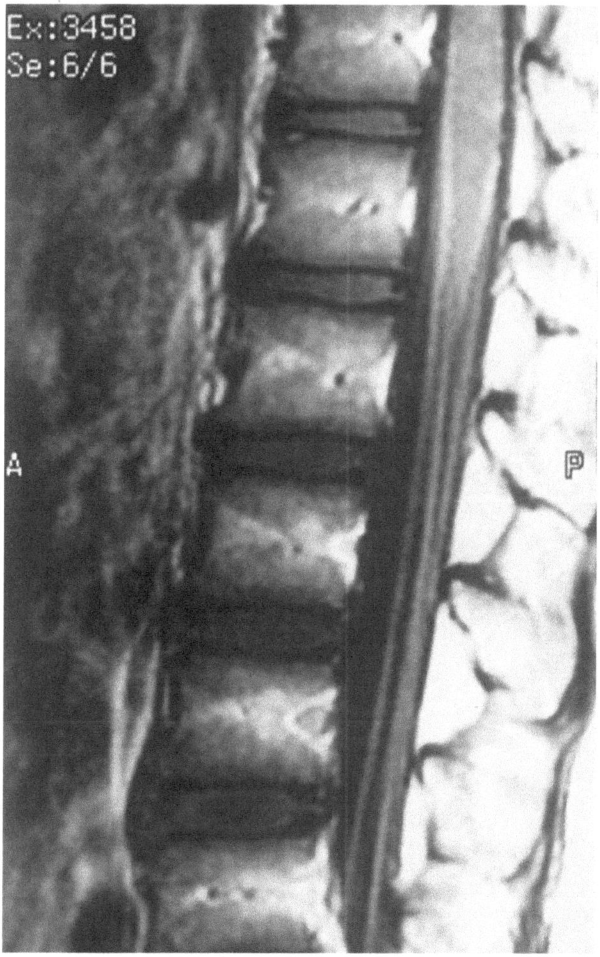

Fig. 9.3 Contrast-enhanced MRI showing enlargement of the conus medullaris in patient with *Schistosoma mansoni* schistosomiasis (Courtesy of Dr. Francisco X. Carod-Artal, Barcelona, Spain)

attain a large size due to a mechanism of hydropic degeneration by which the CSF enters through the parasitic membrane and causes enlargement of the vesicle. Spinal cysticerci may be found at either the cord parenchyma or the subarachnoid space. Individual variations in the location of parasites and in the severity of the inflammatory reaction against cysticerci explain the vast clinical pleomorphism of the disease. Some parasites escape the host's immune detection, while others evoke an intense immune response causing both destruction of cysticerci and damage of the surrounding tissues. Common pathological lesions in the latter include astrocytic gliosis, brain swelling, arachnoiditis, hydrocephalus, and angiitis of small- and medium-sized intracranial arteries [32].

Seizures (particularly late-onset seizures) are the most common clinical manifestation of neurocysticercosis. They often occur in patients with parenchymal brain cysts or calcifications. Focal neurological signs usually follow a subacute or chronic course, although they may occur abruptly in patients who develop a cerebral infarct as a

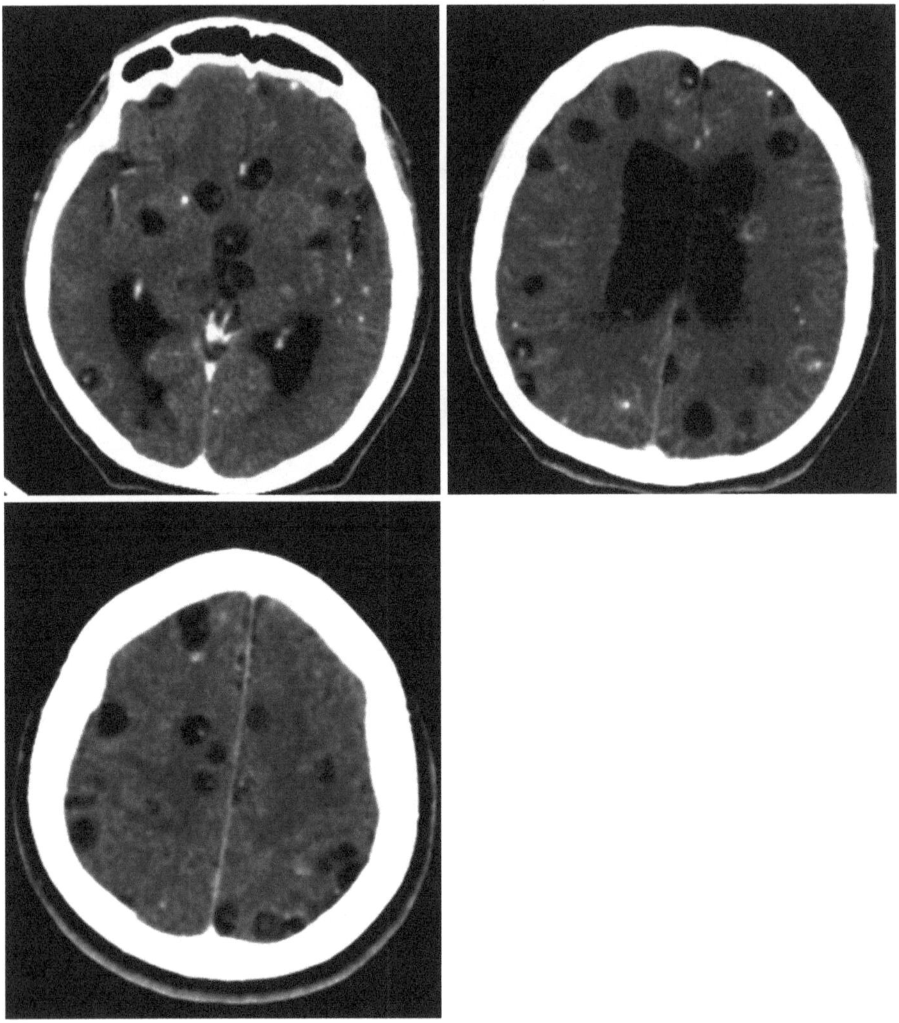

Fig. 9.4 Contrast-enhanced CT of patient with heavy non-encephalitic cysticercosis. Cysts appear as well-defined hypodense lesions with no edema and no abnormal enhancement. The scolex can be visualized in the interior of some of these lesions as a brilliant dot

complication of angiitis. Increased intracranial pressure is the result of hydrocephalus, ventricular cysts, or cysticercotic encephalitis. The latter is a severe form of the disease that occurs in patients who develop a severe immune response against massive cysticerci infection of the brain parenchyma. Clinical manifestations of spinal neurocysticercosis are also nonspecific [15]; spinal arachnoiditis is characterized by root pain and weakness of subacute onset, and cysts in the cord parenchyma are associated with motor and sensory deficits that vary according to the level of the lesion.

Neuroimaging studies provide proper localization of cysticerci and reveal the activity of the disease. Cystic lesions showing the scolex (Fig. 9.4) and

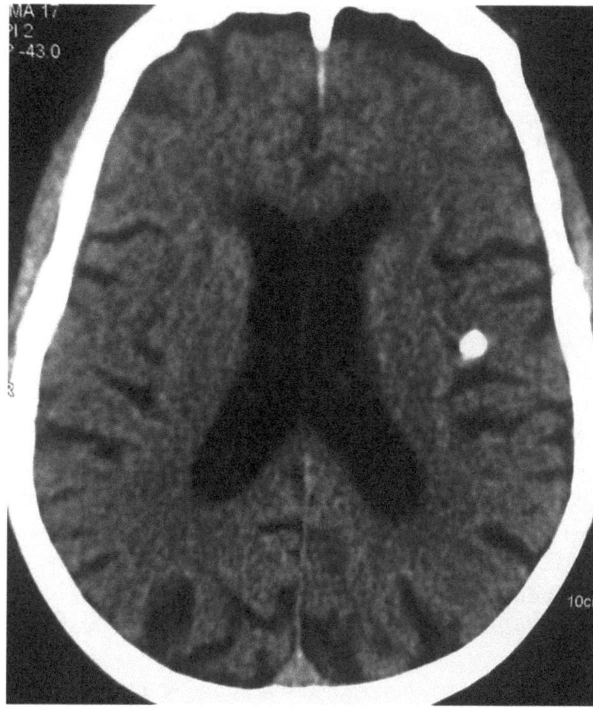

Fig. 9.5 Plain CT showing a single parenchymal brain calcification. This is the most common – though nonspecific – neuroimaging finding in neurocysticercosis

parenchymal brain calcifications (Fig. 9.5) are the most characteristic findings of neurocysticercosis. Ring-enhancing lesions, hydrocephalus, and abnormal enhancement of the leptomeninges are non-pathognomonic and represent a diagnostic challenge. Immune diagnostic tests should never be used by themselves to exclude or confirm the disease. The most effective is the serum immunoblot; however, some disappointing results have been reported in patients with a single brain lesion. A set of diagnostic criteria based on objective clinical, radiological, immunological, and epidemiological information has been proposed to allow physicians to diagnose neurocysticercosis [14]. Four categories of criteria – absolute, major, minor, and epidemiological – are stratified according to their individual diagnostic strength and allow two categories of diagnostic certainty for NCC, definitive and probable.

Patients with parenchymal brain or subarachnoid cysts must be treated with cysticidal drugs (albendazole or praziquantel). These drugs result in disappearance of most cysts as well as in better control of seizures and improvement in focal neurological deficits. Patients with calcifications alone should only receive symptomatic treatment. Ventricular cysts should be better resected by neuroendoscopy to avoid risks related to enlargement of those cysts as the result of cysticidal drug therapy. Also, medical treatment may favor the occlusion of a blood vessel in patients with subarachnoid cysts or may worsen the brain edema accompanying cysticercotic encephalitis; corticosteroids are advised for the prevention of such complications. Therapeutic priorities, i.e., ventricular shunt for hydrocephalus, must be considered before the use of cysticidal drugs in patients with mixed forms of the disease [20].

Echinococcosis (Hydatid Disease)

There are two main forms of hydatid disease: cystic hydatid disease, caused by the larval stage of *E. granulosus*, and alveolar hydatid disease, caused by the larval stage of *E. multilocularis*. In addition, some cases of cystic hydatid disease have been recently attributed to *E. vogeli* infections [36]. Canids are definitive hosts for *Echinococcus* spp., and sheep or rodents are intermediate hosts. Humans may become accidental intermediate hosts after the ingestion of food contaminated with eggs of these cestodes. Echinococcal cysts grow in the liver, the lungs, the heart, and the CNS. In the latter, the cysts may grow primarily or secondarily from metastatic dissemination of a visceral cyst.

E. granulosus cysts are single, spherical, and well demarcated from the surrounding tissues. In contrast, *E. multilocularis* cysts tend to group in clusters, expand rapidly, elicit a severe immune reaction from the host, and tend to metastasize. In both species the larva may be found within the cysts. Both forms of hydatid disease may course with seizures and intracranial hypertension; however, clinical manifestations are more severe in patients with alveolar hydatid disease. Patients with cystic hydatid disease of the orbit develop unilateral proptosis and diplopia. Spinal cord involvement may be observed in both forms of the disease; usual manifestations include root pain and motor or sensory deficits. Primary hydatid cysts of the heart may embolize and occlude an intracranial artery with the subsequent development of a brain infarct.

Cystic hydatid disease is seen on neuroimaging studies as a large, spherical, nonenhancing, liquid-filled vesicle, which is well demarcated from the surrounding brain parenchyma. Cysts are most often located within the brain parenchyma although extradural cysts with bone erosion may occur. In contrast, alveolar hydatid disease is associated with multiple and confluent lesions that show abnormal contrast enhancement. Diagnosis by ELISA or immunoblot is not accurate due to cross-reactions with other parasites [6].

Hydatid cysts have been traditionally resected by surgery using the Dowling's technique. However, albendazole may destroy these cysts, obviating the hazards of transoperative cyst rupture. Albendazole is effective against both *E. granulosus* and *E. multilocularis* and may be used in patients who are not candidates for surgical resection of lesions, as prophylactic therapy for those who have a perioperative risk of accidental rupture of the cysts, or to treat recurrent cystic hydatid disease after surgery [6]. Praziquantel has protoscolicidal activity and may have a role in the prevention of secondary reactions related to accidental spillage of protoscolices during surgery.

Other Cestodes

Coenurosis

This disease is caused by *Coenurus cerebralis*, the larval stage of *Taenia multiceps*. The definitive host is often a canid, and sheep or other herbivorous mammals are the natural intermediate hosts. Humans become accidentally infected after ingestion of dogs' feces contaminated with *T. multiceps* eggs. *C. cerebralis* is a cystic vesicle that includes multiple scolices. Cysts may lodge in subcutaneous tissues, skeletal muscles, and the CNS. In the latter, they are most often located at the base of the skull where they induce arachnoiditis with obstructive hydrocephalus. Parenchymal brain involvement may also occur; seizures and focal signs occur in these cases. Neuroimaging studies show hydrocephalus and cystic or ring-enhancing lesions in the brain parenchyma or CSF cisterns. Diagnosis is done by biopsy of a brain lesion. There is no known medical therapy for cerebral coenurosis [26].

Sparganosis

This disease is caused by the second-stage larva of cestodes of the genus *Spirometra*. Dogs and cats are definitive hosts, cyclops are the first intermediate hosts, and frogs and snakes are the second intermediate hosts. Humans acquire the infection by drinking water contaminated with cyclops harboring the larva or by eating infected frog or snake. The sparganum migrates to skeletal muscles or subcutaneous tissue where it further develops into granulomas. Further migration through the foramina of the skull base and vertebral column is associated with involvement of the CNS, including the brain parenchyma, the subarachnoid space, and the spinal canal. Inflammatory changes and focal necrosis along the tracks of migration of these larvae are common findings. Patients with parenchymal brain sparganosis present with seizures or focal neurological signs. Neuroimaging findings are usually confined to one cerebral hemisphere and include multifocal areas of low density within the subcortical white matter, focal cortical atrophy, ipsilateral ventricular enlargement, spotty calcifications, and enhancing nodules that may change in location on sequential scans. Definitive diagnosis depends on the visualization of the parasite from a brain biopsy. Surgical resection of the parasite is the treatment of choice [26].

References

1. Antinori A, Larussa D, Cingolani A, Lorenzini P, Bossolasco S, Finazzi MG, et al. Prevalence, associated factors, and prognostic determinants of AIDS-related toxoplasmic encephalitis in the era of advanced highly active antiretroviral therapy. Clin Infect Dis. 2004;39:1681–91.
2. Bando Y, Takahashi T, Uehara H, Kagegi T, Nagahiro S, Izumi K. Autopsy case of amebic granulomatous meningoencephalitis caused by *Balamuthia mandrillaris* in Japan. Pathol Int. 2012;62:418–23.

3. Beare NA, Taylor TE, Harding SP, Lewallen S, Molyneux ME. Malarial retinopathy: a newly established diagnostic sign in severe malaria. Am J Trop Med Hyg. 2006;75:790–7.
4. Bhattacharjee P, Dubey S, Gupta VK, Agarwal P, Mahato MP. The clinicopathologic manifestations of *Plasmodium vivax* malaria in children: a growing menace. J Clin Diagn Res. 2013;7:861–7.
5. Bravo FG, Seas C. *Balamuthia mandrillaris* amoebic encephalitis: an emerging parasitic infection. Curr Infect Dis Rep. ;14:391–6.
6. Brunetti E, Kern P, Vuitton DA. Expert consensus for the diagnosis and treatment of cystic and alveolar echinococcosis in humans. Acta Trop. ;114:1–6.
7. Bruschi F, Brunetti E, Pozio E. Neurotrichinellosis. In: Garcia HH, Tanowitz HB, Del Brutto OH, editors. Handbook of clinical neurology, vol. 114 (3rd series). Amsterdam: Elsevier B.V.; 2013;114:243–9.
8. Budge PJ, Lazensky B, Van Zile KW, Elliot KE, Dooyema CA, Visvesvara GS, Beach MJ, Yoder JS. Primary amebic meningoencephalitis in Florida: a case report and epidemiological review of Florida cases. J Environ Health. 2013;75:26–31.
9. Carod-Artal FJ. Neuroschistosomiasis. Expert Rev Anti Infect Ther. 2010;8:1307–18.
10. Carod-Artal FJ. American trypanosomiasis. In: Garcia HH, Tanowitz HB, Del Brutto OH, editors. Handbook of clinical neurology, vol. 114 (3rd series). Amsterdam: Elsevier B.V.; 2013. p. –23.
11. Carod-Artal FJ, Gascon J. Chagas disease and stroke. Lancet Neurol. 2010;9:533–42.
12. Chai J-Y. Paragonimiasis. In: Garcia HH, Tanowitz HB, Del Brutto OH, editors. Handbook of clinical neurology, vol. 114 (3rd series). Amsterdam: Elsevier B.V.; 2013. p. –96.
13. Del Brutto OH. Neurocysticercosis. Continuum (Minneap Minn). 2012;18:1392–416.
14. Del Brutto OH. Diagnostic criteria for neurocysticercosis, revisited. Pathog Glob Health. 2012;106:299–304.
15. Del Brutto OH, Garcia HH. Intramedullary cysticercosis of the spinal cord: a review of patients evaluated with MRI. J Neurol Sci. 2013;331:114–7.
16. Dondorp A, Nosten F, Stepniewska K, Day N, White N. Artesunate versus quinine for treatment of severe falciparum malaria: a randomized trial. Lancet. 2005;366:717–25.
17. Ferrari TCA, Moreira PRR. Neuroschistosomiasis: clinical symptoms and pathogenesis. Lancet Neurol. 2011;10:853–64.
18. Flores-Chávez M, Fernández B, Puente S, Torres P, Rodríguez M, Monedero C, Cruz I, Gárate T, Cañavate C. Transfusional Chagas disease: parasitological and serological monitoring of an infected recipient and blood donor. Clin Infect Dis. 2008;46:e44–7.
19. Graeff-Teixeira C, da Silva AC, Yoshimura K. Update on eosinophilic meningoencephalitis and its clinical relevance. Clin Microbiol Rev. 2009;22:322–48.
20. Gonzales I, Garcia HH. Current status and future perspectives on the medical treatment of neurocysticercosis. Pathog Glob Health. 2012;106:305–9.
21. Halonen SK, Weiss LM. Toxoplasmosis. In: Garcia HH, Tanowitz HB, Del Brutto OH, editors. Handbook of clinical neurology, vol. 114 (3rd series). Amsterdam: Elsevier B.V.; 2013. p. –45.
22. Kazacos KR, Jelicks LA, Tanowitz HB. Baylisascaris larva migrans. In: Garcia HH, Tanowitz HB, Del Brutto OH, editors. Handbook of clinical neurology, vol. 114 (3rd series). Amsterdam: Elsevier B.V.; 2013. p. –62.
23. Keiser P, Nutman T. *Strongyloides stercoralis* in the immunocompromised population. Clin Microbiol Rev. 2004;17:208–17.
24. Kim MK, Cho BM, Yoon DY, Nam ES. Imaging features of intradural spinal paragonimiasis: a case report. Br J Radiol. 2011;84:e72–4.
25. Lejon V, Bentivoglio M, Franco JR. Human African trypanosomiasis. In: Garcia HH, Tanowitz HB, Del Brutto OH, editors. Handbook of clinical neurology, vol. 114 (3rd series). Amsterdam: Elsevier B.V.; 2013. p. –81.
26. Lescano AG, Zunt J. Other cestodes: sparganosis, coenurosis and Taenia crassiceps cysticercosis. In: Garcia HH, Tanowitz HB, Del Brutto OH, editors. Handbook of clinical neurology, vol. 114 (3rd series). Amsterdam: Elsevier B.V.; 2013. p. –45.

27. Lopez C, Budge P, Chen J, Bilyeu S, Mirza A, Custodio H, Irazuzta J, Visvesvara G, Sullivan KJ. Primary amebic meningoencephalitis: a case report and literature review. Pediatr Emerg Care. 2012;28:272–6.
28. Manzella A, Borba-Filho P, Brandt CT, Oliveira K. Brain magnetic resonance imaging findings in young patients with hepatosplenic schistosomiasis mansoni without overt symptoms. Am J Trop Med Hyg. 2012;86:982–7.
29. Medeiros MB, Guerra JA, Lacerda MV. Meningoencephalitis in a patient with acute Chagas disease in the Brazilian Amazon. Rev Soc Bras Med Trop. ;4:520–1.
30. Nicoletti A. Toxocariasis. In: Garcia HH, Tanowitz HB, Del Brutto OH, editors. Handbook of clinical neurology, vol. 114 (3rd series). Amsterdam: Elsevier B.V.; 2013. p. –28.
31. Pereira-Chioccola VL, Vidal JE, Su C. Toxoplasma gondii infection and cerebral toxoplasmosis in HIV-infected patients. Future Microbiol. 2009;4:1363–79.
32. Pittella JEH. Pathology of CNS parasitic infections. In: Garcia HH, Tanowitz HB, Del Brutto OH, editors. Handbook of clinical neurology, vol. 114 (3rd series). Amsterdam: Elsevier B.V.; 2013. p. –88.
33. Postels DG, Birbeck GL. Cerebral malaria. In: Garcia HH, Tanowitz HB, Del Brutto OH, editors. Handbook of clinical neurology, vol. 114 (3rd series). Amsterdam; Elsevier B.V.; 2013. p. –102.
34. Shyam babu C, Satishchandra P, Mahadevan A, Pillai Shibu V, Ravishankar S, Sidappa N, Udaykumar R, Ravi V, Shankar SK. Usefulness of stereotactic biopsy and neuroimaging in management of HIV-1 Clade C associated focal brain lesions with special focus on cerebral toxoplasmosis. Clin Neurol Neurosurg. 2013;115:995–1002.
35. Singer OC, Conrad F, Jahnke K, Hattingen E, Auer H, Steinmetz H. Severe meningoencephalitis due to CNS-toxocariasis. J Neurol. 2011;258:696–8.
36. Stojkovic M, Junghanss T. Cystic and alveolar echinococcosis. In: Garcia HH, Tanowitz HB, Del Brutto OH, editors. Handbook of clinical neurology, vol. 114 (3rd series). Amsterdam: Elsevier B.V.; 2013. p. –34.
37. Thanaviratananich S, Thanaviratananich S, Ngamjarus C. Corticosteroids for parasitic eosinophilic meningitis. Cochrane Database Syst Rev. 2012;10:CD009088. doi:10.1002/14651858.CD009088.pub2.
38. Trabelsi H, Dendana F, Sellami A, Sellami H, Cheikhrouhou F, Neji S, Makni F, Ayadi A. Pathogenic free-living amoebae: epidemiology and clinical review. Pathol Biol. 2012;60:399–405.
39. Wang QP, Wu ZD, Wei J, Owen RL, Lun ZR. Human *Angiostrongylus cantonensis*: an update. Eur J Clin Microbiol Infect Dis. 2012;31:389–95.

Chapter 10
Infections of the Spinal Cord

Francisco Javier Carod-Artal

Abstract Infectious myelopathies can be caused by viral, bacterial, fungal, and parasitic agents. In this chapter, the most common causes of infectious and tropical myelopathies will be reviewed. HIV and HTLV-1 retroviruses have been associated with subacute and chronic myelopathy; herpesviruses may cause radiculomyelitis and transverse myelitis; enterovirus and flavivirus seem to have a tropism for the anterior horns of the spinal cord. Paralytic poliomyelitis can occur as a complication of poliovirus infection in around 1–2 % of cases. Enterovirus 71 has been identified as the etiologic agent of a poliomyelitis-like syndrome. The *Flaviviridae* family includes some mosquito-borne virus such as dengue, Japanese encephalitis, West Nile and Murray Valley viruses, and tick-borne virus and has also been associated with a flaccid poliomyelitis-like syndrome. Tuberculous myelopathy may develop as a secondary extension of vertebral body tuberculosis (Pott disease), as a downward extension of tuberculous meningitis, and even as a primary tuberculous lesion. Spinal schistosomiasis is a common cause of acute myelopathy in tropical regions, and acute transverse myelitis, conus medullaris syndrome, and lower limb myeloradiculopathy are the most common spinal syndromes. Other parasitary diseases that may affect the spinal cord include gnathostomiasis, cysticercosis, hydatid disease, and paragonimiasis. Invasive fungus may provoke a spinal cord compression syndrome from osteomyelitis, epidural abscess, or paravertebral lesions.

Keywords Gnathostomiasis • Epidural abscess • HTLV-1 virus • Infectious myelopathy • Poliomyelitis • Schistosomiasis • Spinal cord infection • Tropical spastic paraparesis • Vacuolar myelopathy • Viral myelitis

---

F.J. Carod-Artal, MD, PhD
Health Sciences and Medicine Faculty, Universitat Internacional de Catalunya (UIC), Barcelona, Spain

Department of Neurology, Raigmore Hospital,
Old Perth Road, Inverness, Highlands IV2 3UJ, UK
e-mail: fjcarod-artal@hotmail.com, javier.carodartal@nhs.net

J.C. García-Moncó (ed.), *CNS Infections*,
DOI 10.1007/978-1-4471-6401-2_10, © Springer-Verlag London 2014

Table 10.1 Acute transverse myelitis diagnostic criteria

Bilateral, not necessarily symmetric, spinal cord dysfunction affecting sensory, motor, and autonomic systems
Clearly defined sensory level
Progression to nadir of clinical symptoms between 4 h and 21 days after the onset of symptoms
Detection of an inflammatory process of the spinal cord in the CSF and/or MRI:
(a) Pleocytosis on the CSF with lymphocytic predominance
(b) Spinal cord MRI showing an enhancing spinal cord lesion
Exclusion of other etiologies including compressive, tumor, vascular, and postirradiation causes

CSF cerebrospinal fluid, *MRI* magnetic resonance imaging

Introduction

Infectious myelopathies can be caused by viral, bacterial, fungal, and parasitic agents. In addition, several infectious tropical diseases are an important cause of myelopathy in endemic regions and also a potential etiology of spinal cord dysfunction in returned travelers [1].

Some viral infections may preferentially involve the anterior horns of the spinal cord leading to a syndrome of acute flaccid paralysis, whereas others may cause an acute transverse myelitis syndrome with focal inflammation, functional transection of the spinal cord, and motor and sensory dysfunction below the level of the injury [2].

Myelitis is a medical emergency and prognosis depends on rapid suspicion, diagnosis, and therapy. Spinal cord magnetic resonance imaging (MRI) is a very helpful diagnostic technique that may reveal the location and extension of the inflammatory and infectious process. Cerebrospinal fluid (CSF) analysis should be performed to differentiate between viral, bacterial, parasitic, and other inflammatory causes such as multiple sclerosis. In this chapter, the most common causes of infectious and tropical myelopathies will be reviewed.

Parainfectious Myelitis

Acute transverse myelitis is a segmental or focal spinal cord damage provoked by an acute inflammatory process and is characterized by the presence of acute or subacute sensory, motor, and autonomic dysfunction including urinary, intestinal, and sexual sphincter abnormalities [3]. A systemic infection process or vaccination may precede acute transverse myelitis in 50 % of cases. This condition has been called parainfectious transverse myelitis, and its diagnostic criteria are summarized in Table 10.1. Probable pathogenic mechanisms include the activation of the host's immune system through molecular mimicry and the development of autoantibodies against pathogen proteins cross-reacting with host antigens located in the spinal cord. Between half and one third of these patients may develop severe sequela in spite of rapid treatment. Pulses of intravenous steroids are the mainstay of treatment, although some refractory cases have been treated with intravenous immunoglobulins, plasma exchange, and even cyclophosphamide or rituximab.

Viral Myelitis

Although viral infections may cause a parainfectious acute transverse myelitis, some viruses are indeed neuroinvase and may provoke a myelopathy. Retroviruses such as human immunodeficiency virus (HIV) and human T-cell leukemia/lymphoma virus type 1 (HTLV-1) have been associated with subacute and chronic myelopathy, whereas Herpesvirus family more commonly causes white matter inflammation and transverse myelitis, and enterovirus and flavivirus seem to have a neurothropic affinity for the anterior horns of the spinal cord.

Retroviruses

Human Immunodeficiency Virus

HIV primary infection has been associated with several neurological disorders including mononeuropathy, inflammatory demyelinating polyneuropathy, motor neuron disease, polymyositis, mononeuritis multiplex, HIV-associated neuromuscular weakness syndrome, immune reconstitution inflammatory syndrome, meningoencephalitis, and acute transverse myelitis [4]. Pathogenic mechanism of HIV acute transverse myelitis is not fully understood, although direct cytopathic HIV effect and immune-mediated toxicity have been proposed. A rapid improvement of HIV primary infection-related myelopathic symptoms has been observed after starting highly active antiretroviral therapy and steroids [5].

HIV can also cause a chronic progressive myelopathy called HIV-associated vacuolar myelopathy, which is clinically characterized by progressive – frequently symmetric – leg weakness, lower limb paresthesias, gait disturbance, and bladder and bowel sphincter dysfunction. Lower limb spasticity is more prominent than muscle weakness and in some cases gait ataxia, and lower limb dyssynergy can be observed. Pathological brisk reflexes in both upper and lower limbs, extensor plantar responses, and impairment of vibratory and position sense are usually found. Increased reflexes may not be found when a coexistent peripheral neuropathy is present. HIV-associated vacuolar myelopathy predominates in the middle and lower thoracic spinal cord and is characterized pathologically by loss of myelin and microvacuolation due to intramyelin swelling [6]. Lateral and posterior columns are usually much more involved than the anterior horns. Axons are usually preserved whereas intranuclear viral inclusions and inflammation are not usually detected [4].

Pathogenesis is unknown. Although the virus is unable to infect neurons directly, it can still injure these structures by a variety of mechanisms, many of which are yet to be elucidated. HIV-associated vacuolar myelopathy can be observed pathologically in approximately half of patients with AIDS, but only 10–20 % may develop clinical symptoms. Nevertheless, since introduction of highly active antiretroviral therapy, the incidence of HIV-associated vacuolar myelopathy has diminished significantly.

Spinal cord MRI may be normal or show some degree of spinal atrophy or even show similar findings to those observed in combined subacute degeneration. Vacuolar myelopathy is a diagnosis of exclusion that should be questioned when the CSF is significantly inflammatory. This chronic myelopathy is not associated with a sensory level or an acute onset, as in acute transverse myelitis, and when found, an alternative diagnosis to vacuolar myelopathy should be ruled out. Differential diagnosis should exclude other causes of HIV-associated myelopathy, including opportunistic infections such as viral (herpes, cytomegalovirus, HTLV-1), bacterial (*Treponema pallidum*, *Mycobacterium tuberculosis*), fungal (*Cryptococcus neoformans*), and parasitic diseases (*Toxoplasma gondii*), and even vascular, neoplasic, inflammatory, and other disorders (cobalamin deficiency) [7, 8].

Human T-Cell Leukemia/Lymphoma Virus Type 1

HTLV-1 is a human type C retrovirus that belongs to the Retroviridae family. At least 20 million people worldwide are infected by the HTLV-1. Sub-Saharan Africa, Middle East, Melanesia, Japan, Central and South America, and the Caribbean region are the main endemic areas. HTLV-II, a related type C retrovirus, affects predominantly American Indians and parenteral drug abusers [9].

HTLV-1 virus has several modes of transmission. It can be transmitted via sexual intercourse, mainly occurring from male to female; from mother to child, due to prolonged breastfeeding; and via contaminated blood products (blood transfusion) and sharing of needles and syringes. Intravenous exposure to blood is the most efficient mode of HTLV-1 transmission [10].

Most of HTLV-1-infected patients may remain lifelong asymptomatic carriers. Nevertheless, between 0.5 and 4 % may develop a progressive spastic paraparesis called tropical spastic paraparesis/HTLV-1-associated myelopathy (TSP/HAM), and an additional 2–5 % may develop adult T-cell leukemia/lymphoma (ATLL). TSP/HAM is at least three to four times more frequent in females and occurs in adults with a mean age at onset of 40–50 years. Incidence of TSP/HAM in endemic areas is around 2 cases/100,000 inhabitants per year. Onset may occur between months and years after the initial infection, and approximately 50 % of TSP/HAM patients may suffer from clinical progression during the first decade after starting symptoms [9].

Classical TSP/HAM is characterized by a slowly and progressive spastic paraparesis with lower limb weakness and sensory symptoms, back pain, sphincter

Table 10.2 Neurological and systemic conditions associated to HTLV-1 infection

Neurological manifestations
Cognitive dysfunction
Tropical spastic paraparesis
Autonomic involvement
Amyotrophic lateral sclerosis-like syndrome
Cerebellar syndrome
Cranial nerve neuropathy (mainly facial palsy)
Axonal sensory-motor neuropathy
Polymyositis
Ophthalmic complications
Retina vasculitis
HTLV-1- associated uveitis
Optic neuritis
Systemic complications
Sjögren syndrome/xerostomy
Arthritis and poly-arthralgias
Periodontal disease
Bronchoalveolitis
Infective dermatitis
Predisposition to helminthic and bacterial infections
Strongyloides stercoralis coinfection

disturbances (neurogenic bladder/bowel), and sexual dysfunction. Patients may present with urinary urgency, incontinence, and urinary retention early in the course of the disease, and in some cases, urinary symptoms and erectile dysfunction may precede the development of TSP/HAM in some years [11]. On neurological exploration, symmetric and proximal weakness of the legs, hypoesthesia and reduced vibration sense, spasticity, hyperreflexia, clonus, and Babinski sign can be detected. More severe patients are wheelchair bound, and disability and falls are common. Clinical spectrum of HTLV-1 infection is much wider than previously thought, and an association between HTLV-1 viral burden and some inflammatory conditions has been observed [11]. A list of systemic and neurological complications associated to HTLV-1 infection is shown in Table 10.2.

Pathogenesis of TSP/HAM may be dependent upon both viral and immunological factors. Its lifelong persistence in CD4+ lymphocytes determines a prolonged interaction between the virus and the host's immune system. HTLV-I proviral DNA and mRNA load are significantly raised in TSP/HAM patients compared to asymptomatic carriers. This antigenic load activates T cells CD8+ specific for Tax-protein, which upregulate pro-inflammatory cytokines [12].

Pathological studies have shown a chronic inflammation with perivascular lymphocytic cuffing and mild parenchymal lymphocytic infiltrates in the spinal cord. There is a predilection of HTLV-1 neuro-inflammation for the lower thoracic spinal cord. Perivascular lymphocytic infiltration with CD4+ lymphocytes can be seen on earlier infiltrates. In advanced stages of the disease, CD8+ T lymphocytes;

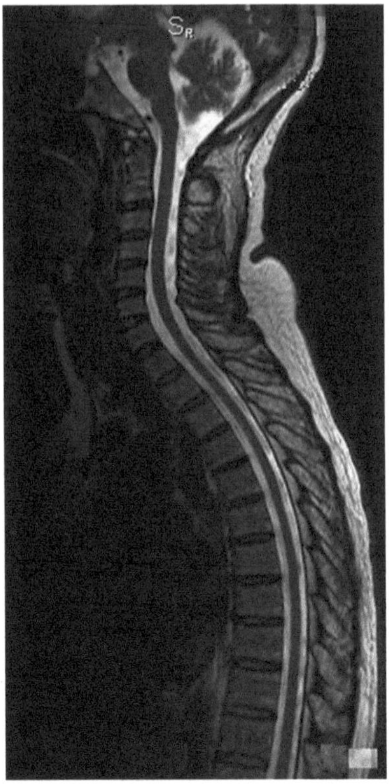

Fig. 10.1 Spinal cord MRI, T2-weighted imaging of a patient affected by HTLV-1 tropical spastic paraparesis. Atrophy of the thoracic spinal cord

pyramidal, spinocerebellar, and spinothalamic tract damage; axonal and myelin degeneration; and spinal cord atrophy predominate [9].

Antibodies directed against HTLV-1 antigens are usually present in both blood and CSF. Enzyme-linked immunosorbent assay (ELISA) is used for screening, and confirmation is done by Western blot technique. CSF may demonstrate a mild lymphocytic pleocytosis, a mild to moderate increase of protein concentration and oligoclonal bands. Peripheral atypical lymphocytes and a high HTLV-1 proviral load can be observed in the blood. Polymerase chain reaction (PCR) in peripheral blood mononuclear cells allows for distinction between HTLV-1 and II and permits the quantification of proviral load.

Spinal cord MRI may show atrophy on the cervical and thoracic regions in the chronic stage (Fig. 10.1). High intensity signal on T2-weighted imaging, and heterogeneous enhancement of gadolinium on T1-weighted imaging, has been observed in the lower cervical and thoracic spinal cord in the initial stages of the disease. Brain MRI may also detect subcortical and periventricular white matter lesions in around 50 % of TSP/HAM patients [11].

Repeated courses of steroids (intravenous methylprednisolone) are used to treat symptoms at initial presentation. Alpha interferon, plasma exchange, intravenous immunoglobulins, danazol, pentoxifilline, zidovudine, lamivudine, monoclonal antibodies (daclizumab), and valproic acid have been used in open trials in a small number of patients. Alpha interferon may cause a reduction in HTLV-I proviral load. Nevertheless, their clinical efficacy is limited, and symptomatic treatment remains the mainstay of therapy. There is an overactivity of the detrusor muscle and a dyssynergy of the bladder sphincter in the TSP/HAM, and urinary tract infections are common and complicated by vesicoureteral reflux. Neurogenic bladder should be managed by means of intermittent catheterization associated with anticholinergic drugs. Constipation, neurogenic pain, and spasticity are other relevant issues that should be treated in the chronic stage of the disease [12].

Enterovirus

Enteroviruses are RNA viruses that belong to the Picornaviridae family. They are transmitted by direct contact as they reproduce in both the gastrointestinal and the upper respiratory tracts [13]. Most enteroviral infections are asymptomatic, but some of them may cause herpangina, myocarditis, pericarditis, and hand-foot-mouth disease. In addition, they are the most common cause of viral meningitis and can also provoke an acute myelitis affecting the anterior spinal cord horn.

Poliovirus

After performing massive worldwide polio immunization campaigns, the number of polio cases has just dropped down dramatically. Global expansion of eradication programs resulted in a reduction of paralytic disease from an estimated annual pre-vaccine level of at least 600,000 cases to fewer than 1,000 cases in 2010 [14]. Nevertheless, poliomyelitis still remains endemic in some regions of Pakistan, Afghanistan and Nigeria, and isolated cases in Central and sub-Saharan African countries have been reported. In addition, polio outbreaks attributed to circulating vaccine-derived poliovirus have been described. Vaccine-derived polioviruses causing paralytic disease have undergone recombination with human enterovirus C species [15, 16].

Paralytic poliomyelitis can occur as a complication of poliovirus infection in around 1–2 % of cases. Most infected people have a mild viral infection and only 5 % may even present with mild systemic symptoms. Several challenges to a final eradication of paralytic poliomyelitis persist today and include the following: (1) the reinfection of polio-free areas, (2) the continued transmission of wild polioviruses in endemic reservoirs, (3) the appearance of outbreaks due to circulating vaccine-derived polioviruses, and (4) the persistent excretion of vaccine-derived poliovirus by a few vaccinees with B-cell immunodeficiency [14].

Poliovirus affects the cells of the anterior horns of the spinal cord and provokes a clinical syndrome of acute and asymmetric flaccid paralysis. On examination, motor weakness, proximal more than distal, areflexia, and fasciculation can be observed, whereas sphincter function and sensory modalities are preserved. Lower limbs are involved more frequently than the upper ones, although a bulbar form of polio has also been described. Risk of developing paralysis is associated with age, with higher risk in adult life, intermediate risk in children, and low risk in infants [13].

After a period of stability subsequent to acute polio infection, some patients have presented an exacerbation of muscle weakness and fatigue. This syndrome has been called post-polio syndrome, and its diagnosis requires the presence of a lower motor neuron disorder and exclusion of other disorders as cause of the new symptoms. It has been hypothesized that the muscle-related effects of post-polio syndrome may be associated with an ongoing process of denervation and reinnervation, reaching a point at which denervation is no longer compensated for by reinnervation. An inflammatory process might be the cause of this denervation. Post-polio patients should be advised to avoid both inactivity and overuse of weak muscles [17].

Enterovirus 71

Enterovirus 71 (EV71) has been identified as the etiologic agent of a poliomyelitis-like syndrome. EV71 infections usually manifest as mild case of hand-foot-mouth disease/herpangina affecting children and have a peak incidence during the summer and seasonal variations. Epidemic outbreaks have happened throughout the world, and mainly in Malaysia, Singapore, Taiwan, and Australia [18]. Severe complications of EV71 infection include shock, cardiopulmonary manifestations such as neurogenic pulmonary edema, cardiac dysfunction, increased vascular permeability, and neurological involvement [19].

Neurological syndromes observed in EV71 infection include meningitis, meningoencephalomyelitis, poliomyelitis-like syndrome, Guillain-Barré syndrome, acute transverse myelitis, cerebellar ataxia, opsoclonus-myoclonus syndrome, and brainstem encephalitis. EV71 may affect the CNS causing an enteroviral encephalomyelitis involving the central midbrain, posterior portion of the medulla oblongata and pons, bilateral dentate nuclei of the cerebellum, and the ventral roots of the cervical spinal cord [20].

Fever exceeding 38 °C and a characteristic mucocutaneous rash can be followed by acute flaccid paraplegia 3–5 days later. Lymphocytic pleocytosis (between 10 and 100 cells/ul) can be found on the CSF. Brain MRI may show hyperintensity lesions on T2-weighted and fluid-attenuation inversion recovery images in the lower brainstem and deep cerebellar nuclei and even on the ventral cervical roots [21]. Bilateral hyperintense lesions in the anterior horn regions of the cord on T2-weighted images can be observed in acute myelitis patients. Fever lasting more than 3 days, peak temperature ≥38.5 °C, and history of lethargy have been identified as independent risk factors for neurological involvement as evidenced by CSF pleocytosis [18]. There is no efficacy therapy for EV71 myelitis; the antiviral drug pleconaril has been used in some cases with modest effects against this virus.

Other Non-polio Enterovirus

Coxsackie A9, B4, and B3 and echovirus 11 and 12 are other common causes of acute flaccid paralysis in the infancy, although Coxsackie meningomyelitis can also happen in elderly people. These non-polio enteroviruses have probably surpassed poliovirus as other causative agents of viral myelitis after starting polio vaccination programs all over the world.

Flavivirus

The *Flaviviridae* family are RNA viruses that include some mosquito-borne virus such as dengue virus, Japanese encephalitis virus, yellow fever virus, West Nile virus (WNV) and Murray Valley encephalitis virus, and tick-borne virus. Flavivirus are a cause of encephalitis in the tropics but they have been associated with a flaccid poliomyelitis-like syndrome [22–24]. These flavivirus may have a special affinity to gray matter including the anterior horn cells. Neurotoxic cytokines are believed to play a role in regional inflammation of the nerve roots in flavivirus polio-like syndrome. MRI of the spinal cord may show marked contrast enhancement of the affected nerve roots in flavivirus polyradiculitis [25]. In some cases, anterior horn cell involvement of the spinal cord has been associated with extensive bilateral thalamic destruction, both of which are well recognized complications of flavivirus infection [22].

Treatment for flavivirus myelitis is supportive, and although several drugs have been used in the acute stage of infection, including ribavirin, steroids, alpha interferon, and intravenous inmunoglobulins, they have not proven any clear effectiveness.

West Nile Virus

West Nile virus is a mosquito-borne flavivirus that is increasingly spread in the Western hemisphere in the last decades. WNV may cause high fever, malaise, headache, backache, arthralgia, myalgias, retro-orbital pain, and a maculopapular rash. Approximately 1 % of infected people may present with meningitis or encephalitic syndrome, and only 10 % of these may have flaccid paralysis [26]. Postmortem examinations of patients with WNV infection have showed a pronounced tropism for the gray matter of the spinal cord, as in other naturally occurring WNV infection in vertebrates, such as monkeys, horses, and birds, causing poliomyelitis [27].

WNV-associated poliomyelitis-like patients may have an acute flaccid and asymmetric paralysis, absent deep tendon reflexes in affected limbs, preserved sensation, bowel or bladder dysfunction, and respiratory failure. These patients usually have associated signs of meningitis, encephalitis, or respiratory distress from involvement of spinal motor neurons supplying the phrenic nerves to the diaphragm. However, acute flaccid paralysis may also occur in the absence of fever or meningoencephalitis [26].

Inflammation of the spinal cord gray matter may extend into the ventral nerve roots and provoke a myeloradiculitis. This fact may explain the appearance of asymmetric acute flaccid paralysis involving one (monoparesis) to four limbs (quadriparesis), seen in many patients with WNV infection. Although isolated radiculopathy is rarer, patients with monoparesis or asymmetric weakness in the arms or legs have been reported.

A positive serum M immunoglobulin (IgM) antibody to WNV indicates a recent infection. CSF may show a positive WNV IgM antibodies, increased leukocytes (usually >200 cells/mm^3) and protein levels, and normal glucose. Around half of WNV meningitis patients may have at least 50 % neutrophils in their initial CSF specimen [28], followed by a shift to lymphocytosis.

Spinal cord MRI may show abnormal signal intensity areas that may be more pronounced in the ventral horns and enhancement around the conus medullaris and cauda equina [29]. In myeloradiculitis cases, MRI may detect enhancement of the ventral nerve roots. A complete resolution of these abnormalities has been observed during MRI follow-up in some patients.

Neurological recovery is usually incomplete with a poorer prognosis for recovery of physical function in patients with acute flaccid paralysis [30].

Dengue Virus

Dengue is a mosquito-borne viral disease that is endemic in almost all tropical and subtropical countries. It is caused by one of four related dengue virus (DENV) serotypes, single-stranded RNA viruses, members of the *Flaviviridae* family. Dengue is the second most common mosquito-borne disease affecting humans after malaria. Although most DENV infections are asymptomatic, symptomatic DENV infections can present as dengue fever and dengue hemorrhagic fever [31].

Spinal cord involvement following DENV infection has been reported during the infectious and post-infectious stages [32, 33]. Direct virus invasion and immune-mediated factors are pathogenic mechanisms involved in each one of these stages, respectively [34]. Post-dengue acute transverse myelitis may present as acute weakness and numbness of the lower limbs and urinary retention. Post-infectious immune-mediated myelitis has been described to occur 1–2 weeks after the onset of dengue symptoms, whereas parainfectious myelitis usually occurs within the first week of infection. CSF intrathecal synthesis of DENV-specific IgG antibodies have been detected in dengue myelitis patients [35]. Spinal cord MRI may be normal or show high-signal areas in T2-weighted imaging. Therapy is supportive.

Herpesvirus

Herpes family viruses include herpes simplex virus 1 (HSV1) and 2 (HSV2), varicella zoster virus (VZV), cytomegalovirus, and Epstein-Barr virus. These viruses may remain latent for years after initial infection. They usually provoke white matter inflammation of the spinal cord and clinically may present as acute transverse myelitis [36].

HSV1 and HSV2

HSV1, HSV2, and VZV establish a latent infection in the dorsal root ganglia for the entire life of the host. HSV1 usually enters the host through oral mucosa. HSV1 can cause encephalitis, corneal blindness, and in some rare cases myelitis in children [36]. HSV2 causes genital herpes and is the causative agent for most HSV-associated myelitis in adults.

After initial infection, HSV2 enters the sensory nerves and reaches the dorsal root ganglia where, once incorporated into cell genoma, it remains latent for years. When reactivated, viral particles transported back to the dermatome may provoke a vesicular rash and asymptomatic shedding of viral particles. During reactivation, newly HSV2 replicated virus can spread axonally into the spinal cord and may cause a lumbosacral myeloradiculitis called Elsberg syndrome [37, 38]. The conus medullaris and lower thoracic cord are predominantly affected. Urinary retention, constipation, erectile dysfunction, back and anogenital dull pain, paresthesias and tingling in lumbosacral dermatomes, and leg muscle flaccid paresis in various combinations can be found. HSV1, VZV, cytomegalovirus, and Epstein-Barr virus can also provoke lumbosacral radiculomyelitis.

A more severe HSV2 ascending necrotizing myelitis has been described in immunosuppressed patients. Diabetes, HIV infection, and neoplasm seem to predispose to cervicothoracic ascension of HSV2 necrotizing myelitis [39]. In these cases, acute flaccid paraplegia with absent reflexes can be found.

The CSF may show mild to moderate lymphocytic pleocytosis, usually less than 200 cell/uL, and elevation of protein. Necrotizing myelitis may also show polymorphonuclear pleocytosis. The diagnosis of HSV infection is based on CSF DNA amplification by PCR and can be complemented by culture from vesicular fluid or less successfully from CSF or by increasing antibody titers.

MRI may show varying degrees of root or lower spinal cord edema with enlargement and hyperintensity on T2-weighted images, accompanied by contrast enhancement in acute infection but may be normal in other cases. MRI reports of HSV sacral radiculitis or radiculomyelitis are sparse [37].

Treatment with intravenous acyclovir for 14 days may shorten the symptomatic period. However, myelopathic deficits may persist despite antiviral treatment. A recurrence of symptoms may occur in up to 30 % of patients during the first year after herpetic meningitis or radiculomyelitis [40].

Varicella Zoster Virus

VZV infection causes chickenpox and herpes zoster. After chickenpox primary infection, VZV can be latent in the cranial nerve or sensory dorsal root ganglia and reactivate several decades later to produce herpes zoster vesicles that involve a specific dermatome. VZV myelitis/myeloradiculitis may occur during reactivation and usually affect elderly, immunocompromised, or AIDS patients [41]. Rare cases of VZV myelitis of the cervical spinal cord in immunocompetent patients have also been reported [42]. Varicella myelitis is very rarely observed in healthy adults [43].

Myelitis may develop several days/weeks after the eruption of vesicles, although VZV myelitis cases without vesicle eruption have been described. A progressive asymmetric paraparesis with lower limb sensory loss affecting pain and temperature sensory modalities and sphincter function impairment are common. Mononuclear pleocytosis and raised proteins can be found on the CSF, and diagnosis can be confirmed by detection of both VZV-DNA on PCR and IgM-type anti-VZV antibodies in the CSF. Detection of anti-VZV antibodies in the CSF is the most sensitive method of diagnosing VZV infection of the CNS. Spinal cord MRI may detect T2 abnormalities on T2-weighted imaging in the spinal level corresponding to the dermatome involved. Symptoms may improve after treatment with parenteral acyclovir [44].

Cytomegalovirus

Cytomegalovirus may cause a lumbosacral polyradiculomyelitis with focal necrosis of the myelin in immunosuppressed patients and mainly in AIDS patients with a CD4 count below 100 cells/uL [45]. Less frequently, a necrotizing myelitis in the absence of radiculitis may happen. Rare cases have also been reported in immunocompetent patients [46, 47]. Polymorphonuclear pleocytosis and elevated protein concentration can be seen on CSF [48]. PCR has been found to be the most reliable method for the diagnosis of CMV myelitis. Spinal cord MRI usually shows spinal cord and roots swelling, adherence of the spinal roots to thecal sac, variable degrees of meningeal thickening, and irregular contrast enhancement. Prognosis is usually poor. Ganciclovir plus foscarnet has been recommended as therapy.

Epstein-Barr Virus

Epstein-Barr virus is the etiologic agent of infectious mononucleosis. Neurological manifestations of EBV infection include encephalitis, cerebellitis, aseptic meningitis, myelitis, and Guillain-Barré syndrome and affect mainly children and young adults. Reactivation on the CNS can occur also in immunosuppressed patients. As EBV does not invade neurons, an immune-mediated mechanism has been proposed. Spinal cord involvement includes myeloradiculitis, encephalomyeloradiculitis, and acute transverse myelitis [49–51].

CSF is usually inflammatory, with mononuclear pleocytosis in 80 % of cases, and 70 % have abnormal MRI findings [52]. The detection of EBV DNA in the CSF by means of PCR technique supports the diagnosis of EBV infection. There is no definitive treatment for EBV myelitis, and steroids and immunoglobulins have been used empirically.

Lyssavirus: Rabies

Rabies is a viral zoonosis that causes approximately 100,000 deaths per year worldwide, and most deaths occur in developing countries. Furious rabies is a life-threatening condition in humans that is provoked by an RNA lyssavirus carried in dogs and bats. The virus is transmitted to humans by infected saliva through the bite of a rabid animal, and the incubation period averages 1–3 months. Dogs are the major vector, especially in developing countries. Once symptoms develop, the disease is invariably fatal [53].

Here are the two classic forms of the disease. The most common is the furious or encephalitic rabies, which is characterized by hyperexcitability, autonomic dysfunction, hydrophobia, and aerophobia. Human paralytic rabies, a form that is not easily identified in clinical practice, may occur in one third of patients. Clinical presentation, a flaccid paralysis in the bitten limb which ascends symmetrically or asymmetrically, resembles Guillain-Barré syndrome or even an acute poliomyelitis and proceeds to encephalopathy [54].

Pathogenic mechanisms responsible for the motor weakness are not clear. Rabies should be ruled out in all patients with a history of animal bite that develop an acute myelopathy or encephalopathy. Rabies diagnosis relies on clinical history, serological antibodies in blood and CSF, and virus amplification and molecular analyses by PCR technique. Molecular analyses of rabies viruses isolated from both furious and paralytic rabies patients have shown only minor genetic variations with no specific patterns in glyco- (G), phospho- (P), and nucleoprotein (N) sequences. Longer survival period in paralytic rabies has been hypothesized to be related to unidentified mechanisms on neuronal gene expression, required for virus transcription/replication and for maintaining neuronal survival [55]. Treatment is supportive.

Bacterial Myelopathies

Spinal Cord Tuberculosis

CNS may be involved in between 1 and 10 % of *Mycobacterium tuberculosis* infections. The most common presentation is tuberculous meningitis, although it also may present as parenchymal tuberculomas, chronic spinal arachnoiditis, intradural spinal granulomas, myelopathy, or even spinal cord infarction. Risk factors of neuro-tuberculosis (TB) are immunosuppression states and chronic malnutrition. Patients coinfected with HIV and tuberculosis may be at higher risk of CNS involvement, although HIV infection does not appear to modify the clinical manifestations of TB radiculomyelitis. In developing countries, neuro-tuberculosis may occur in the context of primary dissemination in young adults, and only half of these patients may present with pulmonary symptoms at onset [56].

Tuberculous myelopathy may develop as a secondary extension of vertebral body tuberculosis (Pott disease), as a downward extension of tuberculous meningitis, and even as a primary TB lesion. In addition, radiculomyelopathy may also develop during appropriate treatment of intracranial TB [57].

Pott disease may be the most frequent cause of TB myelopathy, and bacilli may spread through the vertebral venous system involving the anterior segments of the thoracic and lumbar spine and provoking the collapse of infected vertebral bodies and secondary damage of the spinal roots and spinal cord.

Spinal forms associated to TB meningitis include granulomatous myeloradiculitis, chronic adhesive spinal cord arachnoiditis, intramedullary tuberculomas, intradural extramedullary granulomas, and even spinal cord infarction associated with spinal artery vasculitis [58, 59].

In tuberculous myeloradiculitis, the space between the spinal dura mater and the leptomeninges may be occupied by a thick exudate that may cause encasement of the spinal cord and impingement of the spinal roots. Granulomatous reaction of spinal leptomeninges is associated with vasculitis caseation, histiocyte proliferation, and tubercle formation [60]. Blood vessels may be impaired by necrotizing granulomas or by arteritis. Syringomyelia is another recognized complication.

Epidural tuberculoma and intramedullary tuberculomas may present as a subacute myelopathy depending on the location, level, and extension of the granuloma. TB myeloradiculitis is characterized by a subacute onset of paraparesis that may slowly progress over weeks. Neurological symptoms include root pain, numbness and paresthesias, muscle weakness, and bladder sphincter disturbances; paralysis develops after a few days. Absent reflexes, flaccid weakness of the lower limbs, and extensor plantar response can be found on examination.

Diagnosis of spinal TB is based on clinical and CSF findings, as well as typical CT or MRI appearance. CSF may reveal lymphocytic pleocytosis, hypoglycorrhachia, and high level of proteins as a result of CSF flow block. Around two thirds of patients have positive CSF acid-fast stain and Lowenstein cultures, and less than half may have a positive tuberculin skin test. Sensitivity of these tests in the absence of TB meningitis needs further elucidation.

Spine MRI and myelo-CT in Pott disease may show contrast enhancement with vertebral body collapse and variable degrees of spinal cord compression. Tuberculomas may show a pattern of contrast-enhanced T1 hypointense rings with high signal centrally on T2-weighted image. Granulomatous myeloradiculitis findings include obliteration of the subarachnoid space, loss of the outline in the cervicothoracic spinal cord, matting of the nerve roots in lumbar region, and a nodular, thick, or linear intradural gadolinium-enhanced pattern. In the chronic advanced stage, signs of arachnoiditis such as matted nerve roots and even syringomyelic cavity can be detected [57].

Early diagnosis and treatment is necessary to avoid progression of disability. A four-drug regimen for 2 months followed by 10 months of rifampin and isoniazid is recommended. The value of adjunctive surgery remains uncertain, although localized areas of adhesive arachnoiditis or cord compression from a cyst and instability of vertebral bodies may be surgically treated with good results [61].

Spirochetes: Neurosyphilis and Lyme Borreliosis

The incidence of primary and secondary syphilis has increased over the past decade, and the presenting clinical features have changed since the beginning of the HIV epidemic. *Treponema pallidum* disseminates to the CSF and meninges very early in the infection. Spirochetes can be identified in the CSF in primary syphilis, and in many cases, the spirochetes may be spontaneously cleared from the CSF. Following neuroinvasion, early neurosyphilis may involve the CSF, meninges, and cerebral or spinal cord vasculature. Asymptomatic neurosyphilis is characterized by persistent asymptomatic meningitis with mild abnormalities in the CSF, and spirochetes may or may not be identified in the CSF. Syphilitic meningitis and meningovasculitis are common forms, and vasculitis may affect the spinal cord in some rare cases [62].

Brain and spinal cord parenchyma are affected in the late forms of neurosyphilis that occur years to decades after initial infection. General paresis and *tabes dorsalis* are the classic syndromes of late neurosyphilis, and their incidence has dropped down after the discovery and extensive use of penicillin. *Tabes dorsalis* is a chronic and progressive spinal cord disorder affecting the posterior columns, which is characterized clinically by sensory ataxia, loss of vibration and pain sensation, and bowel and bladder dysfunction. Neurological examination may reveal increased reflexes, insensitivity to deep pain and sensory ataxia, and Charcot joints. Optic atrophy and Argyll-Robertson pupils may also be present. In the last decades, syphilitic meningomyelitis seems to be more common than *tabes dorsalis* [63].

Other less common spinal cord neurosyphilitic syndromes are hypertrophic pachymeningitis, motor neuron disease associated to syringomyelia, and Charcot deformations of the vertebra with compressive spinal cord syndrome.

Diagnosis is based on a positive peripheral serology and CSF assessment. Venereal disease research laboratory (VDRL) and rapid plasma reagin (RPR) tests are sensitive in the early stages of syphilis and may become negative in the late stages. Treponemal-specific test is used for confirmation, and titers remain positive in later stages. A positive serum test requires further confirmation of neurosyphilis by means of CSF analysis. A reactive CSF-VDRL has been considered as diagnostic of neurosyphilis, although this test may be nonreactive in some patients so a negative test does not exclude neurosyphilis diagnosis. The CSF-RPR is as sensitive and specific as the CSF-VDRL. Treponemal tests, such as the fluorescent treponemal antibody-absorbed (FAT-ABS) test, are used to exclude the diagnosis of neurosyphilis. FAT-ABS should be used when CSF-VDRL is negative in spite of a serological evidence for syphilis and a compatible clinical picture [64]. Mild pleocytosis can be found in the CSF. Spinal cord atrophy and high intensity area abnormalities spanning the posterior column of the spine can be found [64].

Tabes dorsalis should be treated with intravenous aqueous penicillin (4 million units every 4 h during 14 days). For those allergic patients, ceftriaxone 2 g intravenously for 14 days has been recommended. Clinical symptoms may worsen when staring antimicrobial therapy due to a sudden increase of spirochete lysis and antigen level rise. This condition is called Jarisch-Herxheimer reaction. A lumbar puncture should be repeated at 6-month interval after therapy, and patients should be retreated if CSF white blood cell count is not normal 6 months after treatment or the CSF-VDRL titer has a fourfold increase. In HIV-infected individuals, the CSF-VDRL may normalize more slowly after treatment [64, 65].

Spinal cord involvement may also occur in Lyme neuroborreliosis, particularly at the level of the affected segment in patients with the so-called Garin-Bujadoux-Bannwarth meningoradiculitis, characterized by severe radicular pain, often mimicking a mechanical radiculopathy, involving one or a few dermatomes, and accompanied by cerebrospinal fluid lymphocytosis. Despite being a painful condition, motor findings with weakness and atrophy are prominent while sensory loss is infrequent.

Spinal Epidural Abscess

Epidural abscess is a medical and neurosurgical emergency that results in severe morbidity and high mortality if diagnosis and treatment are delayed. Incidence of spinal epidural abscess may range between 0.2 and 2.8 per 10,000. Gram-positive bacteria cause epidural abscesses much more frequently than gram-negative. *Staphylococcus aureus* is the most common cause of epidural abscess and occur in between 50 and 70 % of the identified cases, whereas *Streptococcus* species have been isolated in less than 10 % [66]. The most common isolated gram-negative organisms are *Pseudomonas aeruginosa* and *Escherichia coli*.

Infection may originate and spread directly from a near focus of osteomyelitis or hematogeneously from a more distal focus such as skin furuncles, pulmonary and other viscera infections, or surgical instrumentation. These pyogenic infections frequently may seed the anterior epidural space via spread from bone and soft tissue foci, whereas the posterior epidural space via hematogenous dissemination. The thoracic region is the most frequently involved [67].

Risk factors associated with epidural abscess include spinal abnormality, spinal trauma, spinal surgery or procedure, immunosuppression, diabetes mellitus, alcoholism, hemodialysis [68], malignancy, AIDS, bacteremia, and use of intravenous drugs. In around one third of cases, a mild back trauma was identified as preceding clinical symptoms. Fever is present in less than 70 % of cases. Clinical symptoms include focal back pain, motor weakness and spasm, radicular pain, and sensory and sphincter disturbances [69].

Inflammatory biomarkers including C-reactive protein and erythrocyte sedimentation rate are usually elevated, and blood cultures may be positive in around half of the patients. Neuroimaging studies of the spinal cord may show the extension and localization of the epidural abscess. CT scan is useful to assess the degree of bone involvement, whereas spinal MRI usually better describes the extension and degree of compression of the spinal cord (Fig. 10.2). Spinal tap should be not performed to avoid the risk of introducing bacteria into the CSF.

Once diagnosed, patient should perform emergent surgical drainage and debridement, spinal decompression, and prolonged antibiotic therapy for 6–8 weeks.

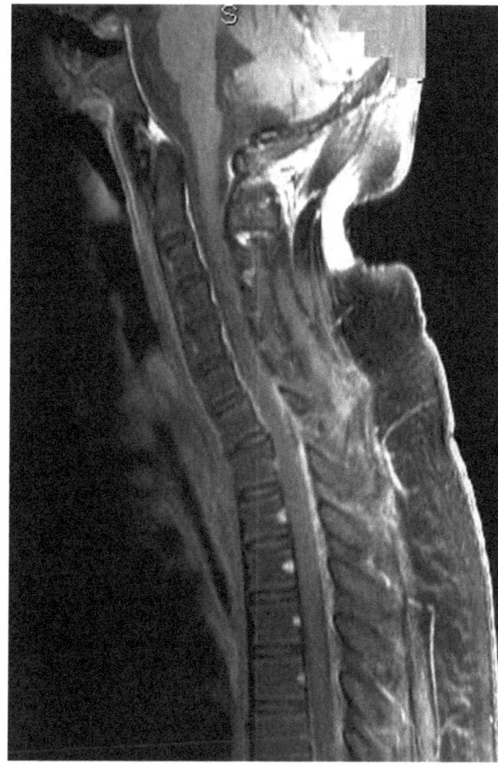

Fig. 10.2 Spinal cord MRI, T1-enhanced weighted imaging. Epidural cervical abscess with diffuse enhancement of contrast

Empiric parenteral antimicrobial therapy should include vancomycin to cover methicillin-resistant *Staphylococcus aureus* and an antibiotic for aerobic gram-negative bacilli such as a cephalosporin with antipseudomonal activity (e.g., ceftazidime or cefepime). Specific antibiotic therapy should be started once cultures were available and on the basis of organisms and susceptibility. In those patients who are critically ill or who have a longitudinal epidural spread, conservative therapy should be considered. Even with best treatment, mortality is still high and may range between 10 and 25 % of cases and has been associated with a delay in surgical therapy. Severity of neurological symptoms at time of surgical drainage has been considered a predictor of mortality and disability [67].

Other Pyogenic Infections of the Spinal Cord

Brucellosis is an infection caused by *Brucella melitensis* that is endemic in the Mediterranean area and Middle East countries. Spondylitis is the most frequent brucellosic vertebral infection in adults, and the lumbar region is more commonly affected; vertebral lesions may occur at several levels in some cases. Brucellosic epidural abscess is a relatively common complication accompanying brucellosis spondylitis. Extradural thoracic and lumbar spinal compression by *Brucella* epidural abscess has been reported [70, 71], and clinical symptoms are unspecific and include fever and lumbar back pain. Epidural abscess may also cause symptoms of myelopathy or radicular pain by compression, and arachnoiditis and multilevel radiculitis due to lumbar epidural abscess may also occur. Differential diagnosis includes other pyogenic spondylitis causes including TB, salmonella, nocardia, and others.

Tropical and Parasitary Myelopathies

Spinal Schistosomiasis

Schistosomiasis is a helminthic infection that affects to more than 230 million people worldwide. *Schistosoma mansoni*, *Schistosoma haematobium*, *Schistosoma japonicum*, *Schistosoma intercalatum*, and *Schistosoma mekongi* are the five species that may infect humans. *S. mansoni* is endemic in South America, the Caribbean region, Africa, and the Middle East. *S. haematobium* is spread in many African and Middle Eastern countries, and *S. japonicum* is endemic in Japan, China, and the Philippines [72].

Schistosomes are blood-dwelling flukes that live in blood vessels of vertebrates including humans and other mammals. Freshwater snails are intermediate host, and cercaria released from snails perforate the skin of human beings and through lymphatic and hematogenous spread settle in the portal circulation. *S. mansoni* and *S. japonicum* inhabit, respectively, the inferior and superior mesenteric vein tributaries whereas *S. haematobium* inhabits the bladder veins. The female worm usually releases hundreds of eggs each day that are excreted in stool (*S. mansoni*) or urine (*S. haematobium*) [73].

Spinal schistosomiasis is a common cause of acute myelopathy in tropical regions. *S. mansoni* and *S. haematobium* are responsible for most cases of spinal schistosomiasis. Around 6 % of neurological patients admitted to a Brazilian hospital with a non-traumatic myelopathy were due to *S. mansoni* spinal schistosomiasis [74]. Schistosomal myelopathy is more common in young people who are exposed to freshwater. Spinal schistosomiasis occurs in the early stage of the infection and systemic symptoms of schistosomiasis are usually absent.

Spinal schistosomiasis occurs as a consequence of the immunogenic interaction between schistosome egg deposition in the spinal cord and the inflammatory response reaction of the host around them. The host's response may vary from a minimal inflammatory reaction to the scattered ova in the absence of neurological manifestations to severe reactions resulting in space-occupying granulomatous mass and spinal cord tissue necrosis. The shape and size of the ova are other factors that may explain the increased frequency of *S. mansoni* infection in spinal

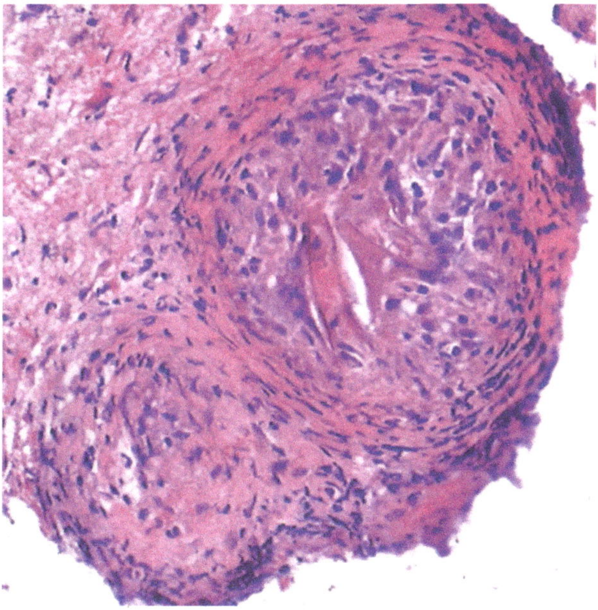

Fig. 10.3 Spinal cord biopsy of a patient with schistosomal myelopathy showing several granulomas around *S. mansoni* eggs

schistosomiasis (Fig. 10.3). *S. mansoni* and *S. haematobium* eggs are larger than the *S. japonicum* ones and are retained much more frequently in the spinal cord. The higher size of *S. mansoni* ova, 60 um in width by 150 um in length, and its lateral spine may limit their progress along the vertebral venous plexus to the brain [73].

The schistosome eggs and even the adult worm may also reach the spinal venous system retrogradely via the Batson's valveless venous plexus that connects the deep iliac veins and the inferior vena cava with the spinal cord's venous system. Schistosomal myelopathy is more frequent in the lumbosacral and lower thoracic regions of the spinal cord. The carriage of the ova into the spinal veins may be facilitated by Valsalva intra-abdominal pressure maneuvers such as defecation and coughing [73].

Schistosomal acute transverse myelopathy, conus medullaris syndrome, and lower limb myeloradiculopathy are the most commonly found syndromes. Schistosome myelitis may start as a flaccid paraplegia with sphincter dysfunction, and lower thoracic spinal cord and conus medullaris are frequently involved [74, 75].

Cauda equina's roots are frequently affected in schistosomal myeloradiculopathy. Granulomatous masses localized in the conus medullaris, lower thoracic level, and spinal lumbar and sacral roots may provoke an asymmetric lower limb weakness, sensory symptoms in lumbosacral dermatomes, and sexual dysfunction and neurogenic bladder. Back pain, tingling, lower limb paresthesias, and urinary retention may appear several days before weakness onset [75].

Less frequent clinical pictures are painful radiculopathy, chronic asymmetric myeloradiculopathy, cervical intramedullary schistosomiasis, and spinal cord compression due to extra-axial granulomas [73].

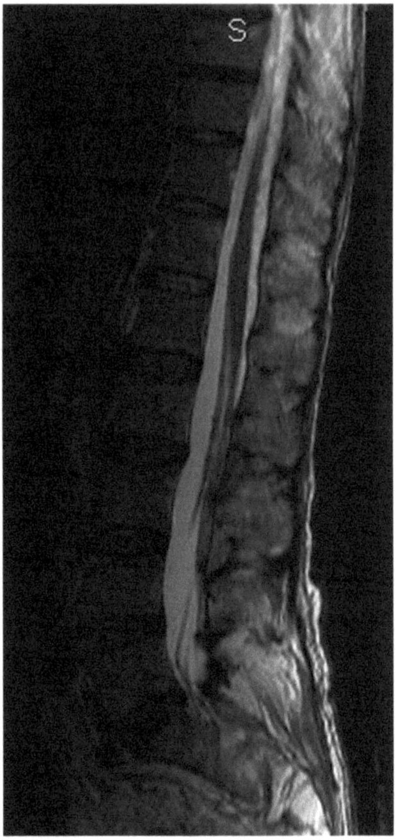

Fig. 10.4 Lumbosacral MRI of a patient affected by a schistosomal myeloradiculopathy showing arachnoiditis and adherence of the lumbar and sacral roots

Swelling of conus medullaris; enlargement of the spinal cord at the thoracic level, usually below T8 level; and thickening of spinal roots and cauda equina can be detected on spinal MRI [76] (Fig. 10.4). Granulomas of conus medullaris heterogeneously enhance gadolinium contrast on T1-weighted imaging. Although enlargement may be evident at the thoracic level, the abnormal T2 high signal may frequently extend to the lumbar and sacral spinal cord, or even to the lower cervical level [77].

Parasitological examinations are of limited value in the diagnosis of schistosomal myelopathy, and schistosome ova may be observed in stool, urine, and/or rectal mucosa (rectal biopsy) in less than 40 % of these patients. A low parasite burden and a day-to-day variation in stool egg count and clustering of eggs within the stool may explain the large number of negative result cases on parasitological examination.

Serological techniques that may detect antibodies against schistosome crude egg and soluble worm antigens in blood and CSF are hemagglutination, indirect immunofluorescence, and ELISA tests. The analysis of the CSF may show lymphocytic pleocytosis, presence of eosinophils, and an increased concentration of proteins

Table 10.3 Clues to the diagnosis of spinal cord schistosomiasis

(a) Person from schistosomiasis endemic area or any returned traveler exposed recently to freshwater in endemic areas who present with acute transverse myelitis, conus medullaris, and/or cauda equine myelopathy
(b) Spinal cord MRI showing swelling of conus medullaris, thickening of spinal roots and cauda equina, and gadolinium enhancement
(c) CSF analysis showing lymphocytic pleocytosis, increased protein concentration, and presence of eosinophils
(d) ELISA, hemagglutination, and/or indirect immunofluorescence tests detect positive antibodies against schistosome
(e) Schistosome eggs are observed in stool and/or rectal biopsy in a person with myelopathy

[72]. In those people living in endemic areas, neither ova detection nor a positive antibody test confirms the schistosomal etiology of a myelopathy. Schistosome antibodies remain positive for life, and a positive immune reaction in endemic regions is considered evidence of exposure. Some clues for the diagnosis of schistosomal myelopathy are summarized in Table 10.3.

Definitive diagnosis can be made in some cases by performing a biopsy of the spinal cord's leptomeninges. Schistosome ova in various stages of evolution, with surrounding inflammatory reaction and demyelination near the ova, can be found on pathological specimens. Schistosome granuloma is characterized by a necrotic center that contains schistosome eggs surrounded by giant cells and lymphocytes and an outer layer of eosinophils, plasma cells, and fibroblasts [74].

Combined therapy with steroids and praziquantel are used to treat acute schistosomal myelopathy [78]. Steroids may reduce the intensity of inflammatory reaction, diminish the edema around granulomas, and suppress granuloma formation. Oxamniquine has also been used to treat *S. mansoni* infection, and artemisinin derivatives may be helpful to kill immature schistosomules.

Although mass exeresis, decompressive laminectomy, and liberation of lumbosacral roots have been used in severe spinal schistosomiasis cases, there is no clinical trial that has compared the efficacy of the best spinal surgical intervention against conventional pharmacological treatment. Surgical decompression should be indicated only in selected cases presenting with rapid deterioration of lower limb strength and evidence of extra-axial spinal cord compression due to tumor-like lesions.

Gnathostomiasis

Gnathostomiasis is a parasitic disease caused by *Gnathostoma spinigerum* which is endemic in Southeast Asia (China, Japan, Korea, and Thailand), Mexico, and Peru. It may be transmitted when human beings eat undercooked fish or poultry and by drinking copepod-contaminated freshwater. The primary intermediate host is the freshwater copepod of the genus Cyclops; secondary intermediate hosts are fish, ducks, pigs, and water snakes. Adult larva inhabits definitive host's stomach. Once ingested raw or undercooked infested fish or poultry, the larvae cross the intestinal wall and migrate to the subcutaneous tissues.

Intermittent, painful, subcutaneous swellings usually occur when humans are infected. Neurological complications of gnathostomiasis include headache, hydrocephalus, seizures, brain hemorrhage, transverse myelitis, and painful radiculomyelitis. *Gnathostoma spinigerum* is not indeed a neurotrophic parasite, although it may accidentally enter into the CNS, migrating on peripheral nerves and spinal roots and provoking a radiculitis and/or radiculomyelitis [79]. Severe neurogenic and radicular pain in the lower limbs and trunk, paraparesis, and neurogenic bladder can occur during this accidental migration. Transverse myelitis can occur as a consequence of larvae's migration and necrosis across the spinal cord and the leptomeningeal inflammation secondary to the host's immunological response.

CSF may show a pattern of eosinophilic meningitis. The CSF usually is xanthochromic, and pleocytosis (500–2,000 white cell count) with predominance of eosinophils (20–70 %), raised proteins (>100 mg/dL), and normal levels of glucose may be a clue for the diagnosis. A positive serological test using the immunoblotting test in the CSF and serum is usually positive for *G. spinigerum*. Spinal cord MRI may show spinal cord swelling, edema, leptomeningeal gadolinium enhancement, and the presence of multiple hemorrhagic tracts [80].

Recovery of the parasite from the tissue provides definitive diagnosis. Patients should be initially treated with steroids to reduce the inflammatory reaction of the spinal cord, and then albendazole or ivermectin. Albendazole alone may exacerbate neurological symptoms as a result of larvae death in the spinal cord, so prednisolone or dexamethasone is used to reduce edema.

Spinal Neurocysticercosis

Cysticercosis is a common parasitic disease, caused by the larval stage of the tapeworm *Taenia solium*. Cysticercosis is endemic in many Central and South American countries, Southeast Asia, and sub-Saharan Africa. Spinal cord involvement may occur in 1–5 % of neurocysticercosis patients and affect much more frequently the subarachnoid space than the medullary parenchyma. Many of these patients may have an already known intracranial neurocysticercosis in which a migration of subarachnoid cyst from the basilar cisterns has occurred. Intramedullary cysts are much less common [1]. Subarachnoid infestation coexists with cyst located on the brain cisterns, a fact that supports the hypothesis of dissemination via the CSF. However, intramedullary cysts may also reach the spinal cord via hematogenous dissemination.

Spinal cord compression by spinal subarachnoid cysts may cause a chronic progressive paraparesis, myeloradiculopathy, or a cauda equina syndrome and may mimic a spinal neoplasm. Spinal cysticercosis may also provoke a chronic adhesive arachnoiditis characterized by neurogenic pain, motor weakness, spasticity, and sphincter disturbances. The rare cases of intramedullary cysticercosis may present as an acute transverse myelitis [81].

CSF may show eosinophilia and increased protein concentration. Spinal cysticercosis should be treated with steroids and albendazole, although decompressive surgery may be needed to treat compressive arachnoiditis [82].

Hydatid Disease

Hydatidosis, the cystic infection caused by the cestoce *Echinococcus granulosus*, may also involve the spinal cord in some exceptional cases. *E. granulosum* is endemic in the Mediterranean area, South America, Middle East, and New Zealand. Humans are infected via fecal-oral route, and once ingested, the eggs hatch and form larvae that migrate across the intestinal wall and will generate large hydatid cysts in the liver. Canines are the definitive hosts.

Case reports of spinal echinococcosis have been described, affecting the extradural or intradural extramedullary space; intramedullary echinococcosis is even rarer [83]. Hydatid disease may affect bones in 0.5–2 % of infected patients, half of them occurring in spinal vertebrae provoking spondylitis mainly in the thoracic (50 %) and lumbar spine. The cysts may grow progressively and provoke a mass effect, bone destruction, and host's inflammatory reaction. Spinal cord MRI may show characteristic cysts, and serological analysis may confirm the diagnosis. Prognosis is poor due to high recurrence index, and treatment is based on albendazole plus spinal decompressive surgery [84].

Other Parasitary Diseases

In China, paragonimiasis can cause myelopathy due to extradural compression or less frequently due to intramedullary granulomas [85]. Paragonimiasis can be acquired on having consumed badly cooked or raw crabs parasited by the larva of *Paragonimus westermani. Toxoplasma gondii* spinal cord abscesses have been described in immunosuppressed patients [86]. Acute disseminated encephalomyelitis associated with acute *Toxoplasma gondii* infection has also been reported in immunocompetent children [87]. Visceral *larva migrans* syndrome due to *Toxocara canis* or *Ascaris suum* infection has been reported to cause myelitis in Japan [88, 89].

Clinically, these parasitic infections of the spinal cord can appear in the shape of a slow and progressive myelopathy, a myeloradicular syndrome, or as an acute transverse myelitis. Medullary inflammation and the host's immune reaction with the formation of granulomas are pathogenic mechanisms. Eosinophils can be detected in the blood or CSF. The analysis of tools and the determination of specific antibodies can help in the diagnosis. MRI may reveal spinal cord swelling with or without gadolinium enhancement.

Fungal Myelopathies

Opportunistic fungi such as *Aspergillus* sp., *Zygomycetes*, or *Candida* sp. may infect mainly immunosuppressed patients suffering hematologic malignancies such as acute myeloid leukemia, lymphoma, or hematopoietic stem cells transplants, AIDS, chronic use of steroids, or after transplantation. Pathogenic fungi (*Cryptococcus neoformans*, *Coccidioides immitis*, *Blastomyces dermatitidis*, *Histoplasma capsulatum*, and *Scedosporium prolificans*) may also provoke CNS infections in immunocompetent people [90].

CNS fungal infections may present as chronic meningitis or focal brain lesions. In these cases, fungi usually reach the CNS via hematogenous dissemination from the lungs, heart (mycotic endocarditis), or skin. Fungal infections of the spinal cord are uncommon and affect more frequently immunocompromised hosts, pregnancy, and patients that underwent cardiovascular surgery. However, fungal chronic epidural abscess and spinal cord infection has been reported also in healthy people.

Most fungus may provoke a spinal cord compression syndrome from osteomyelitis, epidural abscess, or paravertebral lesions. Many cases of spinal cord fungal infections may be related to local invasion of the spinal epidural space from vertebral osteomyelitis or by lesions extending through the intervertebral foramina (Fig. 10.5). Spinal fungal infection may present clinically as epidural abscess, chronic arachnoiditis, myelitis, intramedullary granulomas, or vasculopathy associated with spinal cord infarction. In occasions, the fungi can invade the epidural space provoking granulomatous meningitis with intramedullary or extradural granulomas.

Invasive spinal cord aspergillosis typically occurred in terminal and immunosuppressed patients. Nevertheless, the spectrum of hosts and clinical presentations is increasing, due to better medical treatments that prolong the survival of the patients [91]. Invasive aspergillosis may provoke a meningovascular infiltration and a necrotic endarteritis with thrombosis and ischemia leading to vessel occlusion and spinal cord infarctions. Cases of medullary inflammation and spontaneous cord transection due to invasive spondylitis by *Aspergillus* have been described in both immunosuppressed children (leukemia) and also in immunocompetent ones [92].

Candida albicans can also provoke intramedullary, vertebral, and paravertebral abscesses. Epidural abscess caused by *Candida albicans* has been reported in chronic renal failure patients [93]. However, *Candida albicans* spondylodiscitis and subdural spinal granuloma may occur in healthy people [94, 95].

Cryptococcus neoformans is particularly common in bird feces, such as pigeon droppings. Cases of compressive myelopathy due to cryptococcal granulomas arisen from vertebral osteomyelitis or from another infection spread by contiguity from the intervertebral foramina have been reported. Intra- and/or extra-spinal granulomas may also be the consequence of chronic granulomatous meningitis. Cryptococcosis may mimic spinal tuberculosis and is a diagnostic dilemma in countries with high burden of tuberculosis [96]. Intramedullary cryptococcomas of the spinal cord may resemble a spinal tumor [97]. Cryptococcus myeloradiculitis has also been reported in HIV-infected patients.

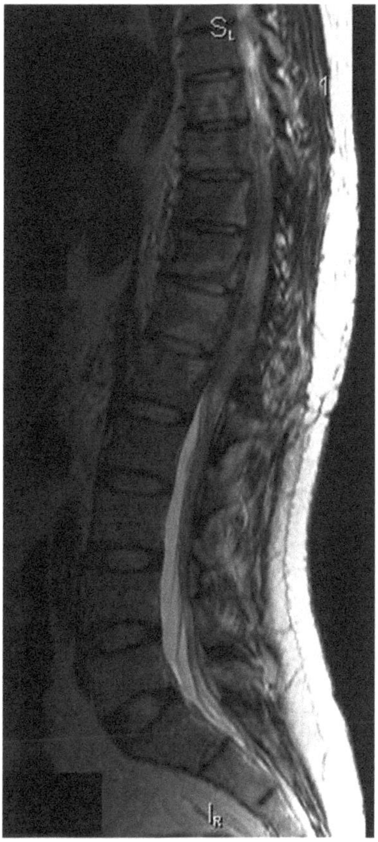

Fig. 10.5 Spinal cord MRI, T2-weighted imaging, of a patient affected by chronic fungal spinal infection due to *Scedosporium prolificans*

Blastomycosis can also imitate vertebral tuberculosis, provoking osteolytic injuries, abscesses, granulomas, and compressive meningitis of the spinal cord [98]. Intramedullary blastomycosis has also been described in children [99]. *Coccidioides immitis* is a dimorphic fungus common in Central and South America. Coccidioides infection can provoke chronic meningitis, tumorlike lesions, hydrocephalus, and spinal arachnoiditis. Coccidioidomicosis can provoke destructive lesions of the vertebral bodies and formation of paraspinal granulomatous masses [100].

Spinal cord fungal infections have high mortality, so aggressive and early treatment should be initiated. Surgical debridement and specific treatment such as intravenous liposomal amphotericin B, 5-fluocytosine, and azoles (voriconazole, posaconazole, itraconazole, fluconazole) have been used with variable results.

Conclusion

Infectious diseases are one of the main causes of acute spinal cord injury. Virus, bacteria, and parasites can provoke acute and chronic infectious myelopathies. Early diagnosis and suspicion is needed to prevent severe sequela and disability.

A detailed neurological examination and assessment of spinal cord syndrome should be followed by a complete spine cord MRI and CSF analysis. Tropical diseases are an emerging etiology of infectious myelopathy, even in non-endemic countries. Teaching programs in neuro-infection and tropical neurology are needed and they should cover this particular topic.

References

1. del Brutto OH, Carod-Artal FJ, Román GC, Sennanayake N. Tropical neurology. Continuum. Philadelphia: American Academy of Neurology; 2002.
2. Brazis PW, Masdeu JC, Biller J. Localization in clinical neurology. 6th ed. New York: Lippincott Williams and Wilkins; 2011.
3. Frohman EM, Wingerchuk DM. Clinical practice. Transverse myelitis. N Engl J Med. 2010;363:564–72.
4. Lyons J, Venna N, Cho TA. Atypical nervous system manifestations of HIV. Semin Neurol. 2011;31:254–65.
5. Hamada Y, Watanabe K, Aoki T, Arai N, Honda M, Kikuchi Y, et al. Primary HIV infection with acute transverse myelitis. Intern Med. 2011;50:1615–7.
6. Petito CK, Navia BA, Cho ES, Jordan BD, George DC, Price RW. Vacuolar myelopathy pathologically resembling subacute combined degeneration in patients with the acquired immunodeficiency syndrome. N Engl J Med. 1985;312:874–9.
7. Garcia-Gubern C, Fuentes CR, Colon-Rolon L, Masvidal D. Spinal cord toxoplasmosis as an unusual presentation of AIDS: case report and review of the literature. Int J Emerg Med. 2010;3:439–42.
8. Schutte C, Townsend T, Van Coller R, Olorunju S. Comparison of HTLV-associated myelopathy (HAM) in HIV-positive and HIV-negative patients at a tertiary South African hospital. S Afr Med J. 2012;103:43–6.
9. Gessain A, Mahieux R. Tropical spastic paraparesis and HTLV-1 associated myelopathy: clinical, epidemiological, virological and therapeutic aspects. Rev Neurol (Paris). 2012;168:257–69.
10. Gonçalves DU, Proietti FA, Ribas JG, Araújo MG, Pinheiro SR, Guedes AC, Carneiro-Proietti AB. Epidemiology, treatment, and prevention of human T-cell leukemia virus type 1-associated diseases. Clin Microbiol Rev. 2010;23:577–89.
11. Carod-Artal FJ, Mesquita HM, Ribeiro Lda S. Neurological symptoms and disability in HTLV-1 associated myelopathy. Neurologia. 2008;23:78–84.
12. Carod-Artal FJ. Immunopathogenesis and treatment of the myelopathy associated to the HTLV-I virus. Rev Neurol. 2009;48:147–55.
13. Cho TA, Vaitkevicius H. Infectious myelopathies. Continuum (Minneap Minn). 2012;18:1351–73.
14. Nathanson N, Kew OM. From emergence to eradication: the epidemiology of poliomyelitis deconstructed. Am J Epidemiol. 2010;172:1213–29.
15. Tyler KL. Emerging viral infections of the central nervous system. Arch Neurol. 2009;66:939–48.
16. Combelas N, Holmblat B, Joffret ML, Colbère-Garapin F, Delpeyroux F. Recombination between poliovirus and coxsackie A viruses of species C: a model of viral genetic plasticity and emergence. Viruses. 2011;3:1460–84.
17. Gonzalez H, Olsson T, Borg K. Management of postpolio syndrome. Lancet Neurol. 2010;9:634–42.
18. Ooi MH, Wong SC, Lewthwaite P, Cardosa MJ, Solomon T. Clinical features, diagnosis, and management of enterovirus 71. Lancet Neurol. 2010;9:1097–105.

19. Chong CY, Chan KP, Shah VA, Ng WY, Lau G, Teo TE, et al. Hand, foot and mouth disease in Singapore: a comparison of fatal and non-fatal cases. Acta Paediatr. 2003;92:1163–9.
20. Hsueh C, Jung SM, Shih SR, Kuo TT, Shieh WJ, Zaki S, et al. Acute encephalomyelitis during an outbreak of enterovirus type 71 infection in Taiwan: report of an autopsy case with pathologic, immunofluorescence, and molecular studies. Mod Pathol. 2000;13: 1200–5.
21. Jang S, Suh SI, Ha SM, Byeon JH, Eun BL, Lee YH, et al. Enterovirus 71-related encephalomyelitis: usual and unusual magnetic resonance imaging findings. Neuroradiology. 2012;54:239–45.
22. Douglas MW, Stephens DP, Burrow JN, Anstey NM, Talbot K, Currie BJ. Murray Valley encephalitis in an adult traveller complicated by long-term flaccid paralysis: case report and review of the literature. Trans R Soc Trop Med Hyg. 2007;101:284–8.
23. Enzinger C, Melisch B, Reischl A, Simbrunner J, Fazekas F. Polyradiculitis as a predominant symptom of tick-borne encephalitis virus infection. Arch Neurol. 2009;66:904–5.
24. Verma R, Praharaj HN, Patil TB, Giri P. Acute transverse myelitis following Japanese encephalitis viral infection: an uncommon complication of a common disease. BMJ Case Rep. 2012.
25. Pfefferkorn T, Feddersen B, Schulte-Altedorneburg G, Linn J, Pfister HW. Tick-borne encephalitis with polyradiculitis documented by MRI. Neurology. 2007;68:1232–3.
26. Leis AA, Stokic DS. Neuromuscular manifestations of west Nile virus infection. Front Neurol. 2012;3:37.
27. Fratkin JD, Leis AA, Stokic DS, Slavinski SA, Geiss RW. Spinal cord neuropathology in human West Nile virus infection. Arch Pathol Lab Med. 2004;128:533–7.
28. Tyler KL, Pape J, Goody RJ, Corkill M, Kleinschmidt-DeMasters BK. CSF findings in 250 patients with serologically confirmed West Nile virus meningitis and encephalitis. Neurology. 2006;66:361–5.
29. Petropoulou KA, Gordon SM, Prayson RA, Ruggierri PM. West Nile virus meningoencephalitis: MR imaging findings. AJNR Am J Neuroradiol. 2005;8:1986–95.
30. Johnstone J, Hanna SE, Nicolle LE, Drebot MA, Neupane B, Mahony JB, et al. Prognosis of West Nile virus associated acute flaccid paralysis: a case series. J Med Case Rep. 2011; 5:395.
31. Carod Artal FJ, Wichmann O, Farrar J, Gascon J. Neurological complications of dengue virus infection. Lancet Neurol. 2013;12:906–19.
32. Seet RC, Lim EC, Wilder-Smith EP. Acute transverse myelitis following dengue virus infection. J Clin Virol. 2006;35:310–2.
33. Chanthamat N, Sathirapanya P. Acute transverse myelitis associated with dengue viral infection. J Spinal Cord Med. 2010;33:425–7.
34. Kunishige M, Mitsui T, Tan BH, et al. Preferential gray matter involvement in dengue myelitis. Neurology. 2004;63:1980–1.
35. Puccioni-Sohler M, Soares CN, Papaiz-Alvarenga R, Castro MJ, Faria LC, Peralta JM. Neurologic dengue manifestations associated with intrathecal specific immune response. Neurology. 2009;73:1413–7.
36. Steiner I, Kennedy PG, Pachner AR. The neurotropic herpes viruses: herpes simplex and varicella-zoster. Lancet Neurol. 2007;6:1015–28.
37. Eberhardt O, Küker W, Dichgans J, Weller M. HSV-2 sacral radiculitis (Elsberg syndrome). Neurology. 2004;63:758–9.
38. Suarez-Calvet M, Rojas-Garcia R, Querol L, Sarmiento LM, Domingo P. Polyradiculoneuropathy associated to human herpesvirus 2 in an HIV-1Yinfected patient (Elsberg syndrome): case report and literature review. Sex Transm Dis. 2010;37:123–5.
39. Wiley CA, Van Patten PD, Carpenter PM, Powell HC, Thal LJ. Acute ascending necrotizing myelopathy caused by herpes simplex virus type 2. Neurology. 1987;37:1791–4.
40. Gobbi C, Tosi C, Städler C, Merenda C, Bernasconi E. Recurrent myelitis associated with herpes simplex virus type 2. Eur Neurol. 2001;46:215–8.
41. Hung CH, Chang KH, Kuo HC, Huang CC, Liao MF, Tsai YT, et al. Features of varicella zoster virus myelitis and dependence on immune status. J Neurol Sci. 2012;318:19–24.

42. Lee CC, Wu JC, Huang WC, Shih YH, Cheng H. Herpes zoster cervical myelitis in a young adult. J Chin Med Assoc. 2010;73:605–10.
43. Takei-Suzuki M, Hayashi Y, Kimura A, Nagasawa M, Koumura A, Sakurai T, et al. Case of varicella myelitis in nursing care worker. Brain Nerve. 2008;60:79–83.
44. Amlie-Lefond C, Jubelt B. Neurologic manifestations of varicella zoster virus infections. Curr Neurol Neurosci Rep. 2009;9:430–4.
45. Corti M, Soto I, Villafañe MF, Bouzas B, Duarte JM, Yampolsky C, Schtirbu R. Acute necrotizing myelitis in an AIDS patient. Medicina (B Aires). 2003;63:143–6.
46. Rigamonti A, Usai S, Ciusani E, Bussone G. Atypical transverse myelitis due to cytomegalovirus in an immunocompetent patient. Neurol Sci. 2005;26:351–4.
47. Karunarathne S, Govindapala D, Udayakumara Y, Fernando H. Cytomegalovirus associated transverse myelitis in an immunocompetent host with DNA detection in cerebrospinal fluid; a case report. BMC Res Notes. 2012;5:364.
48. Haug A, Mahalingam R, Cohrs RJ, Schmid DS, Corboy JR, Gilden D. Recurrent polymorphonuclear pleocytosis with increased red blood cells caused by varicella zoster virus infection of the central nervous system: case report and review of the literature. J Neurol Sci. 2010;292:85–8.
49. Majid A, Galetta SL, Sweeney CJ, Robinson C, Mahalingam R, Smith J, et al. Epstein-Barr virus myeloradiculitis and encephalomyeloradiculitis. Brain. 2002;125:159–65.
50. Sanefuji M, Ohga S, Kira R, Nomura A, Torisu H, Takada H, et al. Epstein-Barr virus-associated meningoencephalomyelitis: intrathecal reactivation of the virus in an immunocompetent child. J Child Neurol. 2008;23:1072–7.
51. Albany C, Psevdos G, Balderacchi J, Sharp VL. Epstein-Barr virus myelitis and Castleman's disease in a patient with acquired immune deficiency syndrome: a case report. J Med Case Rep. 2011;5:209.
52. Doja A, Bitnun A, Jones EL, Richardson S, Tellier R, Petric M, et al. Pediatric Epstein-Barr virus-associated encephalitis: 10-year review. J Child Neurol. 2006;21:385–91.
53. Leung AK, Davies HD, Hon KL. Rabies: epidemiology, pathogenesis, and prophylaxis. Adv Ther. 2007;24:1340–7.
54. Jackson AC. Rabies. Neurol Clin. 2008;26:717–26.
55. Hemachudha T, Wacharapluesadee S, Mitrabhakdi E, Wilde H, Morimoto K, Lewis RA. Pathophysiology of human paralytic rabies. J Neurovirol. 2005;11:93–100.
56. Eisen S, Honywood L, Shingadia D, Novelli V. Spinal tuberculosis in children. Arch Dis Child. 2012;97:724–9.
57. Gómez-Argüelles JM, Florensa J. Spinal cord involvement by tuberculosis. Rev Neurol. 2008;47:599–606.
58. Lee IC, Quek YW, Tsao SM, Chang IC, Sheu JN, Chen JY. Unusual spinal tuberculosis with cord compression in an infant. J Child Neurol. 2010;25:1284–7.
59. Consigilieri G, Kakarla UK, Theodore N. Pott disease in a 13-month-old: case report. Neurosurgery. 2011;68:E1485–90.
60. Hernández-Albújar S, Arribas JR, Royo A, González-García JJ, Peña JM, Vázquez JJ. Tuberculous radiculomyelitis complicating tuberculous meningitis: case report and review. Clin Infect Dis. 2000;30:915–21.
61. Thwaites G, Fisher M, Hemingway C, Scott G, Solomon T, Innes J, British Infection Society. British Infection Society guidelines for the diagnosis and treatment of tuberculosis of the central nervous system in adults and children. J Infect. 2009;59:167–87.
62. Lafond RE, Lukehart SA. Biological basis for syphilis. Clin Microbiol Rev. 2006;19:29–49.
63. Berger JR. Neurosyphilis and the spinal cord: then and now. J Nerv Ment Dis. 2011;199:912–3.
64. Marra CM. Update on neurosyphilis. Curr Infect Dis Rep. 2009;11:127–34.
65. Chilver-Stainer L, Fischer U, Hauf M, Fux CA, Sturzenegger M. Syphilitic myelitis: rare, nonspecific, but treatable. Neurology. 2009;72:673–5.
66. Reihsaus E, Waldbaur H, Seeling W. Spinal epidural abscess: a meta-analysis of 915 patients. Neurosurg Rev. 2000;23:175–204.

67. Tompkins M, Panuncialman I, Lucas P, Palumbo M. Spinal epidural abscess. J Emerg Med. 2010;39:384–90.
68. Wong SS, Daka S, Pastewski A, Kyaw W, Chapnick E, Sepkowitz D. Spinal epidural abscess in hemodialysis patients: a case series and review. Clin J Am Soc Nephrol. 2011;6:1495–500.
69. Liou LM, Shih PY. Epidural abscess of the cervical spine with atypical manifestations: a report of two cases. Neurologist. 2007;13:215–8.
70. Lampropoulos C, Kamposos P, Papaioannou I, Niarou V. Cervical epidural abscess caused by brucellosis. BMJ Case Rep. 2012.
71. Ekici MA, Ozbek Z, Gökoğlu A, Menkü A. Surgical management of cervical spinal epidural abscess caused by Brucella melitensis: report of two cases and review of the literature. J Korean Neurosurg Soc. 2012;51:383–7.
72. Carod-Artal FJ. Neuroschistosomiasis. Expert Rev Anti Infect Ther. 2010;8:1307–18.
73. Carod Artal FJ. Cerebral and spinal schistosomiasis. Curr Neurol Neurosci Rep. 2012;12:666–74.
74. Carod Artal FJ, Vargas AP, Horan TA, Marinho PB, Coelho Costa PH. Schistosoma mansoni myelopathy: clinical and pathologic findings. Neurology. 2004;63:388–91.
75. Peregrino AJ, Puglia PM, Nobrega JP, Livramento JA, Marques-Dias MJ, Scaff M. Schistosomiasis of the spinal cord: analysis of 80 cases. Arq Neuropsiquiatr. 2002;60: 603–8.
76. Henriques-Souza AM, Valença MM. Schistosomal myelopathy in childhood: findings of magnetic resonance imaging in 26 patients. Pediatr Neurol. 2011;45:373–6.
77. Saleem S, Belal AI, El-Ghandour NM. Spinal cord schistosomiasis: MR imaging appearance with surgical and pathologic correlation. AJNR Am J Neuroradiol. 2005;26:1646–54.
78. Doenhoff MJ, Cioli D, Utzinger J. Praziquantel: mechanisms of action, resistance and new derivatives for schistosomiasis. Curr Opin Infect Dis. 2008;21:659–67.
79. Schmutzhard E, Boongird P, Vejjajiva A. Eosinophilic meningitis and radiculomyelitis in Thailand, caused by CNS invasion of Gnathostoma spinigerum and Angiostrongylus cantonensis. J Neurol Neurosurg Psychiatry. 1988;51:80–7.
80. Sawanyawisuth K, Tiamkao S, Kanpittaya J, Dekumyoy P, Jitpimolmard S. MR imaging findings in cerebrospinal gnathostomiasis. AJNR Am J Neuroradiol. 2004;25:446–9.
81. Garcia HH, Del Brutto OH, Cysticercosis Working Group in Peru. Neurocysticercosis: updated concepts about an old disease. Lancet Neurol. 2005;4:653–61.
82. Alsina GA, Johnson JP, McBride DQ, Rhoten PR, Mehringer CM, Stokes JK. Spinal neurocysticercosis. Neurosurg Focus. 2002;12:e8.
83. Prabhakar MM, Acharya AJ, Modi DR, Jadav B. Spinal hydatid disease: a case series. J Spinal Cord Med. 2005;28:426–31.
84. Sengul G, Kadioglu HH, Kayaoglu CR, Aktas S, Akar A, Aydin IH. Treatment of spinal hydatid disease: a single center experience. J Clin Neurosci. 2008;15:507–10.
85. Hughes AJ, Biggs BA. Parasitic worms of the central nervous system: an Australian perspective. Intern Med J. 2002;32:541–53.
86. Pittner Y, Dufour JF, David G, Boibieux A, Peyramond D. Spinal cord toxoplasmosis in HIV infection. Med Mal Infect. 2009;39:401–5.
87. Aksoy A, Tanir G, Ozkan M, Oguz M, Yıldız YT. Acute disseminated encephalomyelitis associated with acute Toxoplasma gondii Infection. Pediatr Neurol. 2013;48:236–9.
88. Osoegawa M, Matsumoto S, Ochi H, Yamasaki K, Horiuchi I, Kira YO, et al. Localised myelitis caused by visceral larva migrans due to Ascaris suum masquerading as an isolated spinal cord tumour. J Neurol Neurosurg Psychiatry. 2001;70:265–6.
89. Umehara F, Ookatsu H, Hayashi D, Uchida A, Douchi Y, Kawabata H, et al. MRI studies of spinal visceral larva migrans syndrome. J Neurol Sci. 2006;249:7–12.
90. Murthy JM. Fungal infections of the central nervous system: the clinical syndromes. Neurol India. 2007;55:221–5.
91. Andaluz N, Zuccarello M. Multidrug-resistant, progressive, invasive diffuse spinal aspergillosis: case report and review of the literature. J Neurosurg Sci. 2008;52:49–53.

92. Karthik K, Shetty AP, Rajasekaran S. Spontaneous cord transection due to invasive aspergillus spondylitis in an immunocompetent child. Eur Spine J. 2011;20 Suppl 2:S188–92.
93. Ozdemir N, Celik L, Oğuzoğlu S, Yildirim L, Bezircioğlu H. Cervical vertebral osteomyelitis and epidural abscess caused by Candida albicans in a patient with chronic renal failure. Turk Neurosurg. 2008;18:207–10.
94. Sakayama K, Kidani T, Matsuda Y, Fujibuchi T, Miyazaki T, Takada K, et al. Subdural spinal granuloma resulting from Candida albicans without immunosufficiency: case report. Spine. 2002;27:E356–60.
95. Joshi TN. Candida albicans spondylodiscitis in an immunocompetent patient. J Neurosci Rural Pract. 2012;3:221–2.
96. Gupta R, Kushwaha S, Behera S, Jaiswal A, Thakur R. Vertebro-cerebral cryptococcosis mimicking tuberculosis: a diagnostic dilemma in countries with high burden of tuberculosis. Indian J Med Microbiol. 2012;30:245–8.
97. Gültaşli NZ, Ercan K, Orhun S, Albayrak S. MRI findings of intramedullary spinal cryptococcoma. Diagn Interv Radiol. 2007;13:64–7.
98. Gottlieb JR, Eismont FJ. Nonoperative treatment of vertebral blastomycosis osteomyelitis associated with paraspinal abscess and cord compression. A case report. J Bone Joint Surg Am. 2006;88:854–6.
99. Parr AM, Fewer D. Intramedullary blastomycosis in a child: case report. Can J Neurol Sci. 2004;31:282–5.
100. Bañuelos AF, Williams PL, Johnson RH, Bibi S, Fredricks DN, Gilroy SA, et al. Central nervous system abscesses due to Coccidioides species. Clin Infect Dis. 1996;22:240–50.

Chapter 11
The Human Borreliosis: Lyme Neuroborreliosis and Relapsing Fever

John J. Halperin and Juan Carlos García-Moncó

Abstract Lyme disease, caused by the tick-borne spirochete *Borrelia burgdorferi*, infects the nervous system in up to 15 % of patients. Involvement can include the peripheral nervous system, with a mononeuropathy multiplex manifest as a radiculopathy, cranial neuropathy, plexopathy, or confluent mononeuropathy multiplex. In most instances, central nervous system involvement is limited to meningitis; rarely the spinal cord or brain parenchyma can be involved. Recent work has shed light on the pathophysiologic sequence that results in neuroborreliosis, including early CNS invasion, CXCL13-stimulated B cell entry into and proliferation within the CNS, and then a prominent immune response that requires ongoing presence of organisms. Pathophysiology of peripheral nerve involvement is not well established although it similarly requires the presence of viable organisms. Future work should focus on the mechanisms of tissue injury. Regardless of the presentation, infection is highly responsive to antimicrobial therapy.

Relapsing fever is another human borreliosis caused by a variety of Borrelia species and transmitted by lice (epidemic form) or ticks (endemic form). Both are characterized by recurrent spirochetemia and can cause neurological complications similar to Lyme neuroborreliosis. Diagnosis is made by the direct observation of the spirochetes in peripheral blood during febrile episodes and by PCR. Tetracycline therapy is used.

Keywords Lyme disease • Neuroborreliosis • Diagnosis • Treatment • Pathophysiology • Garin-Bujadoux-Bannwarth syndrome • Erythema migrans • Relapsing fever • Louse-borne relapsing fever • Tick-borne relapsing fever • *Borrelia recurrentis*

J.J. Halperin, MD
Department of Neurosciences, Overlook Medical Center, Summit, NJ, USA

J.C. García-Moncó, MD (✉)
Department of Neurology, Hospital de Galdakao-Usansolo,
Barrio Labeaga S/N, Galdakao, Vizcaya, 48960, Spain
e-mail: hospit05@sarenet.es

J.C. García-Moncó (ed.), *CNS Infections*,
DOI 10.1007/978-1-4471-6401-2_11,

Introduction

Much like syphilis – and neurosyphilis – which achieved near mythological status during the centuries it ran rampant in Europe, Lyme disease is often thought to be an undiagnosable, incurable illness that will inexorably reduce its unfortunate victims to cognitive cripples. With syphilis, this misperception could be explained by the then very limited understanding of pathophysiology, particularly as it pertained to nervous system diseases. Until the advent of reaginic tests and antibiotics, syphilis was indeed often very difficult to diagnose and virtually impossible to treat. How is it then that in this age of molecular diagnosis and effective antimicrobial therapy so many misperceptions persist concerning Lyme disease – among patients and even many physicians?

To understand Lyme disease – the multisystem infection caused by the tick-borne spirochete *Borrelia burgdorferi* – and its nervous system manifestations, it is important to appreciate not only what has been learned about the illness and its pathogenesis but also the historical context that has resulted in current misperceptions.

History

The term "Lyme disease" was coined to describe what appeared to be an outbreak of juvenile rheumatoid arthritis in Lyme and Old Lyme, Connecticut [1]. Importantly from a historical perspective, the unusual nature of this outbreak was initially recognized not by an astute epidemiologist or physician but by the parents of affected children, who declined to accept their physicians' diagnoses and appealed to both the Yale School of Medicine and the Centers for Disease Control. This then triggered a series of epidemiologic, entomologic, and clinical studies leading to the recognition that the arthritis was associated both with bites by hard-shelled *Ixodes* ticks and the development of an unusual rash. Further studies led to the observation that the same tick bites and rashes could be associated with a neurologic triad [2] and occasionally with heart block. Ultimately this led to the isolation and identification of *B. burgdorferi* as the causative agent [3–5].

Several years before these investigations began, a Wisconsin dermatologist identified the same rash in a patient bitten by a wood tick; recognized the rash as erythema migrans (EM), long described in the European literature; and treated the patient successfully with penicillin [6] as had been customarily done in Europe since the 1950s [7].

The European history of this infection actually goes back to early in the twentieth century, with early characterizations of EM – ironically, perhaps, in a journal of dermatology and syphilology [8]. Of historical importance, the first extracutaneous manifestations recognized were neurological, with the description of a patient with painful radiculitis, meningitis, and EM following a tick bite [9]. The patient had a slightly positive reaginic test for syphilis; the authors conjectured that this was a tick-borne spirochetal infection and treated him successfully with neoarsphenamine. The syndrome was ultimately expanded to include both cranial neuropathies and joint symptoms. The perception from this 1922 report onward was that this was primarily a neurologic disorder.

It was only in the 1980s that the responsible microorganisms were identified as *Borrelia* spirochetes – *B. burgdorferi* sensu stricto in the USA; this species as well as *B. garinii* and *B. afzelii* in Europe (as well as several less commonly seen species) [10].

Disease manifestations appear to differ somewhat depending on the specific *Borrelia* species – although to some extent this perception may be colored by an ascertainment bias since historically Lyme disease has been perceived to be a rheumatologic disease in the USA, while Garin-Bujadoux-Bannwarth syndrome is felt to be a neurologic one in Europe.

Diagnosis

Like syphilis, and unlike most other bacterial infections, diagnosis generally relies on demonstration of an antibody response to the causative organism, as direct microbiologic diagnostics are of limited sensitivity and availability. EM, and occasionally elements of Garin-Bujadoux-Bannwarth syndrome, can occur before a measurable antibody response has developed. In the case of EM, the appearance – in the appropriate context – is sufficiently characteristic that treatment should be initiated without even trying to obtain serologic results – particularly since the latter will be negative in over 50 % of such patients [11]. This seronegativity should not be interpreted as a unique flaw in the laboratory tools available in Lyme disease but rather as the perfectly normal lag between antigen exposure and development of a detectable antibody response.

A number of misconceptions about serologic testing are common and contribute greatly to the "controversy" surrounding this infection. First, with the exception of the normal, very early seronegativity just described, "seronegative Lyme disease" occurs rarely if ever. Early reports of this [12] probably reflected shortcomings of the then available technology. Virtually all patients with symptoms attributable to Lyme disease, who have been ill for more than 4–6 weeks, should have positive serologic results.

Once a patient has developed an antibody response, this will usually continue to be evident for quite some time – reflecting the normal function of the humoral immune response. There is no reason to expect the antibody response to disappear at the end of curative treatment. Hence, the serology cannot be used as a measure of treatment efficacy and treating until the serology becomes negative is illogical. For the same reason, the presence of a positive serology can only be considered evidence of infection at some time in the past and not necessarily current infection. Taking antibiotics at the time the serum sample is obtained has no effect on the test results.

Recommended serologic testing involves a two-tier approach [13]. An initial screening test – typically an enzyme-linked immunosorbent assay (ELISA), but

Table 11.1 Western blot criteria for the serologic diagnosis of Lyme disease, applicable only if ELISA (or IFA) positive or borderline [13]

	IgM	IgG
Bands tested (kD MW)	24, 39, 41	18, 21, 28, 30, 39, 41, 45, 58, 66, 93
# needed for Dx	Any 2 of 3	Any 5 of 10
Applicability	Only in first 4–6 weeks of disease	Required if symptoms > 4–6 weeks duration

occasionally an immunofluorescent assay (IFA) – is used to measure total *B. burgdorferi-reacting* antibody, comparing this immunoreactivity to normal controls. This sensitive screening method can lack specificity. ELISAs to a specific antigen known as C6 have been proposed as an alternative initial test, particularly since the antigen is present in both North American and European *B. burgdorferi* strains [14]. Although the specificity of this as a single test remains unclear, a recent study suggests it may be more useful as a secondary confirmatory test in individuals whose conventional ELISA is borderline or positive [15].

Until this finding is confirmed, though, Western blots – to determine the specific antigens that result in ELISA positivity – remain the recommended confirmatory assay in such individuals. Western blots are rarely informative in patients whose ELISAs are negative – the signal to noise ratio of the background reactivity makes it very difficult to judge the significance of any bands that might be present in such a situation. The criteria for interpretation of Western blots (Table 11.1) are based on statistical analyses of large numbers of samples, to determine which combinations of bands have the greatest positive predictive value for a correct diagnosis. Interpretation is not based on the presence of any single unique bands that in and of themselves make the diagnosis likely.

Western blots are performed separately for IgG and IgM antibodies. Studies have demonstrated that patients with five or more of ten selected IgG bands (Table 11.1) almost certainly have been infected with *B. burgdorferi*. Such IgG bands should be demonstrable in essentially all patients with more than 4–6 weeks of symptomatic infection. IgM blots, interpreted based on the presence of two of three selected bands (Table 11.1), are only meaningful in the first 4–6 weeks, before the serologic response has evolved to produce IgG. IgM generally is far more cross-reactive than IgG. With a requirement of just two bands, there is considerable risk of false positives, particularly in patients with hypergammaglobulinemia due to any inflammatory state. Isolated IgM blot positivity in a patient with many months of symptoms should never be interpreted as evidence of ongoing *B. burgdorferi* infection.

Intrathecal Antibody Production

Although the innate, humoral, and cell-mediated arms of the immune system all play important roles in the host response to this infection, the humoral response is quite prominent. This is particularly apparent when infection involves the central nervous system (CNS). Since normally only a small amount of peripheral blood immunoglobulin enters the CNS, and since the CNS behaves as an immunologically distinct compartment, to which antigen-specific B cells migrate and then proliferate, measurement of CSF antibodies can be quite informative. The prominent intrathecal humoral response often results in an increase in total CSF IgG concentration, reflected in an increased IgG synthesis rate or IgG index. Because this increased synthesis is directed at a small number of antigens, oligoclonal bands may be evident, a finding reported more frequently in patients infected with European strains. This added production of antibodies specific to the antigens of the infecting organisms allows a particularly helpful diagnostic tool. In many patients with CNS infection, the proportion of CSF IgG specific to *B. burgdorferi* exceeds that in serum, allowing a calculation of intrathecal production of specific antibody by comparing CSF and serum immunoreactivity [16–18]. This measure of intrathecal antibody production (ITAb) has high specificity for CNS Lyme disease infection. False positives occur with neurosyphilis, but this can usually be distinguished by measuring CSF reaginic antibodies, such as the VDRL or RPR, which occur rarely if ever in neuroborreliosis. In theory, relapsing fever, another *borrelia* infection, could produce cross-reactions, but there is so little geographic overlap between these infections that this is rarely an issue. The one problematic "false positive" is that apparent ITAb may persist for years after successful eradication of the CNS infection [19], presumably as antibody production in the CNS and the periphery gradually decline in parallel.

The greater concern with this measure is with its sensitivity. European studies, which historically required the presence of ITAb to confirm the diagnosis of CNS neuroborreliosis, not surprisingly find sensitivity to be nearly 100 %. In the USA, small studies of acute neuroborreliosis have reported sensitivity as high as 90 % [20], but with more chronic syndromes estimates have been closer to 50 % [21]. One of the challenges in defining sensitivity is the absence of an alternative, more definitive diagnostic test for CNS neuroborreliosis. As a result, some patients included in these studies may not have actually had CNS infection. Since there is no reason to think ITAb would need to be present in patients with peripheral nerve involvement, or in those with an infection-related encephalopathy, the implications of these observations are unclear.

Clinical Phenomenology

Both EM and the neurologic triad of meningitis, cranial neuritis, and radiculoneuropathy occur commonly in both European and US patients. EM, which occurs in up to 90 % of infected children [22], typically consists of a single erythroderm arising at the site of a tick bite. Unlike an acute allergic reaction to tick saliva, which appears almost immediately, EM appears days to at most a month after the bite. Its hallmark is its slow expansion, day by day, ultimately becoming many inches in diameter (minimum of 2 in. for CDC diagnostic criteria). The rash, which results from spirochetes slowly migrating centrifugally from the initial site of inoculation, can be remarkably asymptomatic. If not in a readily visualized location, it may go unnoticed. In some patients spirochetes disseminate hematogenously from the initial locus, seeding remote cutaneous sites where secondary EMs can develop. This occurs in about a fourth of US patients, a smaller proportion in Europe.

B. afzelii causes an unusual late cutaneous manifestation in European patients, known as acrodermatitis atrophicans, in which the skin, typically of a distal extremity, becomes tissue-paper thin and discolored. This disorder has not been recognized in patients infected in the USA. Even though Bannwarth's paper on this neurologic disorder included the term "rheumatism" in its title [23], joint involvement has been considered the hallmark of US Lyme disease, felt to occur in up to 85 % of patients not treated early in the infection. This arthritis is distinctive in that it preferentially affects single large joints, which spontaneously become red and swollen and then gradually improve. Over the course of the illness, different joints are affected, seemingly at random.

Cardiac involvement, which generally occurs quite early in infection, typically consists of conduction abnormalities. In severe cases it can include complete heart block, requiring a temporary pacemaker. This almost invariably resolves with antibiotic treatment. Occurring in about 5 % of patients in early US series, this is now felt to occur even less commonly.

Neurologic Manifestations

Overall, CNS or peripheral nervous system (PNS) involvement occurs in 10–15 % of infected patients [24] – a number that appears to be similar in both Europe and the USA. The classic three manifestations – meningitis, cranial neuritis, and radiculoneuritis – typically occur quite early in infection [25]. Since ticks feed from spring through fall, this is when these are most likely to present. Each element of the triad presents its own diagnostic challenges. Meningitis, which may occur in isolation or in association with either or both of the other two elements, varies widely in its symptomatology. Some patients have severe headache, photosensitivity, and neck stiffness – with or without inflammation in the cerebrospinal fluid (CSF). Other patients with cranial neuritis may have a substantial CSF pleocytosis with no meningeal symptoms. When abnormal, the CSF typically shows a modest lymphocyte-predominant pleocytosis (up to several 100 WBCs/mm^3), mildly increased protein, and normal glucose. There may be evidence of local production of anti-*B. burgdorferi* antibodies within the CNS – i.e., disproportionately increased *Borrelia*-specific antibodies (ITAb). In patients in whom CNS inflammation has been present for a longer period of time, particularly with European strains of *Borrelia*, there may be sufficient overproduction of immunoglobulins that patients have both increased total IgG in the CSF (increased IgG synthesis rate or IgG index) and even oligoclonal bands.

Since Lyme meningitis and enteroviral meningitis often occur in similar locations at similar times of year, several algorithms have been proposed to try to differentiate between these entities. The common thread is that Lyme meningitis tends to have a more indolent evolution and a more strongly mononuclear cell pleocytosis [26–28]. The most compelling differentiating element is the presence of an associated VII nerve palsy, which virtually never occurs in viral meningitis. Unfortunately, the other criteria overlap so extensively that they are not terribly helpful.

Cranial neuropathies are probably the most common presenting neurologic sign (as meningitis may be asymptomatic). The facial nerve is the most commonly involved; Lyme disease is one of the few disorders associated with bilateral facial nerve palsies (others including sarcoidosis, HIV, other basilar meningitides, Guillain–Barré syndrome). In endemic areas, Lyme disease-associated facial nerve palsy (LAFP) may be the cause of about a quarter of cases of facial nerve palsy [29]. As with meningitis, a number of authors have attempted to develop algorithms to differentiate between LAFP and Bell's palsy; these have emphasized the greater likelihood of a CSF pleocytosis with LAFP [30] and the more frequent co-occurrence of other neurologic signs or symptoms, elements which may be helpful but are not sufficiently compelling to obviate the need for laboratory support for the diagnosis.

Other cranial nerves can be involved in neuroborreliosis, but substantially less commonly. Nerves III, IV, and VI are involved occasionally, as are V and VIII, each causing the expected symptoms. Optic nerve involvement has been reported, but most case reports are not compelling [31]. Involvement of nerves IX–XII is reported rarely.

Peripheral nerve involvement occurs with some frequency. As described by Garin and Bujadoux, this can involve striking radicular pain, mimicking a mechanical radiculopathy, typically involving one or a few dermatomes. Weakness and atrophy can be far more impressive than sensory loss. The frequency of this disorder is difficult to estimate as symptoms are probably frequently misdiagnosed as mechanical in origin and testing not performed. Patients may present as plexopathies, mononeuropathies, mononeuropathy multiplex, or even as an apparent diffuse polyneuropathy. Notably, all – including most cranial neuropathies – probably represent varying manifestations of a mononeuropathy multiplex [32, 33]. Biopsies consistently demonstrate perivascular inflammatory infiltrates with neither vessel wall necrosis nor unambiguous evidence of spirochetes or their antigens [34–38].

Parenchymal CNS involvement occurs rarely and has been reported primarily in patients infected with European strains. Least rare is involvement of the spinal cord at the affected segmental level in Garin-Bujadoux-Bannwarth radiculitis. More rarely patients develop parenchymal brain involvement, presenting with focal symptoms and findings consistent with the location [39, 40]. This disorder appears to affect white matter more often than gray, rarely causes seizures, and can cause MRI abnormalities similar in character to those seen in demyelinating disease, but without the same anatomic predilection [16].

Lyme Encephalopathy

Probably the disorder responsible for more of the confusion and controversy related to Lyme disease than any other is the phenomenon usually referred to as Lyme encephalopathy. Originally described in patients with other clear evidence of Lyme disease, e.g., arthritis, cardiac conduction abnormalities, acute neuroborreliosis, the earliest studies indicated that this was probably not caused by CNS infection but rather was analogous to the "toxic metabolic" encephalopathy occurring in most other infections and inflammatory states – from urinary tract infections and pneumonia to acute flares of rheumatoid arthritis [16, 41, 42]. However, three incorrect assumptions rapidly entered the discussion and have been virtually impossible to eradicate. First was that this disorder – consisting of difficulty with mental processing, memory and other cognitive functions – was indicative of a CNS infection. Second was the sense that this was in some way specific to Lyme disease. Third was the notion that it was sufficiently specific for Lyme disease that these symptoms, in and of themselves, were evidence of active neuroborreliosis in need of treatment, regardless of any other clinical, laboratory, or epidemiologic considerations. The last has, in turn, resulted in the notion of post Lyme disease syndrome, patients who have persisting fatigue and cognitive symptoms following what should be microbiologically curative treatment.

Numerous studies of "Lyme encephalopathy" have shown that intrathecal antibody production or even other, less specific markers of CNS infection such as a CSF pleocytosis are neither necessary nor sufficient for this diagnosis [43]. Unfortunately, the observed lack of ITAb in these patients, coupled with the misperception that this state is necessarily due to CNS infection, probably contributed to the conclusion that ITAb is an insensitive measure of CNS infection. No studies have identified unique biologic or neuropsychologic markers that differentiate between Lyme encephalopathy and other toxic metabolic encephalopathies.

Finally, the notion of post Lyme disease syndrome (or encephalopathy) is itself suspect. While uncontrolled trials emphasize that these symptoms persist in about 40 % of treated patients [44, 45], a number confirmed in some trials that include control groups, the latter studies have found a comparable frequency of symptoms in controls – both in children [46] and in adults [47]. Other controlled trials have found a similar rate of subjective symptoms among patients previously treated for Lyme disease [48], a rate higher than that in the included control group, but no difference in objective abnormalities when these individuals are compared to controls. Others have found lower rates of subjective symptoms in treated patients, with these lower rates indistinguishable from that in controls [49]. Since it is clear that these symptoms occur in large numbers of otherwise healthy individuals [50], and since the popular perception that these symptoms persist following Lyme disease is so ubiquitous, leading patients and others to assume a causal relationship, it seems quite plausible that "post Lyme disease syndrome" is primarily due to ascertainment bias and is not a real entity.

Pathophysiology

Much has been learned about the pathophysiology of neuroborreliosis in recent years. It has long been clear that *B. burgdorferi* can cross the blood-brain barrier very early in infection [51–53]. *B. burgdorferi* bind to brain microvascular endothelial cells [54] and then cross the blood-brain barrier in a process that requires metalloproteinases and plasmin [55]. Strains of *B. burgdorferi* vary in their ability to accomplish this [55]. Once inside the CNS, *B. burgdorferi* appears to trigger the production of CXCL13 in endothelial cells and microglia. This cytokine then induces B cell in-migration and proliferation [56].

One of the conceptual challenges has always been the great difficulty in finding evidence of spirochetes in CSF or tissue from patients with known CNS *B. burgdorferi* infection. Even polymerase chain reaction (PCR)-based techniques only detect spirochetes in a small percentage of CSF samples from patients with known Lyme meningitis [51, 57]. Yet the consistent improvement in symptoms with antibiotic treatment seems to provide compelling if indirect evidence of the requirement for viable organisms in disease pathogenesis. The alternative hypothesis that disease might be due to immune cross reactivity between *B. burgdorferi* and neural antigens [58, 59] has seemed less plausible based both on this rapid improvement with treatment and the corollary observation that patients recover from nervous system disease despite the persistence of most anti-*B. burgdorferi* antibodies. Although some studies have found evidence of *B. burgdorferi* in brain samples of experimentally infected animals [60], these studies have been unconvincing due to the possibility of CSF contamination. More recent work demonstrating organisms in dorsal root ganglia is perhaps the most suggestive evidence to date [61]. Other studies showing that microglia stimulated by *B. burgdorferi* might trigger oligodendroglia apoptosis [62] are intriguing, but the implication of this observation in neuroborreliosis is unclear, given the extreme rarity of CNS parenchymal infection.

Treatment

Fortunately, *B. burgdorferi* remains highly sensitive to widely available antimicrobials. Recommended treatment for cutaneous and other nonnervous system infections consists of oral amoxicillin, cefuroxime axetil, or doxycycline (Table 11.2). Although for many years parenteral penicillin, ceftriaxone, and cefotaxime have been recommended for nervous system infection, numerous European studies support the use of oral doxycycline for Lyme meningitis, cranial neuritis, and radiculoneuritis, with efficacy shown to be comparable to parenteral treatment in multiple controlled trials [63]. Although these studies have not, to date, been replicated in the USA, similar antibiotic sensitivities would strongly suggest efficacy of such regimens in US patients. No studies have addressed treatment specifically in those very rare individuals with parenchymal CNS infections, but by analogy to other brain

Table 11.2 Treatment recommendations [65]

	Adult	Pediatric[a]
Medication, duration		
Parenteral (2–4 weeks)		
Ceftriaxone[b]	2 g/day IV	50–75 mg/kg/day
Cefotaxime	2 g q8/IV	150–200 mg/kg/day in 3–4 divided doses
Penicillin	20–24 million units IV/day	300,000 units/kg/day divided, every 4 h
Oral (3, possibly 4 weeks)		
Doxycycline[c]	100 mg PO b.i.d. to q.i.d.	4 mg/kg/day in 2 divided doses
Limited data but probably effective		
Amoxicillin	500 mg PO t.i.d.	50 mg/kg/day in 3 divided doses
Cefuroxime axetil	500 mg PO b.i.d	30 mg/kg/day in 2 divided doses

Notes:
[a]Pediatric weight-based doses should never exceed the recommended adult dose
[b]Ceftriaxone should not be used late in pregnancy
[c]Doxycycline should not be used in pregnant women or children under the age of 8 years

infections, parenteral treatment would seem the most reasonable. Multiple studies have consistently shown that prolonged treatment – for more than 4 weeks – is rarely needed, but carries significant potential for side effects [14, 64–66].

Relapsing Fever

Relapsing fever (RF) is a multisystemic borreliosis that occurs in epidemic (louse-borne) and endemic (tick-borne) forms and is caused by a variety of Borrelia species. The former is caused *Borrelia recurrentis* and is transmitted by the human body louse *Pediculus humanus*, while the endemic form is transmitted by soft-bodied ticks, mostly of the genus Ornithodoros and caused by several different Old and New World Borrelia species. RF is found in Africa, Asia, Central and South America, southwestern North America, and the Mediterranean basin. Humans are the main reservoir for the epidemic form, while several species of rodents are the reservoirs for the endemic species.

Neurological Manifestations of RF

In contrast to Lyme disease, where spirochetes in the blood are difficult to detect, RF is characterized by a recurrent spirochetemia that coincides with episodes of high fever and constitutional symptoms, such as headache, malaise, and myalgia.

In time, the relapses of spirochetemia become shorter and less frequent. The recurrent nature of these borrelioses is due to a complex interplay of antigenic variation of the organisms and the immune system, notably, the antibody response [67].

The pattern of neurological and ocular manifestations of the relapsing fevers closely parallels and resembles those of Lyme disease [25, 68].

Studies of outbreaks of tick-borne RF have repeatedly shown that the neurological complications dominate the clinical picture. This clinical feature of relapsing fever has been known since the early twentieth century, when studies demonstrated that spirochetes were found in the cerebrospinal fluid of patients, thus providing definitive evidence of nervous system invasion.

The most common neurological manifestations of RF are meningitis and peripheral facial nerve palsy, followed by radiculitis, encephalitis, and psychiatric disturbances [68].

Neurological abnormalities are more common in tick-borne RF than in the epidemic form, with frequencies that greatly vary from one clinical series to another. Almost half of the patients affected by RF caused by *B. dutonii* in Africa presented meningismus [69], as compared with only 9 % in another series [70]. Likewise, a variable degree of pleocytosis was present in the cerebrospinal fluid of 50–100 % of patients with this type of neuroborreliosis [69], further underscoring the variable presentation of the relapsing fevers.

Encephalitis occurs occasionally in RF, sometimes accompanied by seizures and intense somnolence. Focal signs of central nervous system involvement such as hemiplegia and aphasia have been infrequently reported. Cranial nerve palsy, particularly of the seventh nerve, is common in tick-borne RF, usually appearing after the second febrile episode. Cranial palsies usually resolve spontaneously in several weeks, and this feature closely resembles the findings in Lyme disease. Little information is available about the cerebrospinal fluid findings in cranial palsy patients, but increased proteins have been noted. Radicular and spinal cord involvement may also appear, resulting in sciatic pain and sometimes paraplegia. Psychiatric problems include delirium and hallucinations in a variable degree of intensity [68].

Neurophthalmological problems may also occur in tick-borne infections and include optic neuritis and uveitis. Eye involvement may be bilateral and almost always appears after several febrile episodes [71]. Sometimes it follows a relapsing course and may result in residual visual loss.

Diagnosis

The definitive diagnosis of relapsing fever is established by demonstrating the presence of Borrelias in the peripheral blood of febrile patients, in whom spirochetes are found in approximately 70 % of cases by dark field microscopy or in Giemsa- or Wright-stained thick and thin smears [72]. Due to the high rate of antigenic variation of these organisms, serological assays based on antibody production are initially unreliable.

The polymerase chain reaction (PCR) is useful for the diagnosis of relapsing fever. It can be performed on blood samples or culture medium that is growing Borrelia species [73].

Treatment

Antibiotic therapy is employed in RF patients, not only to treat the neurological manifestations of RF but to prevent further febrile episodes. Systemic *louse-borne RF* fever is best treated with a single oral dose of 500 mg of tetracycline or 200 mg of doxycycline. A single oral dose of erythromycin (500 mg) is also effective and is indicated in pregnant women and children, in whom tetracycline should be avoided.

Intramuscular penicillin G procaine is an alternative (400,000–800,000 units). The recurrence rate after antibiotics is less than five percent.

Tick-borne RF fever is treated with oral tetracycline (500 mg every 6 h) or doxycycline (100 mg twice daily) for 10 days, since the relapse rate is higher (20 %) and treatment failures are more common.

Erythromycin is an alternative in intolerant or allergic individuals, at a dose of 500 mg every 6 h for the same period.

When neurological manifestations are present, intravenous antibiotics are indicated, such as penicillin G (three million units every 4 h) or ceftriaxone (2 g once daily or 1 g twice daily) for at least 2 weeks or longer depending on the patient's response.

Rapid removal of large numbers of spirochetes from the circulation after antibiotic treatment requires that patients under therapy be monitored for the frequent appearance of Jarisch-Herxheimer reactions, which occur within 2 h of antibiotic administration and present with fever, shivering, and hypotension.

Pathophysiology

The laboratory mouse has been used to reproduce the neuroborreliosis of relapsing fever experimentally for many years. The presence of large numbers of motile spirochetes in the circulation could be a factor in the breakdown of the blood-brain barrier through waste products or mediators of inflammation so that penetration into the CNS could be achieved more easily. Immunocompetent and immunodeficient mice have been infected successfully with both old and new world species of relapsing fever Borrelia. Infection of mice with subsequent neurological manifestations can be achieved through cutaneous inoculation, the route that reproduces transmission by ticks [74].

The most common neurologic manifestation in mice is meningitis with spirochetes detectable infrequently in the leptomeninges and in the cerebrospinal fluid. Despite the paucity of spirochetes in the brain, there is cerebral microgliosis that is more severe in immunodeficient mice. This finding emphasizes the role of the immune response in the development and severity of relapsing fever. Of note is the vestibular dysfunction of mice infected with relapsing fever Borrelia. While spirochetes have been observed in cranial and peripheral nerves, there are no studies documenting peripheral nerve disease in mice [5].

RF Borrelias are best known for the phenomenon of antigenic variation, which allows them to spontaneously change their serotype by switching the expression of variable major proteins (VMPs) of two sizes, large (Vlp) and small (Vsp). A switch in VMP allows RF Borrelias to escape killing by the host's serotype-specific antibody response. RF Borrelias persist in the brain after they disappear from the blood, a phenomenon known as residual brain infection (RBI) [75].

Borrelia miyamotoi *and Meningoencephalitis*

Borrelia miyamotoi is another spirochete belonging to the RF taxonomic group and transmitted by ixodid ticks and hence potentially concurrent with the Lyme disease agent. It is unclear whether *B. miyamotoi* causes disease in humans, but a recent report suggested that this spirochete was responsible for a meningoencephalitis in an 80-year-old patient immunosuppressed as a result of non-Hodgkin's lymphoma who presented with progressive cognitive decline and weight loss [76]. He had had a previously treated erythema migrans and was resident in an endemic area for Lyme disease. Brain magnetic resonance imaging was normal, but his cerebrospinal fluid examination disclosed pleocytosis and increased proteins, and staining showed the presence of several spirochetes that were identified as *B. miyamotoi* by real-time polymerase chain reaction. Treated with intravenous penicillin, his status improved to normal. The authors concluded that the patient's illness was caused by *B. miyamotoi*. For many years, the relapsing fever Borrelias were thought to be transmitted exclusively by soft ticks, whereas the Lyme Borrelias were transmitted by hard ticks. *B. miyamotoi*, a relapsing fever Borrelia transmitted by a hard tick, suggests that these differences are not as clear-cut as once thought, particularly in areas where RF and Lyme Borrelia coexist [77].

References

1. Steere AC, Malawista SE, Hardin JA, Ruddy S, Askenase W, Andiman WA. Erythema chronicum migrans and Lyme arthritis. The enlarging clinical spectrum. Ann Intern Med. 1977;86:685–98.
2. Reik L, Steere AC, Bartenhagen NH, Shope RE, Malawista SE. Neurologic abnormalities of Lyme disease. Medicine. 1979;58:281–94.
3. Benach JL, Bosler EM, Hanrahan JP, et al. Spirochetes isolated from the blood of two patients with Lyme disease. N Engl J Med. 1983;308:740–2.
4. Burgdorfer W, Barbour AG, Hayes SF, Benach JL, Grunwaldt E, Davis JP. Lyme disease-a tick-borne spirochetosis? Science. 1982;216:1317–9.

5. Steere AC, Grodzicki RL, Kornblatt AN, et al. The spirochetal etiology of Lyme disease. N Engl J Med. 1983;308:733–40.
6. Scrimenti RJ. Erythema chronicum migrans. Arch Dermatol. 1970;102:104–5.
7. Hollstrom E. Successful treatment of erythema migrans Afzelius. Acta Derm Venereol. 1951;31:235–43.
8. Azfellius A. Erythema chronicum migrans. Arch Dermatol Venereol (Stockh). 1921;2:120–5.
9. Garin C, Bujadoux A. Paralysie par les tiques. J Med Lyon. 1922;71:765–7.
10. Asbrink E, Hovmark A, Hederstedt B. The spirochetal etiology of acrodermatitis chronica atrophicans Herxheimer. Acta Derm Venereol. 1984;64:506–12.
11. Nowakowski J, Schwartz I, Liveris D, et al. Laboratory diagnostic techniques for patients with early Lyme disease associated with erythema migrans: a comparison of different techniques. Clin Infect Dis. 2001;33:2023–7.
12. Dattwyler RJ, Volkman DJ, Luft BJ, Halperin JJ, Thomas J, Golightly MG. Seronegative Lyme disease. Dissociation of specific T- and B-lymphocyte responses to Borrelia burgdorferi. N Engl J Med. 1988;319:1441–6.
13. Anonymous. Recommendations for test performance and interpretation from the Second National Conference on Serologic Diagnosis of Lyme Disease. MMWR. 1995;44:590–1.
14. Wormser GP, Schriefer M, Aguero-Rosenfeld ME, et al. Single-tier testing with the C6 peptide ELISA kit compared with two-tier testing for Lyme disease. Diagn Microbiol Infect Dis. 2013;75:9–15.
15. Branda JA, Strle F, Strle K, Sikand N, Ferraro MJ, Steere AC. Performance of United States serologic assays in the diagnosis of lyme borreliosis acquired in Europe. Clin Infect Dis. 2013;57:333–40.
16. Halperin JJ, Luft BJ, Anand AK, et al. Lyme neuroborreliosis: central nervous system manifestations. Neurology. 1989;39:753–9.
17. Hansen K, Cruz M, Link H. Oligoclonal Borrelia burgdorferi-specific IgG antibodies in cerebrospinal fluid in Lyme neuroborreliosis. J Infect Dis. 1990;161:1194–202.
18. Stiernstedt GT, Granstrom M, Hederstedt B, Skoldenberg B. Diagnosis of spirochetal meningitis by enzyme-linked immunosorbent assay and indirect immunofluorescence assay in serum and cerebrospinal fluid. J Clin Microbiol. 1985;21:819–25.
19. Hammers-Berggren S, Hansen K, Lebech AM, Karlsson M. Borrelia burgdorferi-specific intrathecal antibody production in neuroborreliosis: a follow-up study. Neurology. 1993;43:169–75.
20. Halperin JJ, Volkman DJ, Wu P. Central nervous system abnormalities in Lyme neuroborreliosis. Neurology. 1991;41:1571–82.
21. Steere AC, Berardi VP, Weeks KE, Logigian EL, Ackermann R. Evaluation of the intrathecal antibody response to Borrelia burgdorferi as a diagnostic test for Lyme neuroborreliosis. J Infect Dis. 1990;161:1203–9.
22. Gerber MA, Shapiro ED, Burke GS, Parcells VJ, Bell GL. Lyme disease in children in southeastern Connecticut. Pediatric Lyme Disease Study Group. N Engl J Med. 1996;335:1270–4.
23. Bannwarth A. Chronische lymphocytare meningitis, entzundliche polyneuritis und "rheumatismus". Arch Psychiatr Nervenkr. 1941;113:284–376.
24. Bacon RM, Kugeler KJ, Mead PS, Centers for Disease Control, and Prevention. Surveillance for Lyme diseas--nited States, 1992–2006. MMWR Surveill Summ. 2008;57:1–9.
25. Garcia-Monco JC, Benach JL. Lyme neuroborreliosis. Ann Neurol. 1995;37:691–702.
26. Cohn KA, Thompson AD, Shah SS, et al. Validation of a clinical prediction rule to distinguish Lyme meningitis from aseptic meningitis. Pediatrics. 2012;129:e46–53.
27. Garro AC, Rutman M, Simonsen K, Jaeger JL, Chapin K, Lockhart G. Prospective validation of a clinical prediction model for Lyme meningitis in children. Pediatrics. 2009;123:e829–34.
28. Tuerlinckx D, Bodart E, Jamart J, Glupczynski Y. Prediction of Lyme meningitis based on a logistic regression model using clinical and cerebrospinal fluid analysis: a European study. Pediatr Infect Dis J. 2009;28:394–7.
29. Halperin JJ, Golightly M. Lyme borreliosis in Bell's palsy. Long Island Neuroborreliosis Collaborative Study Group. Neurology. 1992;42:1268–70.

30. Bremell D, Hagberg L. Clinical characteristics and cerebrospinal fluid parameters in patients with peripheral facial palsy caused by Lyme neuroborreliosis compared with facial palsy of unknown origin (Bell's palsy). BMC Infect Dis. 2011;11:215.
31. Sibony P, Halperin J, Coyle PK, Patel K. Reactive Lyme serology in optic neuritis. J Neuroophthalmol. 2005;25:71–82.
32. Halperin J, Luft BJ, Volkman DJ, Dattwyler RJ. Lyme neuroborreliosis. Peripheral nervous system manifestations. Brain. 1990;113(Pt 4):1207–21.
33. Logigian EL, Steere AC. Clinical and electrophysiologic findings in chronic neuropathy of Lyme disease. Neurology. 1992;42:303–11.
34. Camponovo F, Meier C. Neuropathy of vasculitic origin in a case of Garin-Bujadoux-Bannwarth syndrome with positive borrelia antibody response. J Neurol. 1986;233:69–72.
35. Elamin M, Alderazi Y, Mullins G, Farrell MA, O'Connell S, Counihan TJ. Perineuritis in acute lyme neuroborreliosis. Muscle Nerve. 2009;39:851–4.
36. England JD, Bohm Jr RP, Roberts ED, Philipp MT. Mononeuropathy multiplex in rhesus monkeys with chronic Lyme disease. Ann Neurol. 1997;41:375–84.
37. Halperin JJ, Little BW, Coyle PK, Dattwyler RJ. Lyme disease: cause of a treatable peripheral neuropathy. Neurology. 1987;37:1700–6.
38. Vallat JM, Hugon J, Lubeau M, Leboutet MJ, Dumas M, Desproges-Gotteron R. Tick-bite meningoradiculoneuritis: clinical, electrophysiologic, and histologic findings in 10 cases. Neurology. 1987;37:749–53.
39. Ackermann R, Rehse-Kupper B, Gollmer E, Schmidt R. Chronic neurologic manifestations of erythema migrans borreliosis. Ann N Y Acad Sci. 1988;539:16–23.
40. Kalina P, Decker A, Kornel E, Halperin JJ. Lyme disease of the brainstem. Neuroradiology. 2005;47:903–7.
41. Halperin JJ, Krupp LB, Golightly MG, Volkman DJ. Lyme borreliosis-associated encephalopathy. Neurology. 1990;40:1340–3.
42. Krupp LB, Masur D, Schwartz J, et al. Cognitive functioning in late Lyme borreliosis. Arch Neurol. 1991;48:1125–9.
43. Logigian EL, Kaplan RF, Steere AC. Chronic neurologic manifestations of Lyme disease. N Engl J Med. 1990;323:1438–44.
44. Eikeland R, Mygland A, Herlofson K, Ljostad U. Risk factors for a non-favorable outcome after treated European neuroborreliosis. Acta Neurol Scand. 2013;127:154–60.
45. Ljostad U, Mygland A. Remaining complaints 1 year after treatment for acute Lyme neuroborreliosis; frequency, pattern and risk factors. Eur J Neurol. 2010;17:118–23.
46. Skogman BH, Glimaker K, Nordwall M, Vrethem M, Odkvist L, Forsberg P. Long-term clinical outcome after Lyme neuroborreliosis in childhood. Pediatrics. 2012;130:262–9.
47. Seltzer EG, Gerber MA, Cartter ML, Freudigman K, Shapiro ED. Long-term outcomes of persons with Lyme disease. JAMA. 2000;283:609–16.
48. Shadick NA, Phillips CB, Sangha O, et al. Musculoskeletal and neurologic outcomes in patients with previously treated Lyme disease. Ann Intern Med. 1999;131:919–26.
49. Cerar D, Cerar T, Ruzic-Sabljic E, Wormser GP, Strle F. Subjective symptoms after treatment of early Lyme disease. Am J Med. 2010;123:79–86.
50. Luo N, Johnson JA, Shaw JW, Feeny D, Coons SJ. Self-reported health status of the general adult U.S. population as assessed by the EQ-5D and Health Utilities Index. Med care. 2005;43:1078–86.
51. Keller TL, Halperin JJ, Whitman M. PCR detection of Borrelia burgdorferi DNA in cerebrospinal fluid of Lyme neuroborreliosis patients. Neurology. 1992;42:32–42.
52. Luft BJ, Steinman CR, Neimark HC, et al. Invasion of the central nervous system by Borrelia burgdorferi in acute disseminated infection. JAMA. 1992;267:1364–7.
53. Garcia-Monco JC, Villar BF, Alen JC, Benach JL. Borrelia burgdorferi in the central nervous system: experimental and clinical evidence for early invasion. J Infect Dis. 1990;161:1187–93.
54. Grab DJ, Perides G, Dumler JS, et al. Borrelia burgdorferi, host-derived proteases, and the blood–brain barrier. Infect Immun. 2005;73:1014–22.

55. Grab DJ, Nyarko E, Nikolskaia OV, Kim YV, Dumler JS. Human brain microvascular endothelial cell traversal by Borrelia burgdorferi requires calcium signaling. Clin Microbiol Infect. 2009;15:422–6.
56. Rupprecht TA, Plate A, Adam M, et al. The chemokine CXCL13 is a key regulator of B cell recruitment to the cerebrospinal fluid in acute Lyme neuroborreliosis. J Neuroinflammation. 2009;6:42.
57. Lebech AM, Hansen K, Brandrup F, Clemmensen O, Halkier-Sorensen L. Diagnostic value of PCR for detection of Borrelia burgdorferi DNA in clinical specimens from patients with erythema migrans and Lyme neuroborreliosis. Mol Diagn. 2000;5:139–50.
58. Sigal LH. Molecular mimicry and Lyme borreliosis. Ann Neurol. 1990;28:195–6.
59. Sigal LH, Tatum AH. Lyme disease patients' serum contains IgM antibodies to Borrelia burgdorferi that cross-react with neuronal antigens. Neurology. 1988;38:1439–42.
60. Pachner AR, Zhang WF, Schaefer H, Schaefer S, O'Neill T. Detection of active infection in nonhuman primates with Lyme neuroborreliosis: comparison of PCR, culture, and a bioassay. J Clin Microbiol. 1998;36:3243–7.
61. Ramesh G, Borda JT, Gill A, et al. Possible role of glial cells in the onset and progression of Lyme neuroborreliosis. J Neuroinflammation. 2009;6:23.
62. Ramesh G, Benge S, Pahar B, Philipp MT. A possible role for inflammation in mediating apoptosis of oligodendrocytes as induced by the Lyme disease spirochete Borrelia burgdorferi. J Neuroinflammation. 2012;9:72.
63. Halperin JJ, Shapiro ED, Logigian E, et al. Practice parameter: treatment of nervous system Lyme disease (an evidence-based review): report of the Quality Standards Subcommittee of the American Academy of Neurology. Neurology. 2007;69:91–102.
64. Fallon BA, Keilp JG, Corbera KM, et al. A randomized, placebo-controlled trial of repeated IV antibiotic therapy for Lyme encephalopathy. Neurology. 2008;70:992–1003.
65. Klempner MS, Hu LT, Evans J, et al. Two controlled trials of antibiotic treatment in patients with persistent symptoms and a history of Lyme disease. N Engl J Med. 2001;345:85–92.
66. Krupp LB, Hyman LG, Grimson R, et al. Study and treatment of post Lyme disease (STOP-LD): a randomized double masked clinical trial. Neurology. 2003;60:1923–30.
67. Barbour AG. Antigenic variation of a relapsing fever Borrelia species. Annu Rev Microbiol. 1990;44:155–71.
68. Cadavid D, Barbour AG. Neuroborreliosis during relapsing fever: review of the clinical manifestations, pathology, and treatment of infections in humans and experimental animals. Clin Infect Dis. 1998;26:151–64.
69. Bergeret C, Raoult A. Notes sur les formes nerveuses de la fievre recurrente & tiques en Afrique Occidentale Franchise. Bulletin Medicale de l'Afrique Occidentale Francaise 1948; 5:271–9.
70. Salih SY, Mustafa D, Abdel Wahab SM, Ahmed MA, Omer A. Louse-borne relapsing fever: I. A clinical and laboratory study of 363 cases in the Sudan. Trans R Soc Trop Med Hyg. 1977;71:43–8.
71. Hamilton J. Ocular complications in relapsing fever. Br J Ophthalmol. 1943;27:68–80.
72. Southern P, Sanford JP. Relapsing fever: a clinical and microbiological review. Medicine. 1969;48:129–50.
73. Brahim H, Perrier-Gros-Claude JD, Postic D, Baranton G, Jambou R. Identifying relapsing fever Borrelia, Senegal. Emerg Infect Dis. 2005;11:474–5.
74. Garcia-Monco JC, Miller NS, Backenson PB, Anda P, Benach JL. A mouse model of Borrelia meningitis after intradermal injection. J Infect Dis. 1997;175:1243–5.
75. Cadavid D, Sondey M, Garcia E, Lawson CL. Residual brain infection in relapsing-fever borreliosis. J Infect Dis. 2006;193:1451–8.
76. Gugliotta JL, Goethert HK, Berardi VP, Telford 3rd SR. Meningoencephalitis from Borrelia miyamotoi in an immunocompromised patient. N Engl J Med. 2013;368:240–5.
77. Arteaga F, Golightly MG, Garcia Perez A, Barral M, Anda P, Garcia-Monco JC. Disparity between serological reactivity to Borrelia burgdorferi and evidence of past disease in a high-risk group. Clin Infect Dis. 1998;27:1210–3.

Chapter 12
Neurosyphilis

Juan C. Salazar

Abstract Syphilis is a sexually transmitted infection caused by the spirochetal bacterium *Treponema pallidum*, subspecies *pallidum*. During early syphilis, the spirochete has the ability to disseminate into the central nervous system and cause both symptomatic and asymptomatic meningitis and in more severe cases vasculitis leading to thrombosis, ischemia, and even death. During tertiary syphilis, the chronic inflammatory responses to the spirochete can severely compromise the brain parenchyma and the spinal cord, leading to paresis and tabes dorsalis. In this chapter we will review the clinical presentation, diagnostic criteria, and treatment modalities for neurosyphilis.

Keywords *Treponema pallidum* • Neurosyphilis • Meningitis • Meningovascular syphilis • Gumma • Paresis • Tabes dorsalis

Introduction

Syphilis is a sexually transmitted infection caused by the spirochetal bacterium *Treponema pallidum*, subspecies *pallidum* [1, 2]. Despite the existence of inexpensive and effective antibiotic treatment regimens, roughly 10.5 million new syphilis cases are estimated to occur yearly throughout the world [3]. The multistage clinical syndrome, generally associated with untreated syphilis, reflects the propensity of *T. pallidum* to disseminate systemically and to induce chronic inflammation in skin, meninges, and various organ tissues [1]. Infection begins soon after the bacterium comes into contact with skin or mucous membranes, multiplying locally over several days, while simultaneously disseminating through blood and lymphatic vessels.

J.C. Salazar, MD, MPH
Department of Pediatrics, Connecticut Children's Medical Center,
282 Washington Street, Hartford, CT, USA
e-mail: jsalaza@connecticutchildrens.org

J.C. García-Moncó (ed.), *CNS Infections*,
DOI 10.1007/978-1-4471-6401-2_12, © Springer-Verlag London 2014

The distinctive painless ulcer (chancre) of primary syphilis typically only appears 2–4 weeks after the initial infection. By this time, organisms have disseminated from the primary site of infection and invaded various organ tissues, most notably the skin, setting the stage for what is classically known as secondary syphilis. This period of the disease characteristically presents with a variety of dermal manifestations as well as a series of systemic signs and symptoms, appearing within 4–10 weeks of the initial infection, and in some cases affecting the central nervous system (CNS). Despite the robust nature of the cellular and humoral immune responses typically associated with this stage of the disease, which include the appearance of high titers of anti-*T. pallidum* antibodies with opsonizing activity and robust mixed cellular infiltrate in skin lesions, several weeks to months may elapse before the host can gain control of the invading bacterial pathogen [4]. The period that follows is generally asymptomatic and referred to as latent syphilis. Classic studies demonstrate that up to 30 % of latent syphilis patients will develop recrudescent and more complex forms of the disease, which are collectively referred to as tertiary syphilis [5]. The tertiary stage may involve any organ system but primarily affects the central nervous system (neurosyphilis) [6], the heart and vascular structures (aortitis/aneurysms) [7], and skin and bones (gummatous syphilis) [7]. These complications can ultimately lead to death. In this chapter we will review the neurologic syndromes associated with both early and late venereal syphilis.

Causative Agent

T. pallidum belongs to one of five genera within the order Spirochaetales. The genera that are pathogenic for man include Leptospira (leptospirosis), Borrelia (Lyme disease and relapsing fever), and Treponema. Four human diseases are caused by members of the genus Treponema: venereal syphilis (caused by *T. pallidum* subspecies *pallidum*), endemic syphilis (*T. pallidum* subspecies *endemicum*), yaws (*T. pallidum*, subspecies *pertenue*), and pinta (*T. carateum*) [6, 8]. The spirochete is a helically shaped microaerophilic bacterium varying from 6 to 20 μm in length and a diameter of 0.10–0.18 μm [8]. This ultrastructural feature places the bacterium below the resolution of conventional light microscopy, thus requiring its visualization by dark-field or phase-contrast microscopy (Fig. 12.1c). The spirochete has a central protoplasmic cylinder bounded by a cytoplasmic membrane with an overlying thin layer of peptidoglycan and a very interesting outer membrane [9]. Two or three flagella, the organelles that allow the spirochete to move, originate at each end of the bacterium and twist around the body of the organism within a very thin periplasmic space. Unlike the outer membranes of typical gram-negative bacteria, that of *T. pallidum* lacks the potent proinflammatory glycolipid lipopolysaccharide (LPS) [10]. The outer membrane of *T. pallidum* contains an extraordinarily low density of integral membrane proteins (OMPs) (Fig. 12.1a, c), and the bacterium's abundant lipoproteins, a major pathogen-associated molecular pattern (PAMP), are located on the cytoplasmic membrane and not the OM [11–13]. The paucity of proteins and prototypical PAMPs on the spirochetal outer membrane is the basis for the bacterium's impressive capacity for immune evasion, thus its well-deserved designation by Radolf as a "stealth pathogen" [1, 2, 11, 12]. *T. pallidum's* genome is a circular chromosome of 1,138,006 base pairs and contains 1,041 open reading frames (ORFs) [10]. The absence of plasmids, pathogenicity islands, transposable elements, and restriction-modification systems point out that the spirochete has little capacity for uptake of exogenous DNA, almost certainly explaining why the bacterium has not yet developed resistance to penicillin.

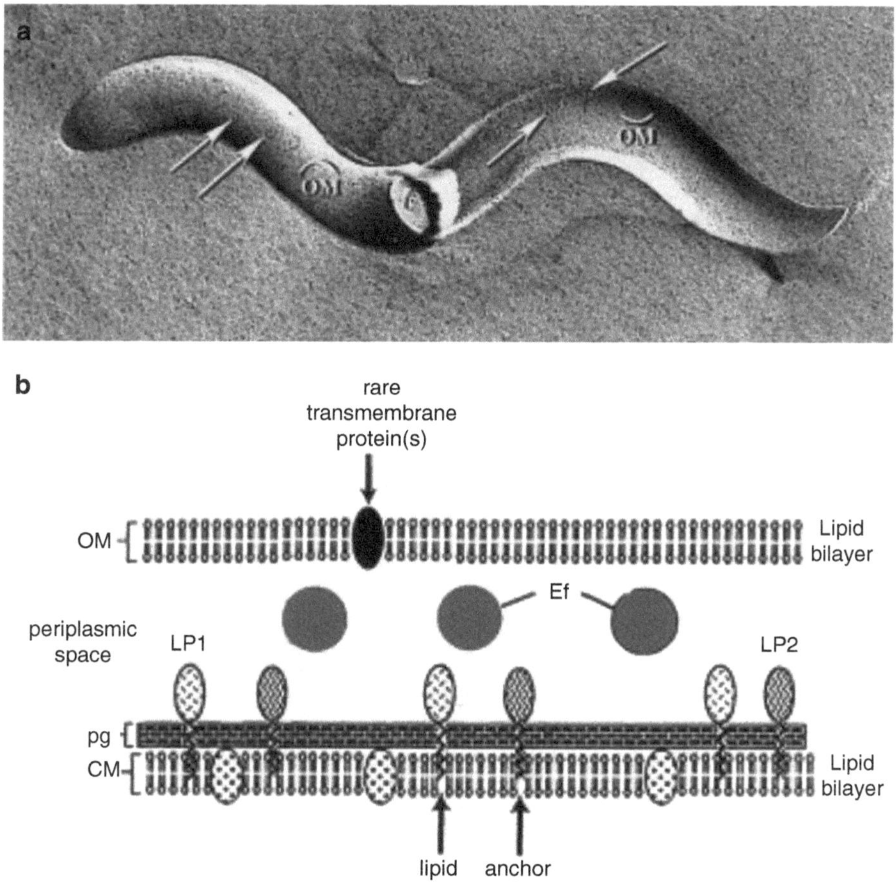

Fig. 12.1 (**a–c**) *T. pallidum* ultrastructure. (**a**) Membrane architecture of *T. pallidum* subspecies *pallidum*, as demonstrated by freeze-fracture electron microscopy. The figure shows the paucity of outer membrane (OM) transmembrane proteins. (**b**) Proposed molecular architecture of *T. pallidum*. The OM is depicted as having rare transmembrane proteins, while major immunogens are lipoproteins (LP1 and LP2) anchored to the periplasmic leaflet of the OM. The bacterium is also shown with periplasmic endoflagellum (*Ef*) and peptidoglycan (*pg*)-cytoplasmic membrane (*CM*) complex (Adapted with permission from Salazar et al. [2]). (**c**) Dark-field microscopy showing a single spirochete with it classic morphology (Courtesy of Karson Karanian)

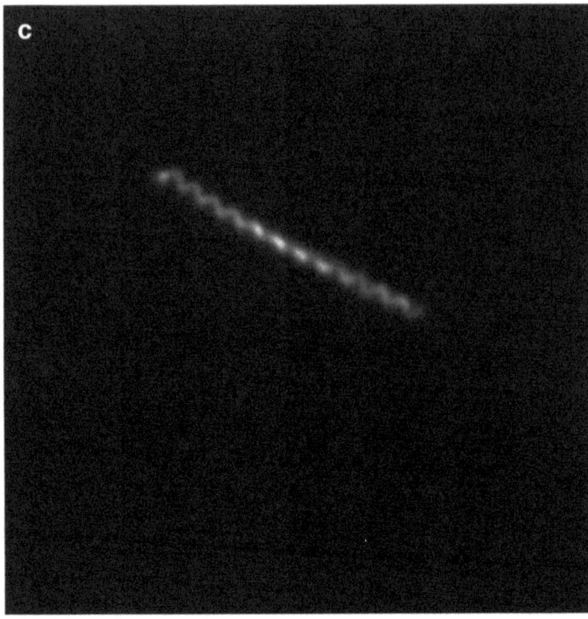

Fig. 12.1 (continued)

Epidemiology

According to the World Health Organization (WHO), in 2008, approximately 11 million people newly acquired syphilis and 36 million were estimated to have active infection (new cases + existing untreated cases) [3]. Although venereal syphilis has recently reemerged in the United States and Europe [14–16], most individuals (>90 %) who acquire syphilis, not surprisingly, reside in underdeveloped and poor regions of the world with poor access to health care [17]. In Western Europe and the United States, syphilis is currently characterized by low-level endemicity with concentration among population subgroups with high rates of partner change, most notably in men who have sex with men (MSM), as well as individuals with poor access to health services and socially marginalized [15, 18]. In Eastern Europe and Russia, the social changes and disruption of medical services which followed the breakup of the Soviet Union, led to important increases in syphilis rates [19]. Prevention strategies subsequently led to a steady decrease in the overall disease burdens in this region of the world. By contrast, in China, a country where syphilis was virtually eradicated in the 1950s, the incidence and prevalence of the disease has more than quadrupled over the last several years [20]. This increase in syphilis rates has been attributed to migration of large segments of the population from rural Chinese communities to large urban centers, limited syphilis screening practices, lack of adequate partner notification, and an overall unwillingness to access to STD health-care services by the general population [21]. In China, as in other parts of the world, the incidence of neurosyphilis tracks the overall prevalence of incidence of venereal syphilis in the general population.

It is important to highlight that the worldwide epidemiology of syphilis has also been greatly influenced by developments in the HIV epidemic [22–24]. Early neurosyphilis is more common than late neurosyphilis and presents most frequently in patients with HIV. Although the association between syphilis and HIV infection does reflect similar behavioral risk factors for their acquisition and transmission, it is now known that complex biologic relationships between these two diseases do contribute to high coinfection rates [24–26]. The presence of a syphilitic chancre can theoretically facilitate HIV transmission either by increasing the host's susceptibility to infection with the virus or the HIV-infected host's infectiousness to discordant sexual partners. The former is associated with the disruption of the protective epithelial and mucosal barriers present in genital chancres and the known enrichment of the lesion with activated lymphocytes, macrophages, and dendritic cells, all of which are potential targets and donors for HIV [27–30] and which differentially increase expression of key HIV co-receptors (i.e., CCR5 and DC-SIGN) in untreated patients [30, 31]. With respect to increased infectiousness, *T. pallidum* is also capable of inducing HIV expression of selective genes which promote viral replication [32]. In line with the proposed coinfection pathogenesis model, in HIV–syphilis-coinfected patients, CD4 counts decrease and HIV viral loads increase in untreated patients [33].

Clinical Syndromes Associated with Neurosyphilis

CNS invasion by the syphilis spirochete can occur during any stage of the disease and can present with a variety of clinical syndromes (Fig. 12.2). Long-term follow-up studies conducted in the pre-antibiotic era provided evidence that up to 1/3 of all untreated syphilis patients developed neurosyphilis [5, 34]. In those individuals who developed neurosyphilis, 30 % were deemed to have asymptomatic meningitis [5, 34], 10 % developed some form of meningovascular syphilis, 30 % had tabes dorsalis, and 10 % had paresis. The remaining patients had other forms of CNS disease, including optic nerve compromise as well as other cranial neuropathies. The reality is that combinations of each of the clinical syndromes associated with neurosyphilis, including asymptomatic and symptomatic meningitis, meningovascular syphilis, and CNS parenchymatous compromise, are more the norm than the exception [35]. These syndromes will be described below.

Asymptomatic Neurosyphilis

Asymptomatic neurosyphilis is classically defined and established by the presence of one or more abnormalities in the spinal fluid of a patient with confirmed venereal syphilis (generally primary or secondary syphilis) and with no symptoms or signs

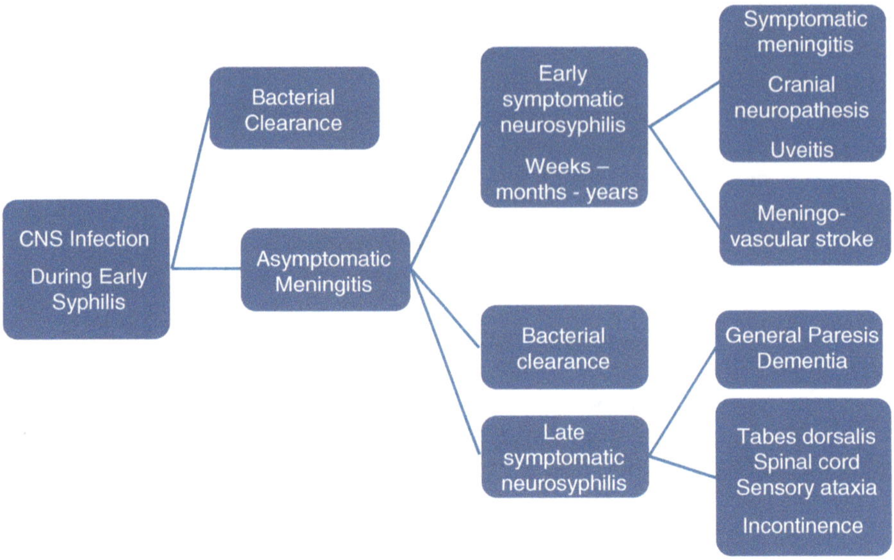

Fig. 12.2 Natural history and clinical syndromes associated with neurosyphilis

of neurologic disease. CSF abnormalities include lymphocytic pleocytosis (typically < 100 cells/μL), elevated protein values (usually < 100 mg/dL), and/or a reactive CSF Venereal Disease Research Laboratory [VDRL] test. Rabbit infectivity (RIT) studies conducted in the 1920s and 1930s [5, 36–38], which were subsequently confirmed in the 1980s and 1990s [39, 40], established definitively that the CSF abnormalities seen in asymptomatic early syphilis patients are indeed associated with CNS invasion by *T. pallidum*. This form of the disease can follow three distinct clinical patterns. In the majority of patients with either early or late venereal syphilis, spinal fluid abnormalities resolve spontaneously; in the remainder, they either persist without development of overt neurologic symptoms or worsen with the eventual appearance of a neurosyphilitic syndrome. Natural history studies indicate that in the case of asymptomatic untreated neurosyphilis, most CSF alterations resolve without treatment [5]. To be sure, Merrit et al. [5] reported that the incidence of late asymptomatic neurosyphilis was no higher than 10 %. These same natural history studies provided evidence that asymptomatic neurosyphilis was indeed a predecessor of meningeal, vascular, and parenchymatous syphilitic neurologic syndromes and that asymptomatic neurosyphilis diagnosed during late syphilis carried a worse prognosis than asymptomatic neurosyphilis during early infection. Not surprisingly, progression from asymptomatic to symptomatic neurosyphilis increased in rough proportion to the extent of CSF abnormalities in these same patients.

Although the clinical importance of diagnosing asymptomatic neurosyphilis was well appreciated in the pre-antibiotic era [37], there was diversity of opinion, as to when lumbar puncture should be done [41, 42]. Europeans argued for later spinal fluid examination to avoid overtreating persons whose CNS infections were going to resolve spontaneously, while the Americans advocated early examination of the spinal fluid to identify persons with severe CSF abnormalities who would benefit from more intensive arsenical therapy. Ironically, the same dilemma has resurfaced today as a result of numerous case reports suggesting that single-dose intramuscular penicillin could lead to CNS relapse in HIV-infected individuals with severe compromise of their immune system [43], in addition to clinical studies suggesting a higher prevalence of asymptomatic neurosyphilis among early syphilis patients coinfected with HIV [44–46]. Regardless of HIV status, the CDC does not recommend performing a spinal tap in individuals with either primary or secondary syphilis and without signs and symptoms of neurologic disease at the time of diagnosis [40].

Symptomatic Syphilitic Meningitis

Syphilitic meningitis most often occurs within the first year after initial infection but can also present several years after the initial infection. Symptomatic syphilitic meningitis can occur as either an early or late manifestation of venereal syphilis. Up to 10 % of symptomatic meningitis cases occur in patients initially diagnosed with secondary syphilis and most cases occur during the first 2 years following the initial infection. Although headache and meningismus are not uncommon in early syphilis, particularly in patients with secondary syphilis, a full-blown meningeal syndrome (headache, confusion, nausea, vomiting, and a stiff neck) is seen in less than 10 % of all cases of neurosyphilis [47]. In their classic series, Merritt and Moore [47] could find only 80 such cases over a 15-year period in three general hospitals, and they estimated that symptomatic meningitis may complicate between 0.3 and 2 % of early syphilis cases. These authors described three distinct clinical presentations: (i) acute hydrocephalus without focal signs unrelated to increased intracranial pressure; (ii) meningitis of the vertex, presenting with seizures, focal neurologic deficits (e.g., hemiplegia, aphasia), and changes in sensorium; and (iii) basilar meningitis with cranial nerve palsies, especially of nerves III, VI, VII, and VIII. Eighth cranial nerve involvement can be unilateral or bilateral and can affect either or both the acoustic and vestibular nerves. In these patients, CSF changes are more intense than those described for patients with asymptomatic meningitis, including more pronounced CSF lymphocytosis (generally between 200 and 400 cells/μl) and higher CSF protein levels (usually between 100 and 200 mg/dL). Neuroimaging studies can show enhancement of the meninges, cranial nerves, and/or spinal roots. The differential diagnosis for this condition is broad and includes viral causes of aseptic meningitis, neuroborreliosis, tuberculous and fungal meningitis, parameningeal processes (e.g., abscess), and noninfectious pathology such as sarcoidosis and carcinomatous meningitis. Reactive serological tests for syphilis in blood and CSF, along with the subacute onset of signs and symptoms typical of meningitis, while complicated, help to distinguish meningeal syphilis from other conditions listed above in the differential diagnosis.

Meningovascular Syphilis

T. pallidum can also induce an infectious arteritis affecting any arterial vessel in the brain or spinal cord, resulting in thrombosis, ischemia, and infarction. Meningovascular syphilis represents an early to late syphilis overlap syndrome, although most patients are diagnosed in the late end of the syphilitic continuum. The spinal cord, brainstem, or cerebrum may be involved separately or together, although the majority of patients typically suffer middle cerebral artery infarctions [5]. Not surprisingly, the most common neurologic findings are contralateral hemiplegia/hemiparesis, homonymous hemianopsia, and aphasia. Death can result from involvement of the posterior cerebral circulation [48]. The relatively young age (30–50 years) of patients with meningovascular syphilis helps to distinguish this syndrome from other forms of vascular stroke (i.e., atherosclerotic). Onset may be sudden, although most patients have prodromal symptoms, such as headache, vertigo, insomnia, irritability, personality, and behavioral changes, weeks to months before the thrombotic event. In the original neurosyphilis series by Merrit et al. [5], only a handful of patients had neurologic deficits suggesting involvement of more than one blood vessel in the brain. The use of MRI and magnetic resonance angiography imaging suggests that most patients have diffuse and often bilateral involvement of the brain [49], as would be expected with any form of systemic CNS vasculitis. Meningovascular syphilis can also involve vessels in the spinal cord, leading to infarction of the anterior or less commonly posterior spinal arteries. The spinal variant lacks prodromal symptoms and is usually sudden in onset. The differential diagnosis of meningovascular syphilis is broad and includes fungal and tuberculous meningitis and rheumatologic causes of cerebral vasculitis, including systemic lupus erythematosus, Wegener's granulomatosis, and polyarteritis nodosa.

The Parenchymatous Syndromes

The parenchymatous syndromes, general paresis and tabes dorsalis, are the last to occur in the neurosyphilis temporal sequence. These two syndromes are thus generally considered "tertiary forms" of neurosyphilis and account for more than 50 % of all cases of neurosyphilis. Both cases are four- to sevenfold more common in men than women. According to Stokes [37], paresis accounted for 11 % of neuropsychiatric admissions in the United States and around 7 % of all cases of mental disease in the French, German, American, and Russian armies. The virtual disappearance of tabes dorsalis, which is disproportionate to the decline in the incidence of paresis, is one of the most striking changes in the epidemiology of neurosyphilis in the modern age. Nevertheless, it is very important that clinicians remain aware for this rare dementing illness, in particular because a substantial degree of reversibility can be seen when paresis is promptly recognized and treated [50–53].

General paresis is a chronic, spirochetal meningoencephalitis, which severely disturbs the structure and function of the cerebral cortices, particularly the frontal and temporal lobes [5]. The typical clinical picture is a slow, often insidious, onset of neuropsychiatric disturbances coupled with progressive deterioration in cognitive function. The presentation, however, may be abrupt. In one case series, the duration of symptoms varied between 24 h and 5 years and approximately 20 % of patients had seizures [54]. As the disease worsens, patients experience loss of motor control to the point of paralysis along with worsening loss of bowel and bladder control. The constellation of signs and symptoms can be remembered with the mnemonic PARESIS: *p*ersonality (emotional lability, paranoia), *a*ffect (carelessness in appearance), *r*eflexes (hyperactive), *e*ye (Argyll Robertson pupils), *s*ensorium (illusions, delusions, especially megalomania, hallucinations), *i*ntellect (decreased recent memory, judgment, insight), and *s*peech (slurred). The dramatic postmortem pathologic findings described by Merrit et al. [5] have been visualized on a number of occasions in patients by MRI, now an essential tool for making the diagnosis [50, 51, 55, 56]. The alterations in personality and behavior and the temporal lobe findings on MRI can lead to an incorrect diagnosis of herpetic encephalitis in some patients [57–60].

Tabes dorsalis is caused by a demyelinating process in the posterior spinal cords, which ultimately leads to the development of an ataxic, wide-based gait and foot slap (Tabetic gait); paresthesias of the lower extremities; shooting or lightning pains (sudden onset, rapid radiation, and disappearance); bladder disturbances; fecal incontinence; impotence; loss of position and vibratory sense; absent ankle and knee jerk reflexes; and loss of deep pain and temperature sensation. The characteristic "lightning" or lancinating pains experienced by at least 75 % of patients are usually present at the outset of the disease, typically affecting the lower extremities and occurring episodically. Ten to 20 % of patients experience visceral crises including recurrent episodes of sudden, agonizing epigastric pain with nausea and vomiting which can last for days and mimic surgical emergencies. Intestinal, rectal, and laryngeal crises also can occur. Decrease or loss of tendon and patellar reflexes with preservation of muscle strength is a common, relatively early, neurologic finding. Ataxia is widely regarded as one of the cardinal symptoms of tabes, and between 50 and 80 % of patients exhibit a positive Romberg sign. Degenerative ocular changes also are common components of the tabetic syndrome. The Argyll Robertson pupil, though not limited to tabes or even syphilis, is a characteristic late feature. Primary optic atrophy occurs over a period of months to years, beginning peripherally and proceeding to the center of the nerve, producing progressive concentric constriction of the visual fields with retention of normal vision, referred to as "gun barrel" sight [61].

CNS Gumma

The CNS gumma, the rarest form of neurosyphilis, was uncommon even in the preantibiotic era [5]. Rare cases continue to appear in the modern literature [62–64]. Because of the likelihood that a CNS gumma will initially be mistaken for a tumor

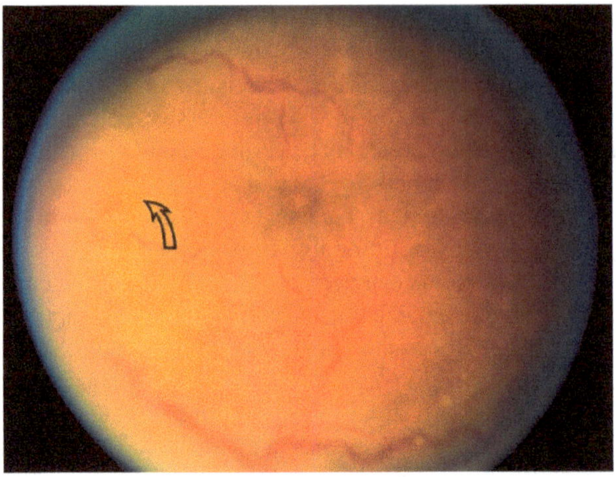

Fig. 12.3 Syphilitic neuroretinitis. Acute syphilitic neuroretinitis in the left eye, with markedly swollen optic nerve (*arrow*) and adjacent retinal edema including the fovea, occlusive retinal arteriolitis involving the inferior central vessels at the optic nerve head, vitreitis, and inferior serous retinal detachment (not shown). Patient was HIV positive with a CD4 cell count of 222 cells/μL (Adapted with permission from Ormerod et al. [107]. ©2001 Infectious Diseases Society of America)

or other type of space occupying lesion (e.g., toxoplasmosis in an AIDS patient), this entity well exemplifies the reputation of syphilis as the great mimicker. The pathologic features of gumma within the CNS are no different than those occurring outside it. Merritt et al. [5] considered gumma of the CNS to be a chronic, localized form of syphilitic meningitis that extends from the pia mater into the adjacent brain or spinal cord. In a recent, comprehensive review of the literature, Fargen et al. [64] found two-thirds of the lesions occurred in the cerebral convexities of which the majority was located in the frontal lobes or frontoparietal region. The pituitary was the most common site outside the cerebral hemispheres.

Ocular Syphilis

Ocular complications may occur as part of a neurosyphilis syndrome or as an isolated manifestation [5, 65]. Anterior or posterior uveitis or panuveitis, the most common abnormalities, can occur during either early or late syphilis and presents with diminished visual acuity (Fig. 12.3). Other ocular syndromes include episcleritis, vitreitis, retinitis, papillitis, interstitial keratitis, acute retinal necrosis, and retinal detachment. Primary optic atrophy is unique to late syphilis and is most associated with tabes dorsalis, which it closely resembles pathologically [5, 61]. The differential diagnosis includes tuberculosis, rheumatoid arthritis, sarcoidosis, toxoplasmosis, histoplasmosis, and ocular *Toxocara canis* infections. The presence of pupillary abnormalities distinguishes syphilis from these other processes. Unless scarring has occurred, improvement with treatment can be dramatic.

Otosyphilis

Syphilis can cause hearing loss via two mechanisms during early or late infection. One is osteitis of the temporal bone with destructive changes in the membranous cochlea and labyrinth. The other, almost certainly more common, is inflammation and atrophy of cranial nerve VIII. Involvement of cranial nerve VIII typically begins with high-frequency hearing loss and progresses to a complete unilateral or bilateral loss of cochlear and vestibular function [66]. Syphilitic labyrinthitis has been known to mimic Ménière's disease. In the post-antibiotic era, otosyphilis has become liberally defined as an unexplained sensorineural hearing loss in the presence of a reactive treponemal serologic test [67, 68]. As noted by Pletcher [69], this definition lacks a clear causal relationship between syphilis and the clinical symptoms. Nevertheless, in such cases, treatment is usually indicated since there are no diagnostic measures that can reliably eliminate the possibility of syphilis.

HIV and Neurosyphilis

Whether coinfection with HIV worsens the manifestations of syphilis and/or accelerates the course of the disease remains a point of contention among experts in the field and public health authorities. A number of case reports and small series have documented ophthalmologic and neurologic complications, as well as unusual or highly destructive non-neurologic syphilis syndromes in HIV-infected patients [43, 70, 71], leading many authorities to conclude that infection with HIV poses a higher risk of complications, particularly neurologic, during active syphilis [24, 70, 71]. Despite these findings, a multicenter prospective, randomized study sponsored by the CDC failed to demonstrate a benefit of enhanced therapy in patients either without or with HIV coinfection [40]. The differences in clinical presentation between HIV-coinfected and HIV-uninfected patients were in fact trivial. While HIV-infected patients with primary syphilis tended to present with more genital ulcers and genital ulcers were present more frequently in HIV-infected patients with secondary syphilis, manifestations of disseminated infection, including neurologic and ophthalmological complications, were not worsened by concomitant HIV infection. Thus, if atypical and aggressive presentations of syphilis do occur more frequently among HIV-infected patients, they likely represent a very small percentage of total cases, an assessment shared by several groups [24, 72, 73]. Three separate studies have suggested that serum RPR titers $\geq$32 or CD4 counts below 350 in HIV-infected patients pose a greater risk of developing asymptomatic neurosyphilis [44, 74, 75]. The long-term benefits of lumbar puncture and the value of more intensive therapy in this patient subset remain unproven [42]. Based on available evidence, the CDC currently does not recommend routine lumbar puncture in patients with early syphilis, regardless of HIV status or CD4 count [76]. Of course, patients with reactive serologies and neurologic symptoms or clinical findings should always undergo lumbar puncture regardless of disease stage or immunologic status [76].

Pathologic Features

Perivascular infiltrates composed of lymphocytes, histiocytes, and plasma cells, accompanied by varying degrees of endothelial cell swelling and proliferation, are the histologic trademarks of syphilis regardless of anatomic site or stage of disease. Spirochetes are abundant in early syphilis lesions and often are observed in and around blood vessels, occasionally even protruding into the lumen in histologic specimens. By contrast, with the exception of paresis, spirochetes are not easily demonstrable in tertiary syphilis lesions. Asymptomatic neurosyphilis and syphilitic meningitis are due to diffuse leptomeningitis [5]. The pathologic features of meningovascular syphilis explain the syndrome's variable mixture of focal neurologic signs with superimposed encephalitis [5, 77, 78]. In this syndrome, there is diffuse thickening and lymphocytic infiltration of the meninges with two kinds of arteritis: (i) *Heubner's* endarteritis, affecting large- and medium-sized arteries, characterized by crescentic collagenous thickening of the intima, thinning of the media, and dense, inflammatory changes (lymphocytes and plasma cells) within the adventitia and (ii) *Nissl–Alzheimer* endarteritis of small vessels, characterized by the proliferation of endothelial and adventitial cells. *Paresis* and *tabes dorsalis* are considered a neurodegenerative processes of brain or spinal cord parenchyma, hence their designation as "parenchymatous." In paresis, diffuse meningovascular inflammatory changes are associated with striking and progressive loss of cerebral cortical neurons, resulting in gross cerebral atrophy (greatest in the frontal and temporal lobes), and proliferation of astrocytes and glial cells. Microglial cells are hypertrophied and elongated. Spirochetes are often readily detectable, usually in the grey matter, with little correlation between the clinical picture and the location and distribution of organisms. Tabes dorsalis is characterized by demyelination of dorsal root ganglia with secondary Wallerian degeneration of the posterior columns of the spinal cord. In early tabes, the leptomeninges and dorsal roots are heavily infiltrated with lymphocytes and plasma cells. These inflammatory changes diminish as the disease becomes chronic, eventually disappearing in so-called burnt out cases.

A gumma is a circumscribed mass of granulation tissue, so named because of its rubbery or gummy gross consistency. The gumma of tertiary syphilis histologically is comprised of a dense infiltrate of lymphocytes, plasma cells, epithelioid cells, and multinucleated giant cells surrounding a caseous, necrotic core; proliferating fibroblasts and fibrosis also may be present [64]. Endarteritis and perivascular inflammation help to distinguish syphilitic gummas from those caused by tuberculosis. Obliterative endarteritis involving the *vasa vasorum*, the nutrient vessels of the aortic adventitia, is the key pathologic lesion in cardiovascular syphilis [79]. The ascending aorta and arch are most frequently affected because the *vasa vasorum* are most plentiful in these regions of the aorta. These changes eventually give rise to intimal thickening and wrinkling patchy medial necrosis, and adventitial scarring with destruction of elastic fibers and weakening of the aortic wall.

Laboratory Diagnosis of Neurosyphilis

No laboratory gold standard exists for the diagnosis of neurosyphilis [80]. Diagnosis of neurosyphilis is thus stage dependent and requires a combination of clinical presentation and serologic and CSF laboratory studies. Because *T. pallidum* cannot be cultivated on artificial medium, laboratory diagnosis relies on direct detection of the pathogen in patient specimens and/or reactivity in serological tests. Confirmation would require inoculation of biologic samples into rabbit testicles, a procedure which is only available in a research environment. Below we will first describe available serologic assays for the diagnosis of venereal syphilis, followed by available CSF studies for the diagnosis of neurosyphilis.

Serological Tests for the Diagnosis of Venereal Syphilis

Venereal syphilis serodiagnosis depends upon the use of two distinctly different types of antibody reactivities, the so-called nontreponemal and treponemal tests [81, 82]. The term "nontreponemal," derived from the long-held belief that the inciting antigens are lipids liberated from inflamed tissues, is probably a misnomer given that cardiolipin is a major phospholipid constituent in *T. pallidum* [83]. The standard nontreponemal test is the VDRL slide test in which heat-inactivated serum is tested for its ability to flocculate or agglutinate a standardized suspension of a cardiolipin–cholesterol–lecithin antigen [82]. Most diagnostic laboratories now use the RPR card test, which uses finely divided charcoal particles as a visualizing agent, for routine screening and following the response to therapy. As a general rule, RPR titers on the same serum specimens tend to be higher than VDRL titers. The TRUST is a macroflocculation assay in which the charcoal is replaced with toluidine red; its sensitivity is equivalent to that of the RPR while its specificity is slightly higher. Nontreponemal tests are reported as the highest dilution giving a fully reactive result. A fourfold change in titer using the same nontreponemal test method is necessary to demonstrate a significant difference and should be performed in the same laboratory and, if possible, on the same day. Sera with extremely high nontreponemal titers may give weakly reactive, atypical, or even negative reaction at low dilutions because antibody excess prevents the agglutination reaction. Most laboratories circumvent this "prozone" phenomenon, which occurs in approximately 1 % of reactive sera [84], by routinely titering all samples to at least 16 dilutions. While one-third of patients diagnosed with primary and tertiary syphilis have nonreactive nontreponemal tests [85], the majority of secondary syphilis patients have a nontreponemal test titers of at least 1:8. A decline in nontreponemal test titers is the only means of monitoring therapeutic response. Treatment success is currently defined as a fourfold decrease in nontreponemal titer no later than 1 year following therapy for early syphilis and 2 years for late latent syphilis [76]. CSF examination to exclude neurosyphilis is indicated for all patients who do not achieve at least a 4-fold decline during the appropriate interval following therapy [42]. The biologic significance of persistent nontreponemal test reactivity in "serofast" persons (i.e., individuals who show a 2 dilution or greater decrease in nontreponemal titer but do not serorevert) is unknown, and there is no evidence that such individuals benefit from lumbar puncture and/or additional therapy [42].

Treponemal tests should always be performed when primary syphilis is suspected because of their greater sensitivity than nontreponemal tests (86 % vs. 70 %) [85]. Treponemal tests also should be performed for suspected tertiary syphilis even when nontreponemal tests are nonreactive. It is important to remember that a reactive treponemal test usually remains reactive for life. There are several specific anti-treponemal serologic assays available [86]. Until recently, the FTA-ABS test was the gold-standard confirmatory treponemal test. In this test, the patient's serum is used to immunolabel treponemes fixed to glass slides. Labeled organisms are visualized using a FITC-conjugated antihuman immunoglobulin antibody, and the sample is scored by the laboratory technician based upon the intensity of the fluorescence. Because of the subjectivity involved in the interpretation of this assay, it is no longer considered the gold-standard treponemal test [87]. The MHA-TP, is a passive hem-agglutination assay of formalinized, tanned erythrocytes sensitized with *T. pallidum* antigen that can be used to test preabsorbed patient sera. The MHA-TP has now been supplanted by the TP-PA test, a modification that uses gelatin particles sensitized with *T. pallidum* antigens to reduce the number of nonspecific interactions. All three tests measure both anti-treponemal IgG and IgM serum antibodies without distinguishing the immunoglobulin class which is responsible for reactivity. Numerous EIAs, which use recombinant *T. pallidum* antigens and detect IgM and IgG, have recently been developed for syphilis diagnosis.

There is now a well-established consensus that serologic tests for syphilis perform well in persons coinfected with HIV and with some cautions can be relied upon for accurate diagnosis in such individuals [76]. HIV-infected individuals may have a higher incidence of false-positive nontreponemal tests [88, 89]. In addition, nontreponemal test titers in HIV-infected individuals tend to be higher at presentation (including prozone phenomena) and can remain persistently elevated posttreatment [40, 90–92]. These serologic findings probably reflect the B-cell dysregulation associated with HIV infection. Lastly, there are well-documented, albeit extremely rare, cases of HIV-infected patients with secondary syphilis with nonreactive syphilis serologies in which a prozone was ruled out [93, 94]. Skin biopsy for histopathological examination as well as direct detection of *T. pallidum* should be performed if serologic test results are negative in an HIV-infected individual with a high suspension of secondary syphilis.

Specific Tests Used in the Diagnostic Algorithm of Neurosyphilis (Table 12.1)

Table 12.1 summarizes specific clinical parameters and laboratory criteria for the diagnosis of neurosyphilis. While a reactive CSF VDRL constitutes definitive evidence for neurosyphilis, a presumptive diagnosis can be based solely on the

Table 12.1 Diagnostic criteria for neurosyphilis

Confirmed (requires 1, 2, *and* either 3, 4, or 5)
1. Clinical signs consistent with neurosyphilis
2. A reactive serum treponemal test
3. A reactive VDRL in CSF
4. Detection of *T. pallidum* DNA in CSF by PCR
5. Identification of treponemes in nervous tissue by silver stain, immunofluorescence (DFA-TP), or immunohistochemical staining
Probable (requires 1, 2, *and* 3)
1. Clinical signs consistent with neurosyphilis
2. A reactive serum treponemal test
3. Elevated CSF protein or leukocyte count in the absence of other known causes

Adapted from the 2010 Sexually Transmitted Diseases Surveillance Case Definitions for Nationally Notifiable Diseases

presence of an elevated CSF protein and/or pleocytosis. Given the limited and conflicting data on performance [95, 96], the CSF RPR is currently not recommended in place of the CSF VDRL. The CSF FTA-ABS has high sensitivity but low specificity because reactivity may be due to the passive transfer of IgG anti-treponemal antibodies across the blood–brain barrier rather than intrathecal production of antibodies [97]. Because of the lack of specificity, the CDC does not recommend performing treponemal tests on CSF. Pleocytosis, long regarded as the hallmark of an active inflammatory process [5, 37], should resolve within weeks to months following appropriate therapy (see below). When positive, the CSF VDRL should be monitored quantitatively but may not normalize. An elevated protein may, likewise, persist indefinitely. Current CDC recommendations do, however, call for lumbar puncture in patients who have non-neurologic forms of tertiary syphilis given that an abnormal CSF would result in a change in treatment regimen (see below).

Treatment Recommendations for Neurosyphilis (Table 12.2)

Parentally administered aqueous penicillin G is the preferred therapy for all forms and stages of syphilis. Table 12.2 presents current CDC guidelines for the treatment of neurosyphilis [76]. Aqueous penicillin G administered as three to four million units IV every 4 h or continuous infusion for 10–14 days is the currently recommended regimen; failures with this regimen are virtually nonexistent. If compliance can be assured, procaine penicillin 2.4 MU IM daily with probenecid 500 mg four times a day for 10–14 days can be considered as an alternative. Though not mandatory, CDC guidelines allow for follow-up of intravenous therapy with three divided doses of IM benzathine penicillin G (BPG) to ensure prolonged penicillinemia comparable to that during treatment of non-neurologic tertiary syphilis. Syphilitic otitis and ocular syphilis, both frequently associated with neurosyphilis, should be treated as neurosyphilis regardless

Table 12.2 Treatment recommendations for neurosyphilis [76]

Drugs of choice
1. Penicillin G three to four million units intravenously every 4 h or 24 million units as a continuous intravenous infusion for 10–14 days OR
2. Penicillin G procaine 2.4 million units IM daily Plus probenecid 500 mg four times daily oral, both for 10–14 days
Alternatives
1. Ceftriaxone 2 g IV once daily for 10–14 days
2. For patients with serious penicillin allergies who refuse desensitization or those who cannot be treated with penicillin and ceftriaxone, an alternative is oral doxycycline (200 mg twice daily) for 21–28 days

Patients allergic to penicillin requiring treatment for neurosyphilis should be desensitized

of the results of lumbar puncture. Penicillin-allergic patients whose compliance with therapy or follow-up is questionable should be desensitized and treated with BPG. Doxycycline and tetracycline have long established track records as alternatives to penicillin with a reasonable amount of published data, some recent and including HIV-infected persons and indicating efficacy comparable to that of BPG [98–103]. Doxycycline is preferred both because of its twice daily dosing, ensuring better compliance, and its lipophilicity, enabling it to cross the blood–brain barrier. Pharmacokinetics data and limited clinic studies suggest that ceftriaxone is effective for treating both early and late syphilis, including neurosyphilis [102, 104–106], although the optimal dose and duration of therapy for either have not been determined.

Unfortunately there is no microbiological test of cure for neurosyphilis. Thus, to establish success of treatment for this disease, the clinician must use a variety of surrogate markers, most importantly resolution or stabilization of clinical abnormalities and by normalization of CSF findings. Both a clinical examination and a lumbar puncture should be performed 3–6 months after the initial treatment and every 6 months thereafter until the CSF VDRL is nonreactive. In general, it is expected that all CSF abnormalities will resolve by 2 years following treatment. Retreatment will be necessary if any follow-up studies show increasing pleocytosis or if there is a fourfold increase in CSF VDRL titer.

References

1. Radolf JD, Hazlett KRO, Lukehart SA. Pathogenesis of syphilis. In: Radolf JD, Lukehart SA, editors. Pathogenic treponemes: cellular and molecular biology. Norfolk: Caister Academic Press; 2006. p. 197–236.
2. Salazar JC, Hazlett KR, Radolf JD. The immune response to infection with *Treponema pallidum*, the stealth pathogen. Microbes Infect. 2002;4:1133–40.
3. WHO. Global incidence and prevalence of selected curable sexually transmitted infections-2008. Geneva: World Health Organization; 2012.

4. Cruz AR, Ramirez LG, Zuluaga AV, et al. Immune evasion and recognition of the syphilis spirochete in blood and skin of secondary syphilis patients: two immunologically distinct compartments. PLoS Negl Trop Dis. 2012;6:e1717.
5. Merritt HH, Adams RD, Solomon HC. Neurosyphilis. New York: Oxford University Press; 1946.
6. Tramont EC. *Treponema pallidum* (syphilis). In: Mandell GL, Bennett JE, Dolin R, editors. Mandell, Douglas and Bennett's principles and practice of infectious diseases. Philadelphia: Churchill Livingstone Elsevier; 2010. p. 3035–53.
7. Tramont EC, Boyajian SS. Learning from history: what the public health response to syphilis teaches us about HIV/AIDS. J Contemp Health Law Policy. 2010;26:253–99.
8. Norris SJ, Paster BJ, Moter A, G'bel UB. The genus *treponema*. In: Dworkin MS, Falkow S, Rosenberg E, Schliefer KH, Stackebrandt E, editors. The prokaryotes: an evolving electronic resource for the microbiological community. New York: Springer; 2001.
9. Izard J, Renken C, Hsieh CE, et al. Cryo-electron tomography elucidates the molecular architecture of *Treponema pallidum*, the syphilis spirochete. J Bacteriol. 2009;191:7566–80.
10. Fraser CM, Norris SJ, Weinstock GM, et al. Complete genome sequence of *Treponema pallidum*, the syphilis spirochete. Science. 1998;281:375–88.
11. Cameron CE. The T, pallidum outer membrane and outer membrane proteins. In: Radolf JD, Lukehart SA, editors. Pathogenic Treponema: molecular and cellular biology. Norwich: Caister Academic Press; 2006. p. 237–66.
12. Cox DL, Luthra A, Dunham-Ems S, et al. Surface immunolabeling and consensus computational framework to identify candidate rare outer membrane proteins of *Treponema pallidum*. Infect Immun. 2010;78:5178–94.
13. Desrosiers DC, Anand A, Luthra A, et al. TP0326, a *Treponema pallidum* beta-barrel assembly machinery A (BamA) orthologue and rare outer membrane protein. Mol Microbiol. 2011;80:1496–515.
14. Fenton KA, Breban R, Vardavas R, et al. Infectious syphilis in high-income settings in the 21st century. Lancet Infect Dis. 2008;8:244–53.
15. Sexually Transmitted Disease Surveillance 2011. U.S. Department of Health and Human Services. 2012. The online version of this report is available at http://www.cdc.gov/std/stats.
16. Mayer KH, Mimiaga MJ. Resurgent syphilis in the United States: urgent need to address an evolving epidemic. Ann Intern Med. 2011;155:192–3.
17. French P, Gomberg M, Janier M, Schmidt B, van Voorst Vader P, Young H. IUSTI: 2008 European Guidelines on the Management of Syphilis. Int J STD AIDS. 2009;20:300–9.
18. European Centre for Disease Prevention and Control. Sexually transmitted infections in Europe 1990–2010. Stockholm: ECDC; 2012. (http://www.ecdc.europa.eu/en/publications/publications/201206-sexually-transmitted-infections-europe-2010.pdf).
19. Scott CM, Flint SR. Oral syphilis–re-emergence of an old disease with oral manifestations. Int J Oral Maxillofac Surg. 2005;34:58–63.
20. Tucker JD, Yin YP, Wang B, Chen XS, Cohen MS. An expanding syphilis epidemic in China: epidemiology, behavioural risk and control strategies with a focus on low-tier female sex workers and men who have sex with men. Sex Transm Infect. 2011;87 Suppl 2:ii16–8.
21. Tucker JD, Cohen MS. China's syphilis epidemic: epidemiology, proximate determinants of spread, and control responses. Curr Opin Infect Dis. 2011;24:50–5.
22. Hutchinson CM, Hook 3rd EW, Shepherd M, Verley J, Rompalo AM. Altered clinical presentation of early syphilis in patients with human immunodeficiency virus infection. Ann Intern Med. 1994;121:94–100.
23. Ansell DA, Hu TC, Straus M, Cohen M, Sherer R. HIV and syphilis seroprevalence among clients with sexually transmitted diseases attending a walk-in clinic at Cook County Hospital. Sex Transm Dis. 1994;21:93–6.
24. Zetola NM, Klausner JD. Syphilis and HIV infection: an update. Clin Infect Dis. 2007;44:1222–8.
25. Fleming DT, Wasserheit JN. From epidemiological synergy to public health policy and practice: the contribution of other sexually transmitted diseases to sexual transmission of HIV infection. Sex Transm Infect. 1999;75:3–17.

26. Wasserheit JN. Epidemiological synergy. Interrelationships between human immunodeficiency virus infection and other sexually transmitted diseases. Sex Transm Dis. 1992;19: 61–77.
27. Tosca A, Lehou J, Hatjivasiliou M, Varelzidis A, Stratigos JD. Infiltrate of syphilitic lesions before and after treatment. Genitourin Med. 1988;64:289–93.
28. Van Voorhis WC, Barrett LK, Koelle DM, Nasio JM, Plummer FA, Lukehart SA. Primary and secondary syphilis lesions contain mRNA for Th1 cytokines. J Infect Dis. 1996;173: 491–5.
29. McBroom RL, Styles AR, Chiu MJ, Clegg C, Cockerell CJ, Radolf JD. Secondary syphilis in persons infected with and not infected with HIV-1: a comparative immunohistologic study. Am J Dermatopathol. 1999;21:432–41.
30. Salazar JC, Cruz AR, Pope CD, et al. *Treponema pallidum* elicits innate and adaptive cellular immune responses in skin and blood during secondary syphilis: a flow-cytometric analysis. J Infect Dis. 2007;195:879–87.
31. Sheffield JS, Wendel Jr GD, McIntire DD, Norgard MV. Effect of genital ulcer disease on HIV-1 coreceptor expression in the female genital tract. J Infect Dis. 2007;196:1509–16.
32. Theus SA, Harrich DA, Gaynor R, Radolf JD, Norgard MV. *Treponema pallidum*, lipoproteins, and synthetic lipoprotein analogues induce human immunodeficiency virus type 1 gene expression in monocytes via NF-κB activation. J Infect Dis. 1998;177:941–50.
33. Jarzebowski W, Caumes E, Dupin N, et al. Effect of early syphilis infection on plasma viral load and CD4 cell count in human immunodeficiency virus-infected men: results from the FHDH-ANRS CO4 cohort. Arch Intern Med. 2012;172:1237–43.
34. Moore JE. Asymptomatic neurosyphilis: a comparison of early and late asymptomatic neurosyphilis. Arch Derm Syphilol. 1928;18:99–108.
35. Nagappa M, Sinha S, Taly AB, et al. Neurosyphilis: MRI features and their phenotypic correlation in a cohort of 35 patients from a tertiary care university hospital. Neuroradiology. 2013;55:379–88. doi: 10.1007/s00234-012-1017-9. Epub 2012 Dec 30.
36. Chesney AM, Kemp JE. Incidence of *Spirochaeta pallidum* in cerebrospinal fluid during early stages of syphilis. JAMA. 1924;22:1725–8.
37. Stokes JH, Beerman H, Ingraham NR. Modern clinical syphilology. 3rd ed. Philadelphia: W.B. Saunders; 1944.
38. Hahn RD, Clark EG. Asymptomatic neurosyphilis; a review of the literature. Am J Syph Gonorrhea Vener Dis. 1946;30:305–16.
39. Lukehart SA, Hook 3rd EW, Baker-Zander SA, Collier AC, Critchlow CW, Handsfield HH. Invasion of the central nervous system by *Treponema pallidum*: implications for diagnosis and treatment. Ann Intern Med. 1988;109:855–62.
40. Rolfs RT, Joesoef MR, Hendershot EF, et al. A randomized trial of enhanced therapy for early syphilis in patients with and without human immunodeficiency virus infection. The Syphilis and HIV Study Group. N Engl J Med. 1997;337:307–14.
41. Marra CM. Update on neurosyphilis. Curr Infect Dis Rep. 2009;11:127–34.
42. Ghanem KG, Workowski KA. Management of adult syphilis. Clin Infect Dis. 2011;53 Suppl 3:S110–28.
43. Collis TK, Celum CL. The clinical manifestations and treatment of sexually transmitted diseases in human immunodeficiency virus-positive men. Clin Infect Dis. 2001;32:611–22.
44. Marra CM, Maxwell CL, Smith SL, et al. Cerebrospinal fluid abnormalities in patients with syphilis: association with clinical and laboratory features. J Infect Dis. 2004;189:369–76.
45. Flood JM, Weinstock HS, Guroy ME, Bayne L, Simon RP, Bolan G. Neurosyphilis during the AIDS epidemic, San Francisco, 1985–1992. J Infect Dis. 1998;177:931–40.
46. Ghanem KG, Moore RD, Rompalo AM, Erbelding EJ, Zenilman JM, Gebo KA. Lumbar puncture in HIV-infected patients with syphilis and no neurologic symptoms. Clin Infect Dis. 2009;48:816–21.
47. Merritt HH, Moore M. Acute syphilitic meningitis. Medicine. 1935;14:119–83.
48. Feng W, Caplan M, Matheus MG, Papamitsakis NI. Meningovascular syphilis with fatal vertebrobasilar occlusion. Am J Med Sci. 2009;338:169–71.

49. Chahine LM, Khoriaty RN, Tomford WJ, Hussain MS. The changing face of neurosyphilis. Int J Stroke. 2011;6:136–43.
50. Kodama K, Okada S, Komatsu N, et al. Relationship between MRI findings and prognosis for patients with general paresis. J Neuropsychiatry Clin Neurosci. 2000;12:246–50.
51. Berbel-Garcia A, Porta-Etessam J, Martinez-Salio A, et al. Magnetic resonance image-reversible findings in a patient with general paresis. Sex Transm Dis. 2004;31:350–2.
52. Luo W, Ouyang Z, Xu H, Chen J, Ding M, Zhang B. The clinical analysis of general paresis with 5 cases. J Neuropsychiatry Clin Neurosci. 2008;20:490–3.
53. Agayeva N, Karli-Oguz K, Saka E. Teaching neuroImages: a neurosyphilis case presenting with atypical neuroradiologic findings. Neurology. 2013;80:e119.
54. Dewhurst K. The neurosyphilitic psychoses today. A survey of 91 cases. Br J Psychiatry. 1969;115:31–8.
55. Russouw HG, Roberts MC, Emsley RA, Truter R. Psychiatric manifestations and magnetic resonance imaging in HIV-negative neurosyphilis. Biol Psychiatry. 1997;41:467–73.
56. Mehrabian S, Raycheva MR, Petrova EP, Tsankov NK, Traykov LD. Neurosyphilis presenting with dementia, chronic chorioretinitis and adverse reactions to treatment: a case report. Cases J. 2009;2:8334.
57. Abdelerahman KT, Santamaria DD, Rakocevic G. Pearls & Oy-sters: neurosyphilis presenting as mesial temporal encephalitis. Neurology. 2012;79:e206–8.
58. Denays R, Collier A, Rubinstein M, Atsama P. A 51-year-old woman with disorientation and amnesia. Lancet. 1999;354:1786.
59. Bash S, Hathout GM, Cohen S. Mesiotemporal T2-weighted hyperintensity: neurosyphilis mimicking herpes encephalitis. AJNR Am J Neuroradiol. 2001;22:314–6.
60. Szilak I, Marty F, Helft J, Soeiro R. Neurosyphilis presenting as herpes simplex encephalitis. Clin Infect Dis. 2001;32:1108–9.
61. Hahn RD. Tabes dorsalis with special reference to primary optic atrophy. Br J Vener Dis. 1957;33:139–48.
62. Horowitz HW, Valsamis MP, Wicher V, et al. Brief report: cerebral syphilitic gumma confirmed by the polymerase chain reaction in a man with human immunodeficiency virus infection. N Engl J Med. 1994;331:1488–91.
63. Seeley WW, Venna N. Neurosyphilis presenting with gummatous oculomotor nerve palsy. J Neurol Neurosurg Psychiatry. 2004;75:789.
64. Fargen KM, Alvernia JE, Lin CS, Melgar M. Cerebral syphilitic gummata: a case presentation and analysis of 156 reported cases. Neurosurgery. 2009;64:568–75; discussion 75–6.
65. Aldave AJ, King JA, Cunningham Jr ET. Ocular syphilis. Curr Opin Ophthalmol. 2001;12:433–41.
66. Smith MM, Anderson JC. Neurosyphilis as a cause of facial and vestibulocochlear nerve dysfunction: MR imaging features. AJNR Am J Neuroradiol. 2000;21:1673–5.
67. Becker GD. Late syphilitic hearing loss: a diagnostic and therapeutic dilemma. Laryngoscope. 1979;89:1273–88.
68. Zoller M, Wilson WR, Nadol Jr JB, Girard KF. Detection of syphilitic hearing loss. Arch Otolaryngol. 1978;104:63–5.
69. Pletcher SD, Cheung SW. Syphilis and otolaryngology. Otolaryngol Clin North Am. 2003;36:595–605, vi.
70. Musher DM. Syphilis, neurosyphilis, penicillin, and AIDS. J Infect Dis. 1991;163:1201–6.
71. Musher DM, Hamill RJ, Baughn RE. Effect of human immunodeficiency virus (HIV) infection on the course of syphilis and on the response to treatment. Ann Intern Med. 1990;113:872–81.
72. Golden MR, Marra CM, Holmes KK. Update on syphilis: resurgence of an old problem. JAMA. 2003;290:1510–4.
73. Farhi D, Dupin N. Management of syphilis in the HIV-infected patient: facts and controversies. Clin Dermatol. 2010;28:539–45.
74. Poliseli R, Vidal JE, Penalva De Oliveira AC, Hernandez AV. Neurosyphilis in HIV-infected patients: clinical manifestations, serum venereal disease research laboratory titers, and associated factors to symptomatic neurosyphilis. Sex Transm Dis. 2008;35:425–9.

75. Libois A, De Wit S, Poll B, et al. HIV and syphilis: when to perform a lumbar puncture. Sex Transm Dis. 2007;34:141–4.
76. Workowski KA, Berman S. Sexually transmitted diseases treatment guidelines, 2010. MMWR Recomm Rep. 2010;59:1–110.
77. Guyure KA. Infections. In: Prayson RA, editor. Neuropathology. Philadelphia: Elsevier/ Churchill Livingstone; 2005. p. 287–338.
78. Brown E, Gray F. Bacterial infections. In: Love S, Louis DN, Ellison DW, editors. Greenfield's neuropathology. London: Hodder Arnold; 2008. p. 1391–445.
79. Jackman Jr JD, Radolf JD. Cardiovascular syphilis. Am J Med. 1989;87:425–33.
80. Ghanem KG. Neurosyphilis: a historical perspective and review. CNS Neurosci Ther. 2010;16:e157–68.
81. Larsen SA, Pope V, Johnson RE, Kennedy EJ. A manual of tests for syphilis. Washington, DC: American Public Health Association; 1998.
82. Larsen SA, Steiner BM, Rudolph AH. Laboratory diagnosis and interpretation of tests for syphilis. Clin Microbiol Rev. 1995;8:1–21.
83. Belisle JT, Brandt ME, Radolf JD, Norgard MV. Fatty acids of *Treponema pallidum* and *Borrelia burgdorferi* lipoproteins. J Bacteriol. 1994;176:2151–7.
84. Post JJ, Khor C, Furner V, Smith DE, Whybin LR, Robertson PW. Case report and evaluation of the frequency of the prozone phenomenon in syphilis serology – an infrequent but important laboratory phenomenon. Sex Health. 2012;9:488–90.
85. Creegan L, Bauer HM, Samuel MC, Klausner J, Liska S, Bolan G. An evaluation of the relative sensitivities of the venereal disease research laboratory test and the *Treponema pallidum* particle agglutination test among patients diagnosed with primary syphilis. Sex Transm Dis. 2007;34:1016–8.
86. Radolf JD, Pillay A, Cox DL. *Treponema* and *Brachyspira*, human host-associated spirochetes. In: Versalovic J, editor. Manual of clinical microbiology. 10th ed. Washington, D.C.: American Society for Microbiology; 2011. p. 941–63.
87. CDC. Discordant results from reverse sequence syphilis screening-five laboratories, United States, 2006–2010. MMWR Morb Mortal Wkly Rep. 2011;60:133–7.
88. Hernandez-Aguado I, Bolumar F, Moreno R, et al. False-positive tests for syphilis associated with human immunodeficiency virus and hepatitis B virus infection among intravenous drug abusers. Valencian Study Group on HIV Epidemiology. Eur J Clin Microbiol Infect Dis. 1998;17:784–7.
89. Augenbraun MH, DeHovitz JA, Feldman J, Clarke L, Landesman S, Minkoff HM. Biological false-positive syphilis test results for women infected with human immunodeficiency virus. Clin Infect Dis. 1994;19:1040–4.
90. Hutchinson CM, Rompalo AM, Reichart CA, Hook 3rd EW. Characteristics of patients with syphilis attending Baltimore STD clinics. Multiple high-risk subgroups and interactions with human immunodeficiency virus infection. Arch Intern Med. 1991;151:511–6.
91. Geisler WM. The prozone phenomenon in syphilis testing. South Med J. 2004;97:327–8.
92. Ghanem KG, Erbelding EJ, Wiener ZS, Rompalo AM. Serological response to syphilis treatment in HIV-positive and HIV-negative patients attending sexually transmitted diseases clinics. Sex Transm Infect. 2007;83:97–101.
93. Hicks CB, Benson PM, Lupton GP, Tramont EC. Seronegative secondary syphilis in a patient infected with the human immunodeficiency virus (HIV) with Kaposi sarcoma. A diagnostic dilemma. Ann Intern Med. 1987;107:492–5.
94. Kingston AA, Vujevich J, Shapiro M, et al. Seronegative secondary syphilis in 2 patients coinfected with human immunodeficiency virus. Arch Dermatol. 2005;141:431–3.
95. Marra CM, Tantalo LC, Maxwell CL, Ho EL, Sahi SK, Jones T. The rapid plasma reagin test cannot replace the venereal disease research laboratory test for neurosyphilis diagnosis. Sex Transm Dis. 2012;39:453–7.

96. Castro R, Prieto ES, da Luz Martins Pereira F. Nontreponemal tests in the diagnosis of neurosyphilis: an evaluation of the Venereal Disease Research Laboratory (VDRL) and the Rapid Plasma Reagin (RPR) tests. J Clin Lab Anal. 2008;22:257–61.
97. Jaffe HW, Larsen SA, Peters M, Jove DF, Lopez B, Schroeter AL. Tests for treponemal antibody in CSF. Arch Intern Med. 1978;138:252–5.
98. Schroeter AL, Lucas JB, Price EV, Falcone VH. Treatment for early syphilis and reactivity of serologic tests. JAMA. 1972;221:471–6.
99. Zenker PN, Rolfs RT. Treatment of syphilis, 1989. Rev Infect Dis. 1990;12 Suppl 6:S590–609.
100. Ghanem KG, Erbelding EJ, Cheng WW, Rompalo AM. Doxycycline compared with benzathine penicillin for the treatment of early syphilis. Clin Infect Dis. 2006;42:e45–9.
101. Wong T, Singh AE, De P. Primary syphilis: serological treatment response to doxycycline/tetracycline versus benzathine penicillin. Am J Med. 2008;121:903–8.
102. Spornraft-Ragaller P, Abraham S, Lueck C, Meurer M. Response of HIV-infected patients with syphilis to therapy with penicillin or intravenous ceftriaxone. Eur J Med Res. 2011;16:47–51.
103. Long CM, Klausner JD, Leon S, et al. Syphilis treatment and HIV infection in a population-based study of persons at high risk for sexually transmitted disease/HIV infection in Lima, Peru. Sex Transm Dis. 2006;33:151–5.
104. Shann S, Wilson J. Treatment of neurosyphilis with ceftriaxone. Sex Transm Infect. 2003;79:415–6.
105. Marra CM, Boutin P, McArthur JC, et al. A pilot study evaluating ceftriaxone and penicillin G as treatment agents for neurosyphilis in human immunodeficiency virus-infected individuals. Clin Infect Dis. 2000;30:540–4.
106. Hook 3rd EW, Roddy RE, Handsfield HH. Ceftriaxone therapy for incubating and early syphilis. J Infect Dis. 1988;158:881–4.
107. Ormerod LD, et al. Syphilitic posterior uveitis: correlative findings and significance. Clin Infect Dis. 2001;32(12):1661–73. doi:10.1086/320766.

Chapter 13
Drug-Induced Aseptic Meningitis and Other Mimics

Germán Morís and Juan Carlos García-Moncó

Abstract In addition to viruses, several drugs have been associated with the development of aseptic meningitis, most of them belonging to the group of nonsteroidal anti-inflammatory drugs (NSAIDs, mainly ibuprofen), antibiotics, immunosuppressants, and antiepileptic drugs. Although the pathophysiology of drug-induced meningitis (DIAM) remains obscure, hypersensitivity reactions seem implicated. A sizeable group of DIAM patients (50 % in cases of NSAID-related and 41 % in antibiotic-related meningitis) have an underlying process predisposing to meningitis development, most frequently systemic lupus erythematosus (SLE). DIAM and infectious meningitis, including pyogenic meningitis, are indistinguishable based on clinical characteristics and cerebrospinal fluid analysis; thus, a thorough history on prior drug intake is key to avoid expensive diagnostic procedures or lengthy and unnecessary antibiotic treatments. Besides DIAM, several systemic and neurological disorders, including SLE, sarcoidosis, Behçet disease, Sjögren's syndrome, and primary angiitis of the central nervous system may also mimic infectious meningitis, making the etiological diagnosis and management of these patients challenging.

Keywords Meningitis • Drugs • Antibiotics • Monoclonal antibodies • Immune globulins • Nonsteroidal anti-inflammatory drugs • Systemic lupus erythematosus

G. Morís, MD
Department of Neurology, Hospital Universitario Central de Asturias, Oviedo, Asturias, Spain

J.C. García-Moncó, MD (✉)
Department of Neurology, Hospital de Galdakao-Usansolo, Barrio Labeaga S/N, Galdakao, Vizcaya, 48960, Spain
e-mail: hospit05@sarenet.es

J.C. García-Moncó (ed.), *CNS Infections*,
DOI 10.1007/978-1-4471-6401-2_13,

Introduction

Aseptic meningitis is a clinical syndrome that encompasses leptomeningeal inflammation of the brain and is characterized by fever and meningeal symptoms with lymphocytic cerebrospinal fluid (CSF) pleocytosis and sterile cultures.

Aseptic meningitis is mainly caused by viruses and less commonly by noninfectious conditions, including several systemic diseases and drugs. The latter produce direct meningeal irritation when the drug is given intrathecally, but in the last years an increasing list of drugs has been recognized as potential agents to produce meningitis when administered in oral or intravenous preparations. Therefore, the condition of aseptic meningitis is no longer tantamount to viral meningitis, even though the two terms often are used interchangeably.

Drug-Induced Meningitis (DIAM)

Several drugs can induce meningitis, which constitutes a diagnostic and therapeutic challenge. The situation becomes more complex if the offending drug is an antibiotic, where the decision of withdrawing the drug needs to be weighed against the risk of missing the treatment of an underlying infectious disorder. Furthermore, these drugs are often used to treat disorders that in turn may cause meningitis. Therefore, physicians should obtain a careful drug history in every case of meningitis that could obviate inappropriate therapies such as prolonged antimicrobial therapy or high dose of immunosuppressants.

The incidence of DIAM is unknown because cases are underreported, and perhaps because many DIAM are included in reports of viral meningitis. Recent series and case reports have increased the number of drugs capable of inducing a meningeal inflammation. Three groups of drugs have been associated with drug-induced aseptic meningitis (Table 13.1): nonsteroidal anti-inflammatory drugs (NSAIDs), antibiotics, immunosuppressive–immunomodulatory drugs (IS–IM), and antiepileptic drugs, mainly lamotrigine.

When a patient develops meningitis in possible relation with any drug, the clinical syndrome should meet the criteria of DIAM:

(a) Temporal relationship with the drug intake (including a positive reintroduction test when it is possible)
(b) CSF pleocytosis
(c) Negative testing for microorganisms
(d) Absence of other explanation and complete resolution following discontinuation of the drug [1]

Table 13.1 Drugs involved in DIAM

Drug group	No. of reported cases	Drugs involved (no. of cases)	Sex	Age range (mean ± SD)	Range of latency (median)	Prior exposure to drug (%)
NSAIDs	76	Ibuprofen (47)	62 % female	21–73 (39 ± 15)	30 min–4 months (8 h)	35
		Sulindac (7)				
		Naproxen (7)				
		Tolmetin (1)				
		Diclofenac sodium (3)				
		Ketoprofen (1)				
		Celecoxib (1)				
		Dexibuprofen (1)				
		Piroxicam (1)				
		Ketorolaco (1)				
		Rofecoxib (6)				
Antibiotics	69	Sulfamethizole (1)	59 % female	1–90 (46 ± 23)	10 min–3 months (6 h)	33
		TMP–SMX (32)				
		TMP (11)				
		Isoniazid (1)				
		Ciprofloxacin (2)				
		Penicillin (1)				
		Metronidazole (3)				
		Cephalosporin (2)				
		Pyrazinamide (1)				
		Sulfisoxazole (1)				
		Amoxicillin (8)[a]				
		Fumagillin (1)				
		Minocycline (1)				
		Ornidazole (1)				
		Rifampicin (1)				
		Valacyclovir (2)				

(continued)

Table 13.1 (continued)

Drug group	No. of reported cases	Drugs involved (no. of cases)	Sex	Age range (mean ± SD)	Range of latency (median)	Prior exposure to drug (%)
Immunosuppressive or immunomodulatory agents	17	Adalimumab (1)	53 % female	31–78 (51 ± 11)	3 h–5 months (48 h)	26
		Cetuximab (5)				
		Efalizumab (2)				
		Infliximab (4)				
		Leflunomide (1)				
		Methotrexate (1)				
		Salazopyrin (2)				
		Sulfasalazine (1)				
SLE group	28	Ibuprofen (17)	89 % female	21–73 (38 ± 14)	20 min–2 weeks (3.5 h)	32
		Tolmetin (1)				
		Sulindac (1)				
		Naproxen (1)				
		Diclofenac (1)				
		TMP–SMX (3)				
		TMP (1)				
		Sulfisoxazole (1)				
		Dexibuprofen (1)				
		Rifampicin (1)				

The SLE group comprises all the patients with systemic lupus irrespective of the offending drug (see text)
One patient can develop various DIAM episodes in relation with more than one drug
Abbreviations: *TMP–SMX* trimethoprim–sulfamethoxazole, *IS–IM* immunosuppressive or immunomodulatory agents, *NSAIDs* nonsteroidal anti-inflammatory drugs, *SLE* systemic lupus erythematosus
[a]Five patients were on amoxicillin plus clavulanic acid

Table 13.2 Clinical signs and symptoms (%) of drug-induced aseptic meningitis

	Total
Fever	83
Headache	82
Meningeal signs	67
Nausea–vomiting	44
Rash	11
Abdominal pain	4
Arthromyalgias	30
Hypotension	8
Facial edema	18
Abnormal consciousness*	43
Focal neurologic deficit	12
Seizures	7
Papilledema	4
Lymphadenopathies	5
Abnormal liver function	11
Photophobia	27

*Includes somnolence–coma and confusional states

Clinical Characteristics and CSF Profiles of Patients of DIAM

The majority of patients with DIAM, irrespective of the offending drug, are present with headache, fever, meningismus, and mental status abnormalities (Table 13.2). This presentation is also characteristic of infectious meningitis and therefore does not help in differentiating DIAM from infectious meningitis. Other less frequently reported findings include rash, arthralgias, myalgias, facial edema, lymph nodes, and liver tests abnormalities, which occasionally occur in infectious meningitis, particularly of viral origin.

There are minimal differences in the presentation of the meningitides induced by the different drugs that would suggest a specific drug as the culprit. Seizures are recorded in patients with antibiotic-induced meningitis, but can, in turn, be provoked also by antibiotics (particularly beta-lactams at high doses in a setting of renal failure), and are present in up to 7 % of patients with bacterial meningitis, irrespective of therapy. Thus, it seems more likely that seizures in DIAM are related to the meningitis and not to the offending drug [2].

The presentation of NSAID-induced meningitis is rather stereotypical in that it is more common in women (62 % of the patients, Table 13.1), with an autoimmune disorder and prior exposure to the drug, who develop a neutrophilic meningitis with normal-to-low glucose level and increased proteins. The preponderance of ibuprofen reports likely reflect the popularity of nonprescription ibuprofen products, but drug-specific factors may also be at play.

Antibiotic-induced DIAM shows a similar profile to NSAIDs, and 41 % of the patients have an underlying disorder (Table 13.3). Most cases develop after

Table 13.3 Underlying disorder (%) in patients with drug-induced aseptic meningitis

Drug group	Underlying	Condition
	Common (>10 %)	Uncommon (<10 %)
NSAID (*n*=38) 50 %	Systemic lupus erythematosus (*n*=22) 58 %	Undifferentiated connective tissue disease (*n*=1) 3 %
N total=76	Mixed connective tissue disease (*n*=7) 18 %	Isolated rheumatoid factor and antibodies to the SS-A antigen positivity of uncertain origin (*n*=1) 3 %
		Isolated positive antinuclear antibodies of uncertain origin (*n*=1) 3 %
		Ankylosing spondylitis (*n*=1) 3 %
		Rheumatoid arthritis (*n*=2) 5 %
		Sjögren's syndrome (*n*=1) 3 %[a]
		Dermatomyositis (*n*=1) 3 %[a]
		Seronegative acute oligoarthritis (*n*=1) 3 %
		Autoimmune thyroiditis (*n*=1) 3 %
Antibiotics (*n*=28) 41 %	HIV infection (*n*=7) 25 %	Sjögren's syndrome (*n*=2) 7 %
N total=69	Systemic lupus erythematosus (*n*=6) 21 %	Crohn's disease (*n*=1) 3 %
		Rheumatoid arthritis (*n*=1) 3 %
		Interstitial cystitis (*n*=1) 3 %
		Type 1 diabetes mellitus (*n*=1) 3 %
		Type 2 diabetes mellitus (*n*=1) 3 %
		Autoimmune hypothyroidism (*n*=1) 3 %
		Rhizomelic pseudopolyarthritis (*n*=1) 3 %
		Temporal arteritis (*n*=1) 3 %
		G6PD deficiency (*n*=1) 3 %[b]
		Acute nonlymphoblastic leukemia (*n*=1) 3 %
		Bladder cancer and chronic renal insufficiency (*n*=1) 3 %
		Trisomy 21 (*n*=1) 3 %
		Kidney transplantation
Immunomodulators/ immunosupressors (*n*=17)	Rheumatoid arthritis (*n*=5) 29 %[b]	Recurrent laryngeal squamous cell carcinoma (*n*=1) 6 %
N total=17	Non-small cell lung cancer (*n*=2) 12 %	Advanced tonsil squamous cell carcinoma (*n*=1) 6 %
	Psoriasis (*n*=2) 12 %[c]	Squamous maxillary cancer (*n*=1) 6 %
	Crohn's disease (n=2) 12 %	Ulcerative colitis (*n*=1) 6 %
		Unclassified oligoarthritis (*n*=1) 6 %
		Undifferentiated spondyloarthritis (*n*=1) 6 %

The different underlying conditions were arbitrarily split into common (>10 % of cases) and uncommon (<10 %)

G6PD deficiency: glucose-6-phosphate dehydrogenase deficiency

[a]The patient suffered from dermatiomyositis and Sjögren's syndrome

[b]One patient suffered from rheumatoid arthritis and mixed type III cryoglobulinemia. Another patient suffered from rheumatoid arthritis and epilepsy

[c]One patient suffered from psoriasis and Graves' disease

trimethoprim (TMP) exposure, with or without sulfamethoxazole (SMX), followed by amoxicillin. Cephalosporins are rarely linked to aseptic meningitis, with only two reports in the literature: a healthy 66-year-old woman exposed to three different cephalosporins (cefalexin, cefazolin, and ceftazidime) and a 1-year-old boy with trisomy 21 receiving cefotaxime and ceftriaxone [3, 4]. This paucity of reports support the use of third-generation cephalosporins as the first choice in suspected DIAM patients before negative microbacterial studies are obtained. TMP–SMX-associated meningitis is frequent in HIV-infected patients, in part due to the widespread prophylactic use of this drug in this population, but may also reflect the fact that chronic HIV patients are prone to sulfonamide-induced hypersensitivity reactions.

Despite its frequent use, acyclovir has not been related to aseptic meningitis. A few isolated cases of DIAM associated to metronidazole, valacyclovir, fumagillin, ornidazole, minocycline, and rifampicin have been reported in isolated case reports [5–12].

The clinical profile of IS–IM-induced meningitis is similar to the other drug groups although with less female predominance. The first monoclonal antibody associated with aseptic meningitis was OKT3, a murine IgG2a antibody introduced for kidney transplant induction therapy in the early 1980s, which resulted in aseptic meningitis in 1–5 % of patients [13]. Because of its side effects and declining usage, OKT3 was removed from the market. Other IS–IM drugs were later associated with DIAM, including infliximab, efalizumab, cetuximab, adalimumab, and a monoclonal antibody against TNF-alpha.

Four cases of aseptic meningitis after efalizumab, a humanized monoclonal antibody against CD11 molecule on the T-cell surface, have been reported [14–16]. Cetuximab, a chimeric monoclonal antibody against epidermal growth factor receptor approved for the treatment of diverse cancers, has been associated with a few cases of DIAM [17–20].

DIAM has also been described with other drugs prescribed for autoimmune diseases, including leflunomide, methotrexate, salazopyrin, and sulfasalazine. The latter cross-reacts with sulfamethoxazole, and both likely share a common pathogenic mechanism [21–26].

Mild headache is present in 5–80 % of patients following immunoglobulins (IVIGs) administration. However, aseptic meningitis is a much less common complication, with a prevalence of 1–11 % [27, 28]. Fast infusion rates, poor hydration, and a history of migraine headaches may predispose to meningitis development.

The interval between drug intake and the development of meningitis varies between minutes and 4 months for all the drug groups, and prior exposure to the drug is present in 30 % of patients irrespective of the group (Table 13.1). This low rate is striking, considering the high prescription rate of NSAIDs and antibiotics, and the fact that IS–IM drugs are employed periodically to treat autoimmune disorders or neoplasms. There is no relation between DIAM development and the dose of the drug employed, usually within the therapeutic range.

The CSF of DIAM shows pleocytosis of several hundred to several thousand cells per mm^3, normal-to-low glucose values and increased proteins (Table 13.4).

Table 13.4 CSF characteristics of patients with drug-induced aseptic meningitis

Drug group	Cells/mm^3 median (range)	Predominant cells (% of patient)	Median glucose value (range), mmol/L	Median protein value (range), g/L
NSAID	230 (8–5000)	Lymphocytes (26 %) Neutrophils (69 %) Eosinophils (2 %)[a]	3.2 (1.5–6.0)	1.2 (0.49–8.57)
Antibiotics	125 (5–19000)	Lymphocytes (43 %) Neutrophils (51 %)[b]	3.33 (2–8.65)	1.04 (0.27–3.90)
Immunomodulators/ immunosuppressants	160 (18–2300)	Lymphocytes (29 %) Neutrophils (65 %)[c]	2.6 (1.4–3.4)	0.91 (2.12–0.44)
Lupus	282 (8–5000)	Lymphocytes(23 %) Neutrophils (77 %)	3.1 (1.5–6)	1.25 (0.5–8.57)

[a]In two cases, there were macrophages and histiocytes in CSF smear
[b]There were two cases with monocytes representing 95, and 24 % of the total cell count, and two cases with plasma cells and eosinophils representing 57, and 14 % of the total cell count
[c]There was one case with monocytes representing 39 % of the total cell count

The number of cells and protein values is higher in the NSAIDs group. There is a characteristic neutrophilic predominance, with a percentage over the total cell count ranging from 65 to 69 % in NSAIDs and IS–IM and 51 % in antibiotics. Eosinophils are noted in patients from the NSAIDs group (13–60 % of the total cell count) [29, 30], in the antibiotic group (2–24 %) [31–33], and in patients receiving intravenous immunoglobulins (<5 %) [27]. Due to technical difficulties in recognizing CSF eosinophils, it is likely that their presence in the CSF is underreported [29].

Polymorphonuclear leukocytes are the first cells recruited in inflammatory processes, including the acute phase of meningitis, which may justify the neutrophilic pleocytosis present in these patients. The presence of increased levels of interleukin-8, granulocyte colony-stimulating factor, and macrophage inflammatory protein 1-alpha in the subarachnoid space contributes to their accumulation in the CSF. Differences in the CSF profile of DIAM induced by different drugs or even among patients who took the same drug could be partly justified by the different timing at which spinal tap was performed.

The opening CSF pressure is normal, except for a few reports that found a pressure reaching 46 cm H_2O [34, 35].

The presence of eosinophils in the CSF is more common in DIAM than in infectious meningitis, except for those of parasitic origin, and their presence reinforces the allergic condition of DIAM.

When performed, neuroimaging is normal in all but a few patients. Diffuse hemispheric enhancement has been reported in two patients as a likely reflection of blood–brain barrier breakdown [36, 37] and one patient with NSAID-induced meningitis had reversible small, non-enhancing hyperintense lesions involving the supratentorial grey matter, basal ganglia, and cerebellar hemispheres as shown by MRI [38].

Underlying Conditions in Patients with DIAM

SLE stands as the single most frequent underlying condition associated with DIAM (Table 13.3). The analysis of the clinical and CSF profiles of this group of patients is not shared any special or typical characteristic. The predominance in females is marked (90 %) as expected for lupus, but there are no other obvious differences from the rest of parameters (Tables 13.1, 13.2, and 13.4).

Although migraine has been suggested as a predisposing condition to DIAM and reported in several patients [27, 39], the retrospective analysis of these heterogeneous case reports does not allow for the determination of the exact prevalence of prior, potentially predisposing, conditions such as migraine. To further complicate matters, the high prevalence of migraine in the normal population (6–12 %) [40] and its even higher prevalence in populations also prone to DIAM such as SLE patients should be considered [41].

Recurrent DIAM

There are 48 patients with recurrent DIAM in the literature, totaling 115 episodes. Their clinical and CSF characteristics are shown in Table 13.5. Meningitis was associated with NSAIDs in 16 patients (18 episodes) and with antibiotics in 23 (43 episodes). Less often, it was associated with IS–IM drugs or antiepileptics. The highest number of episodes reported in a single patient is 5 [42, 43]. There is female predominance (71 %) with an age range of 2–82 years (mean 45).

An underlying disorder was present in 31 patients (65 %), with SLE being the most frequent (10 patients), followed by Sjögren's syndrome (3), and a variety of different disorders (Table 13.5).

The CSF analysis reveals a neutrophilic pleocytosis of similar magnitude across the different episodes. The latency from exposure to recovery was similar between episodes.

Differential Diagnosis

One of most important problem in DIAM is assessing the causal relationship between drug intake and meningitis development, a probability that is based on clinical judgment, although there are scales to establish the causality of an adverse event and drug exposure, the most popular being the Naranjo's drug-adverse-reaction scale. This scale is composed by ten items and provides a probability category of definite, probable, possible, or doubtful [44]. The only confirmatory test of DIAM, however, would be drug rechallenge, occasionally reported in the literature in inadvertent cases but ethically unjustified.

Table 13.5 CSF characteristics in recurrent episodes of DIAM

	Latency range (median)	Cells/mm^3 median (range)	Predominant cells (%)	Glucose mg/dl median (range)	Protein mg/dl median (range)	Time to recovery median (range)
1st episode ($n=48$)	15 min–4 months (24 h)	145 (8–3600)	Lymphocytes (26 %) Neutrophils (74 %)	3.16 (1.5–5.5)	1.5 (1.14–76)	48 h (24–336 h)
2nd episode ($n=48$)	15 min–14 days (4 h)	208 (9–5440)	Lymphocytes (27 %) Neutrophils (71 %)[a]	3.16 (3.1–6.2)	0.55 (1.17–5.9)	48 h (12–384 h)
3rd episode ($n=15$)	30 min–14 days (5 h)	200 (20–2050)	Lymphocytes (36 %) Neutrophils (64 %)	3.33 (1.6–11.9)	1.22 (0.86–4.67)	48 h (24–336 h)

[a]There was one case with 99 monocytes representing 99 % of the total cell count

Differentiating DIAM from bacterial meningitis, as mentioned, is difficult, particularly considering the similar CSF profile and clinical presentation [45]. Even more problematic is the case of a patient treated with an antibiotic that develops meningitis and in whom the possibility of partially treated meningitis needs to be weighed against antibiotic-related DIAM. Again, these entities cannot be distinguished on clinical and CSF grounds alone. Of help may be to consider the type of antibiotic (Table 13.1). In cases where bacterial meningitis is a possibility, we suggest to treat the patient with a third-generation cephalosporin, only rarely linked to DIAM, and active against the most likely organisms of community-acquired meningitis.

Recovery upon drug discontinuation is the rule; hence, chronic infectious meningitis (tuberculosis, fungi, etc.) would only rarely pose a diagnostic problem. If such is the case, appropriate CSF studies (culture in appropriate media and adequate stains) will be necessary. Meningitis due to parasites may need to be ruled out in those cases with CSF eosinophilia that occur in the appropriate epidemiological context.

Viral aseptic meningitis is another important consideration in terms of frequency, although less critical in terms of prognosis and management. Clinically, it is marked by fever (76–100 %), nuchal rigidity, and headache that may be accompanied by vomiting, rash, diarrhea, pharyngitis, arthralgias, and myalgias [46]. Neutrophils may occasionally dominate the CSF profile early in the infection (particularly with mumps), although there is usually a shift to lymphocytic predominance over the first 48 h. CSF glucose levels are usually normal (may be low in mumps). Again, clinical and CSF overlapping with DIAM occur. It could also be argued whether certain cases of DIAM would in fact correspond to viral meningitis considering the difficulty of making a definitive diagnosis in viral infections. The time to recovery after drug withdrawal may be of help, since it is rapid in DIAM (1–5 days) but usually takes 10–14 days in viral meningitis.

Many other, noninfectious causes of aseptic meningitis exist, an important fact considering that many patients with DIAM harbor underlying systemic disorders that may cause meningitis and that can also predispose them to neurological infections by diverse organisms. In the setting of SLE, DIAM needs to be distinguished from lupus aseptic meningitis. Although signs of meningeal inflammation are present in 18 % of autopsied SLE patients, aseptic meningitis is infrequently diagnosed, since the clinical presentation can be overwhelmed by other neuropsychiatric manifestations. Unlike DIAM, the cellular infiltrate of the CSF in lupus meningitis is usually lymphocytic (less than 50 cells) and is accompanied by other data consistent with a lupus flare-up. In turn, DIAM could mimic a drug-induced exacerbation in SLE if accompanied by systemic manifestations. The rapid onset and resolution of the signs and symptoms as well as the lack of data of SLE activity, especially a fall in serum complement levels, argue against an exacerbation of SLE [47–49].

Antibiotics are probably underrecognized as etiologic agents of recurrent meningitis and must be considered also in their differential diagnosis together with anatomical skull defects, parameningeal infectious foci, immunodeficiencies, and Mollaret's disease [50].

The abrupt onset in some patients with DIAM may suggest an intracranial vascular event, especially in patients with predisposing disease such as idiopathic thrombocytopenic purpura. Neuroimaging helps rule out a vascular lesion [51, 52].

CSF pleocytosis may occasionally accompany migraine, but the cell profile is lymphocytic and rarely exceeds 100 cells per mm^3. NAIDs are commonly used to treat migraines and therefore could play a role in producing migraine pleocytosis, but this aspect has never been systematically assessed. Patients with the syndrome of transient headache and neurological deficits with cerebrospinal fluid lymphocytosis (HaNDL), characterized by focal neurological deficits, headache, fever, and lymphocytic pleocytosis, should also be considered in the differential. The presence of lymphocytic pleocytosis and focal neurologic deficits helps to differentiate this entity from DIAM. As for migraine, the hypothetical role of drugs, such as NSAIDs, should be assessed in this disorder [53].

Pathogenesis

The pathogenic mechanisms of DIAM are not fully understood, but there is evidence to suggest that they may be diverse, perhaps different for the various types of drugs. Most of the authors invoke a hypersensitivity mechanism (especially type 1 and 3) for NSAID-, IS–IM-, and antibiotic-related cases. However, it is striking that such reactions are mainly or exclusively confined to the CSF compartment.

NSAID-Induced Meningitis

In the case of NSAIDs, it seems clear that inhibition of the cyclooxygenase pathway is not involved. Patients can tolerate other NSAIDs both before and after the meningitis episode, and not all drugs in this group lead to meningitis [29, 36, 54–56]. In addition, rofecoxib and celecoxib, selective cyclooxigenase-2 (COX-2) inhibitors, have been also associated with cases of aseptic meningitis [52, 57]. In these cases, the mechanism may be an idiosyncratic reaction to CNS to COX-2 inhibitors. The short latency period after rechallenge argues against accumulation of the NSAID or its metabolites within the CNS. In addition, development of NSAIDs-induced meningitis is irrespective of drug dosage.

Some data point to a type 1 hypersensitivity reaction in the pathogenic mechanism of NSAID-induced meningitis: (a) the temporal relationship between drug intake and the development of meningitis, (b) prior exposure to the offensive drug and disappearance of symptoms after drug discontinuation, (c) the presence of accompanying "allergic" signs such as facial edema and conjunctivitis and rash, (d) and more severe symptoms upon drug reexposure.

Latency after drug intake, however, is not shorter with reexposure. In those patients who developed meningitis upon their first exposure to the NSAIDs, it has been suggested that a prior contact with a cross-reactive chemical could mediate the sensitization [56]. A few patients have developed meningitis after the intake of different NSAIDs or of several unrelated drugs, which suggests individual predisposition [43, 58, 59]. That was the case of a patient with aseptic meningitis induced by naproxen, ibuprofen, and rofecoxib [60].

Based on the findings of increased CSF immune complexes and evidence of intrathecal IgG production, some authors have concluded that ibuprofen-induced meningitis is an antigen-specific immune process confined to the CNS, where the drug, and not a metabolite, would potentiate the activity of a preexisting autoantibody, resulting in complement fixation and development of an acute meningitis [61, 62]. Moreover, an interaction between the drug and a CSF or meningeal protein which acts as a hapten, leading to an inflammatory response in the meninges has been proposed [55].

Taken together, the available data suggest that NSAID-related meningitis develops in individuals rendered susceptible by an underlying autoimmune disorder who were previously sensitized or had a natural immunity to the drug. The confinement of this reaction to the CNS is intriguing.

Antibiotic-Induced Meningitis

Similar mechanisms as those described for NSAIDs have been suggested, but data are contradictory. Evidence of type 1 or 3 hypersensitivity reaction in amoxicillin-induced aseptic meningitis was not supported by the normal values of specific IgE or the absence of immune complexes in serum or CSF of one patient [63]. Conversely, a report of a CSF plasma cell population appearing during a DIAM related to amoxicillin and disappearing with drug withdrawal suggests type III hypersensitivity involvement in drug-induced aseptic meningitis [64].

Immune complex deposition in the choroid plexus inducing a necrotizing small-vessel vasculitis resulting in an aseptic meningitis has also been invoked [3, 42, 65], as has been an underlying defect of the meninges [65, 66].

Immunosuppressive or Immunomodulatory (IS–IM) Agents

While the underlying mechanism is unclear, a serum sickness-like reaction with immune complex-derived allergic reaction has been suspected (hypersensitivity type III reaction) in infliximab cases, although serum antibodies to infliximab have not been detected and infliximab hardly crosses the blood–brain barrier due to high molecular weight [67–71].

Possible mechanisms include hypersensitivity to stabilizing agents of the commercial preparations (unlikely, since this syndrome developed in the same patients who received other prior immunoglobulin preparations), hypersensitivity caused by the direct entry of the immunoglobulins into the CSF compartment, interaction of pooled IgG (allogenic) with antigenic determinants on the endothelial cells of the meningeal vasculature, and activation of the complement system triggered by immunoglobulin macroaggregates [72]. Intriguingly, aseptic meningitis does not occur in patients receiving a standard replacement dose of IVIGs for a congenital immunodeficiency.

Lamotrigine and Antiepileptic Drugs

Lamotrigine is a phenyltriazine derivative with anticonvulsant and mood-stabilizing properties. Forty cases of suspected lamotrigine-associated aseptic meningitis have been reported to the Food and Drug Administration (FDA), although only 25 patients had objective evidence of meningitis through CSF profiles [73]. Outside the USA, five additional cases of CSF pleocytosis after lamotrigine intake have been published [74–77]. The clinical picture is similar to other DIAMs, and symptoms develop hours to more than 1 month after the first dose (ranging from 12.5 to 150 mg). The CSF also shows neutrophilic pleocytosis in two-thirds of patients (around 100 cells/mm^3). Complete recovery in several days after drug discontinuation is the rule. One patient died, but death was not attributable to lamotrigine [73], and another patient developed an abducens palsy [77].

The mechanism of lamotrigine-induced meningitis is unclear and may differ from the other drugs. The clinical picture resembles an acute hypersensitivity reaction based on the greater severity of symptoms upon subsequent exposure.

Four patients have been reported who developed meningitis after carbamazepine therapy, one of them with Sjögren's syndrome and trigeminal neuralgia, two with manic–depressive syndrome, and another with isolated trigeminal neuralgia. The clinical picture was indistinguishable from other DIAM, although one patient had myoclonus with normal carbamazepine levels.

Other Agents Associated with DIAM

Aseptic meningitis is a complication of chemotherapy, including pemetrexed [78] and cytarabine; [79, 80] the latter may also associate cerebellar dysfunction [81].

DIAM has also been reported with salicylate overdose [82], hepatitis B vaccination [83], phenazopyridine [84], dexchlorpheniramine [85], pentoxifylline [86], vitamin B complex [87], ranitidine [88, 89], and allopurinol [90, 91].

Intrathecal Agents

Pyogenic meningitis occasionally occurs after intrathecal drug administration. More frequent, however, is the development of aseptic meningitis. The group of offending drugs is large and heterogeneous and includes radiological contrasts, steroids, anesthetics, chemotherapeutic agents, aminoglycosides, and baclofen [92–94]. A direct chemical irritation of the meninges is the most plausible mechanism. Most patients recover fully in days without sequelae.

Vaccines

The association of aseptic meningitis and vaccination is well known, particularly with measles–mumps–rubella vaccine. All commercially available mumps vaccines contain live attenuated virus, and the incidence of meningitis ranges from 1 in 1.8 million doses to as high as 1 in 1,000 vaccine recipients.

The syndrome is usually observed within the third week after immunization [95].

Other Mimics Associated with Aseptic Meningitis

Aside from drug-induced cases, aseptic meningitis may appear as part of the spectrum of diverse noninfectious conditions (Table 13.6).

Systemic Lupus Erythematosus (SLE)

Neuropsychiatric involvement in SLE is broad and is present in 14–75 % of patients. About 1 % of lupus patients develop aseptic meningitis, which is usually transient and occurs early in the course of SLE, often during flare-ups [49, 96]. In a study of a LES population, 1.63 % of the patients developed meningitis, and in 40 % of the

Table 13.6 Leading noninfectious cause of aseptic meningitis

Drug-induced aseptic meningitis
Neoplastic meningitis
Primary angiitis central nervous system meningitis
Vogt–Koyanagi–Harada syndrome
Headache associated with neurologic deficits and CSF lymphocytosis syndrome
Systemic conditions
(a) Systemic lupus erythematosus
(b) Sarcoidosis
(c) Systemic lupus erythematosus
(d) Sjögren's syndrome
(e) Sarcoidosis
(f) Behçet disease
(g) Wegener's granulomatosis

episodes, no microorganisms were identified. None of the patients was taking any of the drugs related to DIAM, and most of them had a high SLE activity index. The median CSF cell count was 142 per mm^3 (range: 20–1,440), with a mean CSF/plasma glucose ratio of 0.33 [48]. SLE-induced aseptic meningitis may also be associated with myelopathy or brain vasculitis [97]. The pathogenesis of aseptic meningitis in patients with SLE is unclear and could be due to meningeal irritation secondary to SLE activity or to inflammation of brain small vessels. Due to the coexistent SLE activity, steroids might speed patients' recovery.

Sjögren's Syndrome

Sjögren's syndrome (SS) is an autoimmune disease characterized by inflammatory infiltration and secondary chronic dysfunction of exocrine glands. Patients present xerostomia and xerophthalmia (sicca syndrome). Extraglandular manifestations of the disease occur in one-third of the patients, including a wide spectrum of peripheral and central neurological disorders. Aseptic meningitis has been described in around 20 % of the patients with CNS involvement [98] and was recurrent in a few cases [99]. CSF analysis shows a moderate lymphocytic pleocytosis, increased proteins, normal glucose, and oligoclonal bands. Steroid therapy usually leads to disappearance of the symptoms [100].

Sarcoidosis

Sarcoidosis is an inflammatory multisystem disorder of unknown cause. Five percent of the patients have involvement of the nervous system, either central or peripheral, usually during the first 2 years of disease. Cranial nerve abnormalities are the most common neurological complications due to basal meningeal involvement. Aseptic meningitis may occur and the CSF shows lymphocytic pleocytosis, increased proteins and normal glucose (low in 20 % of patients), intrathecal synthesis of IgG, and oligoclonal bands. Steroid therapy is the mainstay of therapy [101, 102].

Behçet Disease

Behçet disease is a multisystem disorder of unknown etiology characterized by recurrent oral and genital ulcers, and uveitis presenting at the age of 20–40. Neurologic involvement ranges from 5 to 10 % of the patients. Cerebral venous sinus thrombosis may occur, as well as posterior fossa parenchymal lesions. CSF analysis shows a lymphocytic pleocytosis (a few hundred cells per mm^3), increased proteins, normal glucose, and intrathecal IgG synthesis. Aseptic meningitis as the sole manifestation of Behçet disease has been reported [103, 104]. Steroids are used to treat exacerbations [105].

Primary Angiitis Central Nervous System Meningitis

Primary angiitis of the central nervous system is an idiopathic vasculitis confined to the CNS. The mean age of onset is 50 years, with male predominance. Vascular involvement is segmental, with predilection for small- and medium-sized leptomeningeal and intracranial vessels. Clinical presentation includes headaches, focal neurologic deficits, and confusion. The CSF analysis is abnormal in up to 90 % of patients, with moderate lymphocytic pleocytosis (<250 cells per mm^3) and protein increase and normal glucose. Neuroimaging is suggestive of vasculitis, and leptomeningeal biopsy is required for diagnosis. Immunosuppressive therapy should be initiated after diagnosis [106, 107].

Neoplastic Meningitis

Involvement of the leptomeninges by metastatic cells is present in 5–15 % of cancer patients, including solid (lung cancer, breast cancer, melanoma) and hematological neoplasms (acute lymphoblastic leukemia and non-Hodgkin lymphoma). It occurs in <2 % of patients with primary brain tumors. CSF in neoplastic meningitis shows mononuclear pleocytosis, increased CSF proteins, and low glucose. Gadolinium-enhanced MRI may suggest the diagnosis, which requires cytological examination of several CSF samples (each containing >10 ml) [108]. Flow cytometry analysis of the CSF is helpful in patients with leukemia or lymphoma [68, 69].

Wegener's Granulomatosis

Wegener's granulomatosis is a necrotizing vasculitis affecting the CNS, respiratory tract, and kidneys. Lymphocytic aseptic meningitis with normal glucose is occasionally present [109].

Vogt–Koyanagi–Harada Syndrome

Vogt–Koyanagi–Harada syndrome is a diffuse granulomatous disease characterized by uveitis, skin involvement (alopecia, poliosis, and vitiligo), and dysacusis. It is caused by a T-cell-mediated autoimmune response against melanocytes in predisposed Caucasian people.

Aseptic meningitis is present in 72–100 % of patients, with a polynuclear pleocytosis in the CSF with decreased glucose [110]. Although treatment is controversial, high-dose corticosteroids that are gradually tapered remain the mainstay of initial therapy.

HaDNL Syndrome

HaDNL syndrome is a self-limited syndrome characterized by 1–21 episodes of sudden onset of headache with temporary neurologic deficit and CSF lymphocytosis. Most patients have nonspecific infectious symptoms several weeks prior to presentation (cough, rhinitis, diarrhea, and malaise). Neurologic deficits last between 5 min and 1 week and include sensory symptoms, language disorders, and hemiparesis. Meningeal signs are not found [111]. When the CSF is studied, CSF opening pressure is elevated in more than 50 % of cases, glucose is normal, and there is a lymphocytic pleocytosis (around 200 cells/mm^3) with increased proteins. There is no IgG synthesis and oligoclonal bands are absent. Complete recovery is the rule and no specific treatment is needed [112, 113].

Other Mimics

Anecdotal causes of aseptic meningitis of noninfectious etiology include rupture of dermoid, epidermoid, or neuroepithelial cysts; dural arteriovenous fistula; vein of Galen aneurysm; cryopyrin-associated periodic syndrome; hypertrophic pachymeningitis; endocarditis; relapsing polychondritis; Fabry disease; subarachnoid hemorrhage; and parameningeal infections [114–121].

References

1. Jolles S, Sewell WA, Leighton C. Drug-induced aseptic meningitis: diagnosis and management. Drug Saf. 2000;22(3):215–26.
2. Moris G, Garcia-Monco JC. The challenge of drug-induced aseptic meningitis. Arch Intern Med. 1999;159(11):1185–94.
3. Creel GB, Hurtt M. Cephalosporin-induced recurrent aseptic meningitis. Ann Neurol. 1995;37(6):815–7.
4. Nakajima W, Ishida A, Takahashi M, Sato Y, Ito T, Takada G. Aseptic meningitis associated with cephalosporins in an infant with trisomy 21. J Child Neurol. 2007;22(6):780–2.
5. Corson AP, Chretien JH. Metronidazole-associated aseptic meningitis. Clin Infect Dis. 1994;19(5):974.
6. Fobelo MJ, Corzo Delgado JE, Romero Alonso A, Gomez-Bellver MJ. Aseptic meningitis related to valacyclovir. Ann Pharmacother. 2001;35(1):128–9.

7. Mondon M, Ollivier L, Daumont A. Aseptic meningitis ornidazole-induced in the course of infectious endocarditis. Rev Med Interne. 2002;23(9):784–7.
8. Olin JL, Gugliotta JL. Possible valacyclovir-related neurotoxicity and aseptic meningitis. Ann Pharmacother. 2003;37(12):1814–7.
9. Khan S, Sharrack B, Sewell WA. Metronidazole-induced aseptic meningitis during Helicobacter pylori eradication therapy. Ann Intern Med. 2007;146(5):395–6.
10. Lefebvre N, Forestier E, Farhi D, Mahsa MZ, Remy V, Lesens O, Christmann D, Hansmann Y. Minocycline-induced hypersensitivity syndrome presenting with meningitis and brain edema: a case report. J Med Case Rep. 2007;1:22.
11. Tuleja E, Bourgarit A, Abuaf N, Le Beller C, Sereni D. Rifampin-induced severe aseptic meningitis. Rev Med Interne. 2010;31(9):e1–3.
12. Audemard A, Le Bellec ML, Carluer L, Dargere S, Verdon R, Castrale C, Lobbedez T, Hurault de Ligny B. Fumagillin-induced aseptic meningoencephalitis in a kidney transplant recipient with microsporidiosis. Transpl Infect Dis. 2012;14(6):E147–9.
13. Adair JC, Woodley SL, O'Connell JB, Call GK, Baringer JR. Aseptic meningitis following cardiac transplantation: clinical characteristics and relationship to immunosuppressive regimen. Neurology. 1991;41(2(Pt 1)):249–52.
14. Scheinfeld N. Efalizumab: a review of events reported during clinical trials and side effects. Expert Opin Drug Saf. 2006;5(2):197–209.
15. Kluger N, Girard C, Gonzalez V, Guillot B, Bessis D. Efalizumab-induced aseptic meningitis. Br J Dermatol. 2007;156(1):189–91.
16. Rivas-Rodriguez R, Romero-Alonso MM, Gabella-Bazarot E, Sanchez-Gomez E. Efalizumab-induced aseptic meningitis. Farm Hosp. 2007;31(1):70–1.
17. Baselga J, Pfister D, Cooper MR, Cohen R, Burtness B, Bos M, D'Andrea G, Seidman A, Norton L, Gunnett K, Falcey J, Anderson V, Waksal H, Mendelsohn J. Phase I studies of anti-epidermal growth factor receptor chimeric antibody C225 alone and in combination with cisplatin. J Clin Oncol. 2000;18(4):904–14.
18. Feinstein TM, Gibson MK, Argiris A. Cetuximab-induced aseptic meningitis. Ann Oncol. 2009;20(9):1609–10.
19. Nagovskiy N, Agarwal M, Allerton J. Cetuximab-induced aseptic meningitis. J Thorac Oncol. 2010;5(5):751.
20. Emani M, Zaiden Jr R. Aseptic meningitis: a rare side effect of cetuximab therapy. J Oncol Pharm Pract. 2013;19(2):178–80.
21. Merrin P, Williams IA. Meningitis associated with sulphasalazine in a patient with Sjogren's syndrome and polyarthritis. Ann Rheum Dis. 1991;50(9):645–6.
22. Alloway JA, Mitchell SR. Sulfasalazine neurotoxicity: a report of aseptic meningitis and a review of the literature. J Rheumatol. 1993;20(2):409–11.
23. Cohen J-D, Jorgensen C, Sany J. Leflunomide-induced aseptic meningitis. Joint Bone Spine. 2004;71(3):243–5.
24. Hawboldt J, Bader M. Intramuscular methotrexate-induced aseptic meningitis. Ann Pharmacother. 2007;41(11):1906–11.
25. Houitte R, Abgueguen P, Masson C. Salazopyrin-induced aseptic meningitis. Joint Bone Spine. 2009;76(2):216–7.
26. Tay SH, Lateef A, Cheung PP. Sulphasalazine-induced aseptic meningitis with facial and nuchal edema in a patient with spondyloarthritis. Int J Rheum Dis. 2012;15(4):e71–2.
27. Sekul EA, Cupler EJ, Dalakas MC. Aseptic meningitis associated with high-dose intravenous immunoglobulin therapy: frequency and risk factors. Ann Intern Med. 1994;121(4):259–62.
28. Stangel M, Kiefer R, Pette M, Smolka MN, Marx P, Gold R. Side effects of intravenous immunoglobulins in neurological autoimmune disorders–a prospective study. J Neurol. 2003;250(7):818–21.
29. Quinn JP, Weinstein RA, Caplan LR. Eosinophilic meningitis and ibuprofen therapy. Neurology. 1984;34(1):108–9.

30. Weksler BB, Lehany AM. Naproxen-induced recurrent aseptic meningitis. DICP. 1991; 25(11):1183–4.
31. Asperilla MO, Smego Jr RA. Eosinophilic meningitis associated with ciprofloxacin. Am J Med. 1989;87(5):589–90.
32. Tunkel AR, Starr K. Trimethoprim-sulfamethoxazole-associated aseptic meningitis. Am J Med. 1990;88(6):696–7.
33. Jurado R, Carpenter SL, Rimland D. Case reports: trimethoprim-sulfamethoxazole-induced meningitis in patients with HIV infection. Am J Med Sci. 1996;312(1):27–9.
34. Rodriguez SC, Olguin AM, Miralles CP, Viladrich PF. Characteristics of meningitis caused by Ibuprofen: report of 2 cases with recurrent episodes and review of the literature. Medicine (Baltimore). 2006;85(4):214–20.
35. Repplinger MD, Falk PM. Trimethoprim-sulfamethoxazole-induced aseptic meningitis. Am J Emerg Med. 2011;29(2):242.e3–5.
36. Yasuda Y, Akiguchi I, Kameyama M. Sulindac-induced aseptic meningitis in mixed connective tissue disease. Clin Neurol Neurosurg. 1989;91(3):257–60.
37. Eustace S, Buff B. Magnetic resonance imaging in drug-induced meningitis. Can Assoc Radiol J. 1994;45(6):463–5.
38. Obermoser G, Bellmann R, Pfausler B, Schmutzhard E, Sepp N. Aseptic meningo-encephalitis related to dexibuprofen use in a patient with systemic lupus erythematosus: a case report with MR findings. Lupus. 2002;11(7):451–3.
39. Lorino GD, Hardin Jr JG. Sulindac-induced meningitis in mixed connective tissue disease. South Med J. 1983;76(9):1185–7.
40. Smitherman TA, Burch R, Sheikh H, Loder E. The prevalence, impact, and treatment of migraine and severe headaches in the United States: a review of statistics from national surveillance studies. Headache. 2013;53(3):427–36.
41. Weder-Cisneros ND, Tellez-Zenteno JF, Cardiel MH, Guibert-Toledano M, Cabiedes J, Velasquez-Paz AL, Garcia-Ramos G, Cantu C. Prevalence and factors associated with headache in patients with systemic lupus erythematosus. Cephalalgia. 2004;24(12):1031–44.
42. Joffe AM, Farley JD, Linden D, Goldsand G. Trimethoprim-sulfamethoxazole-associated aseptic meningitis: case reports and review of the literature. Am J Med. 1989;87(3):332–8.
43. Cano Vargas-Machuca E, Mondejar-Marin B, Navarro-Munoz S, Perez-Molina I, Garrido-Robres JA, Alvarez-Tejerina A. Recurrent aseptic meningitis secondary to taking ibuprofen and ketorolac. Rev Neurol. 2006;42(4):217–9.
44. Naranjo CA, Busto U, Sellers EM, Sandor P, Ruiz I, Roberts EA, Janecek E, Domecq C, Greenblatt DJ. A method for estimating the probability of adverse drug reactions. Clin Pharmacol Ther. 1981;30(2):239–45.
45. van de Beek D, de Gans J, Tunkel AR, Wijdicks EF. Community-acquired bacterial meningitis in adults. N Engl J Med. 2006;354(1):44–53.
46. Logan SA, MacMahon E. Viral meningitis. BMJ. 2008;336(7634):36–40.
47. Widener HL, Littman BH. Ibuprofen-induced meningitis in systemic lupus erythematosus. JAMA. 1978;239(11):1062–4.
48. Baizabal-Carvallo JF, Delgadillo-Marquez G, Estanol B, Garcia-Ramos G. Clinical characteristics and outcomes of the meningitides in systemic lupus erythematosus. Eur Neurol. 2009;61(3):143–8.
49. Kim JM, Kim KJ, Yoon HS, Kwok SK, Ju JH, Park KS, Cho CS, Kim HY, Park SH. Meningitis in Korean patients with systemic lupus erythematosus: analysis of demographics, clinical features and outcomes; experience from affiliated hospitals of the Catholic University of Korea. Lupus. 2011;20(5):531–6.
50. Ginsberg L, Kidd D. Chronic and recurrent meningitis. Pract Neurol. 2008;8(6):348–61.
51. Kressebuch H, Schaad UB, Hirt A, Bianchetti MG. Cerebrospinal fluid inflammation induced by intravenous immunoglobulins. Pediatr Infect Dis J. 1992;11(10):894–5.
52. Bonnel RA, Villalba ML, Karwoski CB, Beitz J. Aseptic meningitis associated with rofecoxib. Arch Intern Med. 2002;162(6):713–5.

53. Cifelli A, Vaithianathar L. Syndrome of transient Headache and Neurological Deficits with cerebrospinal fluid Lymphocytosis (HaNDL). BMJ Case Rep. 2011.
54. Samuelson Jr CO, Williams HJ. Ibuprofen-associated aseptic meningitis in systemic lupus erythematosus. West J Med. 1979;131(1):57–9.
55. Bernstein RF. Ibuprofen-related meningitis in mixed connective tissue disease. Ann Intern Med. 1980;92(2 Pt 1):206–7.
56. Ballas ZK, Donta ST. Sulindac-induced aseptic meningitis. Arch Intern Med. 1982;142(1):165–6.
57. Papaioannides DH, Korantzopoulos PG, Giotis CH. Aseptic meningitis possibly associated with celecoxib. Ann Pharmacother. 2004;38(1):172.
58. Ruppert GB, Barth WF. Tolmetin-induced aseptic meningitis. JAMA. 1981;245(1):67–8.
59. Davis BJ, Thompson J, Peimann A, Bendixen BH. Drug-induced aseptic meningitis caused by two medications. Neurology. 1994;44(5):984–5.
60. Ashwath ML, Katner HP. Recurrent aseptic meningitis due to different non-steroidal anti-inflammatory drugs including rofecoxib. Postgrad Med J. 2003;79(931):295–6.
61. Chez M, Sila CA, Ransohoff RM, Longworth DL, Weida C. Ibuprofen-induced meningitis: detection of intrathecal IgG synthesis and immune complexes. Neurology. 1989;39(12):1578–80.
62. Gilbert GJ, Eichenbaum HW. Ibuprofen-induced meningitis in an elderly patient with systemic lupus erythematosus. South Med J. 1989;82(4):514–5.
63. Kastenbauer S, Pfister HW, Wick M. No evidence of type 1 or type 3 hypersensitivity mechanism in amoxicillin/clavulanic acid induced aseptic meningitis. J Neurol Neurosurg Psychiatry. 2003;74(5):690–1.
64. Thaunat O, Gilquin J, Lazareth I, Priollet P. Amoxicillin-induced aseptic meningo-encephalitis. Allergy. 2003;58(7):687–8.
65. Derbes SJ. Trimethoprim-induced aseptic meningitis. JAMA. 1984;252(20):2865–6.
66. de la Monte SM, Hutchins GM, Gupta PK. Aseptic meningitis, trimethoprim, and Sjogren's syndrome. JAMA. 1985;253(15):2192.
67. Marotte H, Charrin JE, Miossec P. Infliximab-induced aseptic meningitis. Lancet. 2001;358(9295):1784.
68. Hegde N, Gayomali C, Rich MW. Infliximab-induced headache and infliximab-induced meningitis: two ends of the same spectrum? South Med J. 2005;98(5):564–6.
69. Hegde U, Filie A, Little RF, Janik JE, Grant N, Steinberg SM, Dunleavy K, Jaffe ES, Abati A, Stetler-Stevenson M, Wilson WH. High incidence of occult leptomeningeal disease detected by flow cytometry in newly diagnosed aggressive B-cell lymphomas at risk for central nervous system involvement: the role of flow cytometry versus cytology. Blood. 2005;105(2):496–502.
70. Tissot B, Visée S, Pilette C, Prophette B, Puechal X. Lymphocytic meningitis with infliximab for ulcerative colitis. Gastroenterol Clin Biol. 2006;30(12):1420–2.
71. Manthey C, Lohse AW, Pace A. Case report of aseptic meningitis in a patient with Crohn's disease under infliximab therapy. Inflamm Bowel Dis. 2011;17(2):E10.
72. Orbach H, Katz U, Sherer Y, Shoenfeld Y. Intravenous immunoglobulin: adverse effects and safe administration. Clin Rev Allergy Immunol. 2005;29(3):173–84.
73. Simms KM, Kortepeter C, Avigan M. Lamotrigine and aseptic meningitis. Neurology. 2012;78(12):921–7.
74. Kilfoyle DH, Anderson NE, Wallis WE, Nicholls DW. Recurrent severe aseptic meningitis after exposure to lamotrigine in a patient with systemic lupus erythematosus. Epilepsia. 2005;46(2):327–8.
75. Lee SH, Yang M, Kim T, et al. Lamotrigine-induced hypersensitivity syndrome accompanied with aseptic meningitis. J Asthma Allergy Clin Immunol. 2007;27:140–2.
76. Nesseler N, Polard E, Arvieux C, Coquerel N, Michelet C, Tattevin P. Aseptic meningitis associated with lamotrigine: report of two cases. Eur J Neurol. 2007;14(12):e3–4.
77. Boot B. Recurrent lamotrigine-induced aseptic meningitis. Epilepsia. 2009;50(4):968–9.

78. Shah BK, O'Keefe S. Pemetrexed induced aseptic meningitis. Acta Oncol. 2012;51(3): 399–400.
79. Flasshove M, Schutte HJ, Kellner R, Hoffken K, Seeber S. Meningeal fluid granulocytosis after cytarabine. Eur J Cancer. 1992;28(1):243.
80. Pease CL, Horton TM, McClain KL, Kaplan SL. Aseptic meningitis in a child after systemic treatment with high dose cytarabine. Pediatr Infect Dis J. 2001;20(1):87–9.
81. Thordarson H, Talstad I. Acute meningitis and cerebellar dysfunction complicating high-dose cytosine arabinoside therapy. Acta Med Scand. 1986;220(5):493–5.
82. Nair J, Stacy M. Aseptic meningitis associated with salicylate overdose. Psychosomatics. 1993;34(4):372.
83. Heinzlef O, Moguilewski A, Roullet E. Acute aseptic meningitis after hepatitis B vaccination. Presse Med. 1997;26(7):328.
84. Herlihy TE. Phenazopyridine and aseptic meningitis. Ann Intern Med. 1987;106(1):172–3.
85. Lafaurie M, Dixmier A, Molina JM. Aseptic meningitis associated with intravenous administration of dexchlorpheniramine. Ann Med Interne (Paris). 2003;154(3):179–80.
86. Mathian A, Amoura Z, Piette JC. Pentoxifylline-induced aseptic meningitis in a patient with mixed connective tissue disease. Neurology. 2002;59(9):1468–9.
87. Galindo Bonilla PA, Sanchez Rodriguez N, Castro Jimenez A, Munoz-Torrero Rodriguez JJ, Bellon Heredia T, Feo BF. Aseptic meningitis induced by vitamin B complex. J Investig Allergol Clin Immunol. 2012;22(3):225–6.
88. Durand JM, Suchet L, Morange S, Michel B. Ranitidine and aseptic meningitis. BMJ. 1996;312(7035):886.
89. Barbot F, Danan-Causanski S, Chaouat D, Thuong M. Aseptic meningitis after ranitidine treatment for systemic lupus erythematosus. Presse Med. 1999;28(35):1938.
90. Duchene DA, Smith CP, Goldfarb RA. Allopurinol induced meningitis. J Urol. 2000; 164(6):2028.
91. Greenberg LE, Nguyen T, Miller SM. Suspected allopurinol-induced aseptic meningitis. Pharmacotherapy. 2001;21(8):1007–9.
92. Gutknecht DR. Chemical meningitis following epidural injections of corticosteroids. Am J Med. 1987;82(3):570.
93. Bensmail D, Peskine A, Denys P, Bernard L, Bussel B. Aseptic meningitis after intrathecal baclofen injection. Spinal Cord. 2006;44(5):330–3.
94. Tateno F, Sakakibara R, Kishi M, Ogawa E. Bupivacaine-induced chemical meningitis. J Neurol. 2010;257(8):1327–9.
95. Bonnet MC, Dutta A, Weinberger C, Plotkin SA. Mumps vaccine virus strains and aseptic meningitis. Vaccine. 2006;24(49–50):7037–45.
96. Ainiala H, Loukkola J, Peltola J, Korpela M, Hietaharju A. The prevalence of neuropsychiatric syndromes in systemic lupus erythematosus. Neurology. 2001;57(3):496–500.
97. Jennekens FG, Kater L. The central nervous system in systemic lupus erythematosus. Part 1. Clinical syndromes: a literature investigation. Rheumatology (Oxford). 2002;41(6):605–18.
98. Alexander EL, Alexander GE. Aseptic meningoencephalitis in primary Sjogren's syndrome. Neurology. 1983;33(5):593–8.
99. Ishida K, Uchihara T, Mizusawa H. Recurrent aseptic meningitis: a new CSF complication of Sjogren's syndrome. J Neurol. 2007;254(6):806–7.
100. Rossi R, Valeria Saddi M. Subacute aseptic meningitis as neurological manifestation of primary Sjogren's syndrome. Clin Neurol Neurosurg. 2006;108(7):688–91.
101. Hoitsma E, Faber CG, Drent M, Sharma OP. Neurosarcoidosis: a clinical dilemma. Lancet Neurol. 2004;3(7):397–407.
102. Pawate S, Moses H, Sriram S. Presentations and outcomes of neurosarcoidosis: a study of 54 cases. QJM. 2009;102(7):449–60.
103. Benjilali L, Harmouche H, El Bied S, Raffali J, Tazi Mezalek Z, Adnaoui M, Aouni M, Maaouni A. Recurrent meningitis revealing a Behcet's disease. Rheumatol Int. 2008; 29(1):91–3.

104. Sakakibara R, Koide N, Kishi M, Ogawa E, Shirai K. Aseptic meningitis as the sole manifestation of Behcet's disease. Neurol Sci. 2009;30(5):405–7.
105. Siva A, Saip S. The spectrum of nervous system involvement in Behcet's syndrome and its differential diagnosis. J Neurol. 2009;256(4):513–29.
106. Salvarani C, Brown Jr RD, Calamia KT, Christianson TJ, Weigand SD, Miller DV, Giannini C, Meschia JF, Huston 3rd J, Hunder GG. Primary central nervous system vasculitis: analysis of 101 patients. Ann Neurol. 2007;62(5):442–51.
107. Birnbaum J, Hellmann DB. Primary angiitis of the central nervous system. Arch Neurol. 2009;66(6):704–9.
108. Grewal J, Saria MG, Kesari S. Novel approaches to treating leptomeningeal metastases. J Neurooncol. 2012;106(2):225–34.
109. Di Comite G, Bozzolo EP, Praderio L, Tresoldi M, Sabbadini MG. Meningeal involvement in Wegener's granulomatosis is associated with localized disease. Clin Exp Rheumatol. 2006;24(2 Suppl 41):S60–4.
110. Kato Y, Kurimura M, Yahata Y, Tajima K, Kato T. Vogt-Koyanagi-Harada's disease presenting polymorphonuclear pleocytosis in the cerebrospinal fluid at the early active stage. Intern Med. 2006;45(12):779–81.
111. Berg MJ, Williams LS. The transient syndrome of headache with neurologic deficits and CSF lymphocytosis. Neurology. 1995;45(9):1648–54.
112. Gomez-Aranda F, Canadillas F, Marti-Masso JF, Diez-Tejedor E, Serrano PJ, Leira R, Gracia M, Pascual J. Pseudomigraine with temporary neurological symptoms and lymphocytic pleocytosis. A report of 50 cases. Brain. 1997;120(Pt 7):1105–13.
113. Serrano-Castro PJ, Amrani Y, Olivares-Romero J. Cerebral hemodynamics in the syndrome of pseudomigraine with csf-pleocytosis: a transcranial doppler study. Rev Neurol. 2000;31(5):407–11.
114. Collins JJ, Fisher 3rd WS. Vein of Galen aneurysm presenting with recurrent aseptic meningitis and subsequent spontaneous thrombosis. Surg Neurol. 1990;33(5):325–8.
115. Tapiz A, Narberhaus B, Ugarte A, Dorca E. Recurrent aseptic meningitis associated with dural vascular malformation. Rev Neurol. 2000;30(11):1099–100.
116. Pampliega-Perez A, Martin-Estefania C, Caballe-Tura M, Portilla-Sogorb J, Alvarez-Sauco M. Aseptic meningitis caused by the rupture of an epidermoid cyst. Rev Neurol. 2003;37(3):221–4.
117. Kupersmith MJ, Martin V, Heller G, Shah A, Mitnick HJ. Idiopathic hypertrophic pachymeningitis. Neurology. 2004;62(5):686–94.
118. Varona JF. Neurological manifestations as presentation of infectious endocarditis. An Med Interna. 2007;24(9):439–41.
119. Lidove O, Chauveheid MP, Caillaud C, Froissart R, Benoist L, Alamowitch S, Doan S, Szalat R, Baumann N, Alexandra JF, Lavallee P, Klein I, Vuillemet F, Sedel F, Sacre K, Samson Y, Roullet E, Papo T. Aseptic meningitis and ischaemic stroke in Fabry disease. Int J Clin Pract. 2009;63(11):1663–7.
120. Yaguchi H, Tsuzaka K, Niino M, Yabe I, Sasaki H. Aseptic meningitis with relapsing polychondritis mimicking bacterial meningitis. Intern Med. 2009;48(20):1841–4.
121. Kitley JL, Lachmann HJ, Pinto A, Ginsberg L. Neurologic manifestations of the cryopyrin-associated periodic syndrome. Neurology. 2010;74(16):1267–70.

Chapter 14
Central Nervous System Infections in Patients Immunocompromised by Antineoplastic and Other Immune-Modulating Therapies

Amy A. Pruitt

Abstract Central nervous system (CNS) infections in patients receiving immunosuppressive therapy for cancer or other systemic conditions often present complex diagnostic challenges as signs of infection may be absent or atypical. This chapter outlines a systematic clinical approach based on the etiology of immunosuppression, general examination, and presence of concurrent systemic infections. Patients with impaired barrier function, neutropenia, B cell depletion, and T cell abnormalities are included. The laboratory and imaging diagnosis, management, and prognosis of infections such as PML, VZV, human herpesvirus 6, and fungal infections likely to be seen by practicing neurologists are discussed and contrasted with conditions that mimic infection. Infections associated with mycophenolate, cyclosporine, tacrolimus, rituximab, brentuximab, and alemtuzumab are described. Human immunodeficiency virus-associated infections are covered in Chap. 15.

Keywords *Aspergillus* • Corticosteroids • Limbic encephalitis • *Listeria* • Natalizumab • Progressive multifocal leukoencephalopathy • Rituximab • Tacrolimus • Tumor necrosis • Alpha inhibitors • Varicella-zoster virus

Introduction

Despite improved infection prophylaxis and antimicrobial regimens, CNS infections remain significant sources of morbidity and mortality among both cancer patients and a growing, diverse population of patients receiving immune-modulating therapy for nonneoplastic conditions. Major at-risk cancer patient groups include recipients of hematopoietic cell transplants (HCT) or solid organ transplants (SOT), patients

A.A. Pruitt, MD
Department of Neurology, University of Pennsylvania, Perelman School of Medicine, 3400 Spruce St, Philadelphia, PA 19104, USA
e-mail: pruitt@mail.med.upenn.edu

J.C. García-Moncó (ed.), *CNS Infections*,
DOI 10.1007/978-1-4471-6401-2_14, © Springer-Verlag London 2014

with primary and metastatic brain and spinal tumors, and intensively treated patients with leukemia, lymphoma, and other hematologic malignancies. Nonneoplastic conditions whose therapies involve chronic immune modification include both primary neurological diseases and systemic conditions such as rheumatoid arthritis, inflammatory bowel disease, lupus, sarcoidosis, psoriasis, myasthenia gravis, multiple sclerosis, and neuromyelitis optica. Whereas other chapters in this volume are organized by pathogen, this section groups patients by their clinical diagnosis and its degree of disease and drug-associated immunosuppression. Table 14.1 summarizes the patient groups emphasized in this chapter. While some guidelines are offered for antibiotic choice in selected infections, clinicians are encouraged to consult with their own institutional infectious disease departments to assure appropriate coverage based on institutional antibiotic resistance and nosocomial trends.

Table 14.1 Immunocompromised patients: infectious risk factors and syndromes

Patient risk group: type of deficit	Infectious risks	Relevant drugs or other therapies	Special features/ syndromes
Barrier disruption Neurosurgery +/– Shunts Ventricular drains Radiation therapy	Bacteria: skin-derived organisms *S. aureus* *S. epidermidis* *Propionibacterium* *Enterobacteriaceae* *S. bovis* Viruses: HSV CMV VZV Fungi: *Aspergillus* *Candida*	Corticosteroids VEGF inhibitors Radiation therapy	Meningitis lacks classic signs DRESS (increased risk for HSV)
Neutropenia HCT, SOT Intensive chemotherapy without transplant	Bacteria: *S. pneumoniae* GNR Fungi: *Aspergillus* *Mucor* *Candida* Viruses: CMV HSV Adenovirus	Indwelling catheters Chemotherapy	PALE
B-lymphocyte/ immunoglobulin deficits CLL, multiple myeloma splenectomy	Bacteria: *S. pneumoniae* *H. influenzae*, *Klebsiella* Viruses: Measles WNV Enteroviruses	Rituximab Brentuximab Mycophenolate	PML versus IRIS

Table 14.1 (continued)

Patient risk group: type of deficit	Infectious risks	Relevant drugs or other therapies	Special features/ syndromes
T-lymphocyte/ macrophage dysfunction: HCT HIV	Viruses: HHV6, HHV7 VZV CMV EBVPTLD JCV(PML) Fungi: *Cryptococcus* Parasites: *Toxoplasma gondii*: *Strongyloides* Bacteria: *Listeria* *Nocardia* *M. tuberculosis*, *Treponema pallidum* Histoplasmosis Blastomycosis	Donor-derived organisms Corticosteroids Bortezomib Cyclosporine Tacrolimus Alemtuzumab Mycophenolate	PRES Wernicke's encephalopathy
T-lymphocyte/ macrophage dysfunction: SOT	Donor acquired: Rabies, Arenavirus, LCMV WNV, PLUS: organisms listed under HCT	ATG Azathioprine	PTLD, PCNL
Drug- and neurological dysfunction-related deficits: Multiple sclerosis	Bacteria: UTI-related sepsis/meningitis Viruses VZV PML WNV	Neurogenic bladder Corticosteroids Natalizumab Rituximab Fingolimod Dimethyl fumarate	IRIS LTEM: NMO, WNV
Drug-related immune deficits Rheumatoid arthritis SLE Sarcoidosis Psoriasis Myasthenia gravis Uveitis Polymyositis	Viruses VZV PML	Corticosteroids Rituximab Etanercept Mycophenolate Methotrexate Infliximab Adalimumab Alemtuzumab Anakinra	De novo demyelination TNF-alpha Inhibitors VZV EBV JCV (PML)

ATG anti-thymocyte globulin, *CMV* cytomegalovirus, *DRESS* drug rash eosinophilia systemic signs, *EBV* Epstein-Barr virus, *GNR* gram negative rods HCT/SOT hematopoietic cell transplantation/solid organ transplantation, *HSV* herpes simplex virus, *IRIS* immune reconstitution inflammatory syndrome, *JCV/PML* John Cunningham virus/ progressive multifocal leukoencephalopathy, *PCNSL* primary central nervous system lymphoma, *LCMV* lymphocytic choriomeningitis virus, *LTEM* longitudinally extensive transverse myelitis, *NMO* neuromyelitis optica, *PALE* posttransplant acute limbic encephalitis, *PTLD* posttransplantation lymphoproliferative disorder, *SLE* systemic lupus erythematosus, *TNF* tissue necrosis factor, *UTI* urinary tract infection, *VEGF* vascular endothelial growth factor, *VZV* varicella-zoster virus, *WNV* West Nile Virus

Clinical Approach to Potential CNS Infection: Diagnostic Guidelines

1. The *net state of immunosuppression* is a useful construct to remind the consultant to consider all components of infectious risk. These include patient disease and duration, treatment regimen and timing, prophylactic and vaccination exposures, transfusions, community and nosocomial epidemiologic trends, and travel and zoonotic exposures.

   The mnemonic **P-N-E-U-M-O** may help clinicians remember diagnostic pitfalls:

   P: Presentation and course of CNS infections in the types of patients considered in this chapter may differ from those without immunosuppressive therapies [1].

   N: Noninfectious conditions may mimic CNS infection. Examples of such processes include immune reconstitution inflammatory syndrome (IRIS), posterior reversible encephalopathy syndrome (PRES), paraneoplastic processes, and radiation and chemotherapy complications and toxicities, such as demyelination caused by some drugs.

   E: Emerging, **U**nique pathogens and novel syndromes related both to malignancies and to their treatment challenge clinicians' diagnostic acumen.

   M: Multiple infectious pathogens may coexist with or without noninfectious processes.

   O: Ongoing risk of infection extends both before and long past the active cancer or immunomodulating treatment period. A patient's immune system may be impaired at one point in the course of the illness, but dysfunctional during vigorous reconstitution at another point in the disease.
2. *Epidemiology*: A few cancer patient groups account for the majority of CNS infections. Patients with leukemia or lymphoma represent more than a quarter of all cancer patients with any type of CNS infection, and 16 % of patients with CNS infections in series from large cancer centers and tertiary care hospital have primary brain tumors. Three quarters of bacterial or fungal meningitis cases occur in recent neurosurgical patients [2]. Certain drugs, such as natalizumab and alemtuzumab, confer increased risk for specific infections. Table 14.1 correlates both types of immune deficit and notable drug therapy associations with specific infectious pathogens.
3. *Clinical Syndrome*: Physical examination distinguishes two general syndromes that may be of diagnostic value:

   (a) Diffuse meningoencephalitis/encephalitis presentations with headache and altered sensorium are more common with bacterial or viral infections or fungi such as *Candida* or *Cryptococcus*.

   (b) Focal signs and symptoms reflect localized parenchymal process due to such entities as *Toxoplasma gondii*, *Aspergillus* species, or *Nocardia*. Focal cerebral infarction raises suspicion of bacterial or fungal infective endocarditis, varicella-zoster virus (VZV), *Aspergillus*, or *Zygomycetes*. Brainstem syndromes may suggest *Listeria*, WNV, or noninfectious entities such as Wernicke's or osmotic demyelination [3].

Table 14.2 Physical examination: potential localizing clues to underlying pathogen

Mass	Sinusitis	Leukoencephalopathy	Stroke	Limbic	Basal ganglia	Brainstem	Spinal cord
Bacterial abscess	Mucoraceae	PML	VZV	HHV6	WNV	Listeria	VZV
EBV/PCNSL	*Aspergillus*	PRES	IE	HSV1/2	E/WEE	VZV	HSV2
Cysticercosis	*Pseudomonas*	IRIS	Mucor		EBV	WNV	WNV
Mycobacterium tuberculosis		ADEM	*Aspergillus*		Toxo		EBV
ADEM		Drug	Chagas	VGKCC		PRES	=
IRIS		CAA	Vasculitis	Seizures		Wernicke's	RT
RT		Radiation injury	Tumor			Osmotic demyelination	
Tumor		GVHD	Coagulopathy			Whipple's	
			Radiation injury			Anti-Hu	

Blue = infectious causes; Red = noninfectious causes that can mimic infections

ADEM acute disseminated encephalomyelitis, *CAA* cerebral amyloid angiopathy, *E/WEE* eastern/western equine encephalitis, *GVHD* graft versus host disease HHV6 human herpesvirus 6, *HSV* herpes simples virus, *IE* infective endocarditis, *IRIS* immune reconstitution inflammatory syndrome, *PML* progressive multifocal leukoencephalopathy, *PRES* posterior reversible encephalopathy syndrome, *RT* radiation therapy, *VGKC* voltage gated potassium channel antibodies, *VZV* varicella-zoster virus, *WNV* West Nile virus

Ocular pathology occurs with several viruses including cytomegalovirus (CMV), VZV, and Epstein-Barr virus (EBV). Table 14.2 reviews differential diagnostic considerations both infectious and noninfectious based on characteristic focal signs and symptoms. The clinician should be aware that these are not invariable findings and that many atypical combinations of signs and symptoms can occur.

Special Neurodiagnostic Laboratory Considerations

Interpretation of cerebrospinal fluid (CSF) data in immunocompromised hosts can be misleading. Patients who are profoundly pancytopenic may have no pleocytosis even in the presence of bacterial or fungal infection, as may those whose T cell function fails to evoke an inflammatory response to viral pathogens such as varicella-zoster virus (VZV). (See discussion by Aksamit in Chapter One.)

Computed tomography (CT) and magnetic resonance imaging (MRI) in immunocompromised patients also pose several potentially confusing issues:

1. The use of corticosteroids reduces contrast enhancement on both CT and MRI.
2. Diffuse meningeal or dural enhancement can be demonstrated after repetitive seizures, lumbar puncture reaction to calvarial metastases, or neoplastic or chemical meningitis.
3. Increased FLAIR in the subarachnoid space can indicate infection and hemorrhage or can be seen in patients ventilated with high partial pressures of oxygen.
4. Ring-enhancing lesions have an extensive differential diagnosis including metastases, abscesses, primary glial tumors, infarction, contusion, radiation necrosis, demyelination, and sarcoidosis. The use of diffusion-weighted imaging to improve distinction between infections and other processes is discussed in Chap. 2.

At-Risk Patient Populations

Neurosurgical Patients

Patients with primary and secondary brain tumors represent 25 % of CNS infection in patients with cancer. Bacterial meningitis is the most serious infection occurring because of multiple risk factors including barrier disruption, deficits in T cell immunity with prolonged corticosteroids and poor wound healing after steroids, radiation therapy, and repeat craniotomies. Abscesses can occur more than several years after treatment [4]. *Staphylococcus aureus* is the most common pathogen after craniotomy and *Listeria monocytogenes* incidence has declined in a recent Memorial Sloan Kettering Cancer Center series.

Three infectious syndromes occur exclusively among patients treated with surgery and radiation for brain tumors:

1. Carmustine-containing wafers (Gliadel®) are approved for treatment of high-grade astrocytic tumors both at initial diagnosis and at the time of recurrence. They induce a vigorous cerebritis with vasogenic edema. Two radiographic patterns have been described: a ring-enhancing abscess and a "Swiss cheese-like appearance" [5]. External ventricular drains and repetitively accessed Ommaya reservoirs also are associated with meningeal infection.
2. Radiation therapy can complicate wound healing as can bevacizumab and other vascular endothelial growth factor (VEGF) inhibitors, particularly when given within 1 month of surgery, may further raise the risk of wound infection [6].
3. Radiation therapy alone and chemoradiation with temozolomide may predispose patients to herpes simplex virus (HSV) or CMV encephalitis. HSV infection also has been observed during phenytoin- or carbamazepine-initiated hypersensitivity reactions [7, 8] (Fig. 14.1).

Hematopoietic Cell Transplantation and Solid Organ Transplantation (HCT, SOT)

The neurological complications of HCT and OCT have been reviewed recently in detail [9]. Below are highlighted six infectious conditions of clinical importance in the transplant population. Each is discussed in individual chapters in this volume, but the clinical context for transplantation patients is emphasized here. Most clinically significant neurological complications occur within the first 100 days after HCT, but it should be remembered that neurological infectious problems can surface even many years later [10].

Early Posttransplant Period (<30 Days)

HHV6

During the period of neutropenia following HCT, bacterial, viral, fungal, nosocomially acquired, and donor-derived infections are important sources of morbidity as is reactivation of infections such as neurocysticercosis and toxoplasmosis. A syndrome specific to the time of hematopoietic cell engraftment is characterized by rash, fever, and headache about 2–5 weeks posttransplant. This must be differentiated from posttransplant acute limbic encephalitis (PALE) due to HHV6 and characterized by amnesia, hyponatremia, CSF pleocytosis, seizures, and bihippocampal FLAIR abnormality that may be difficult to recognize as it can be quite minimal or

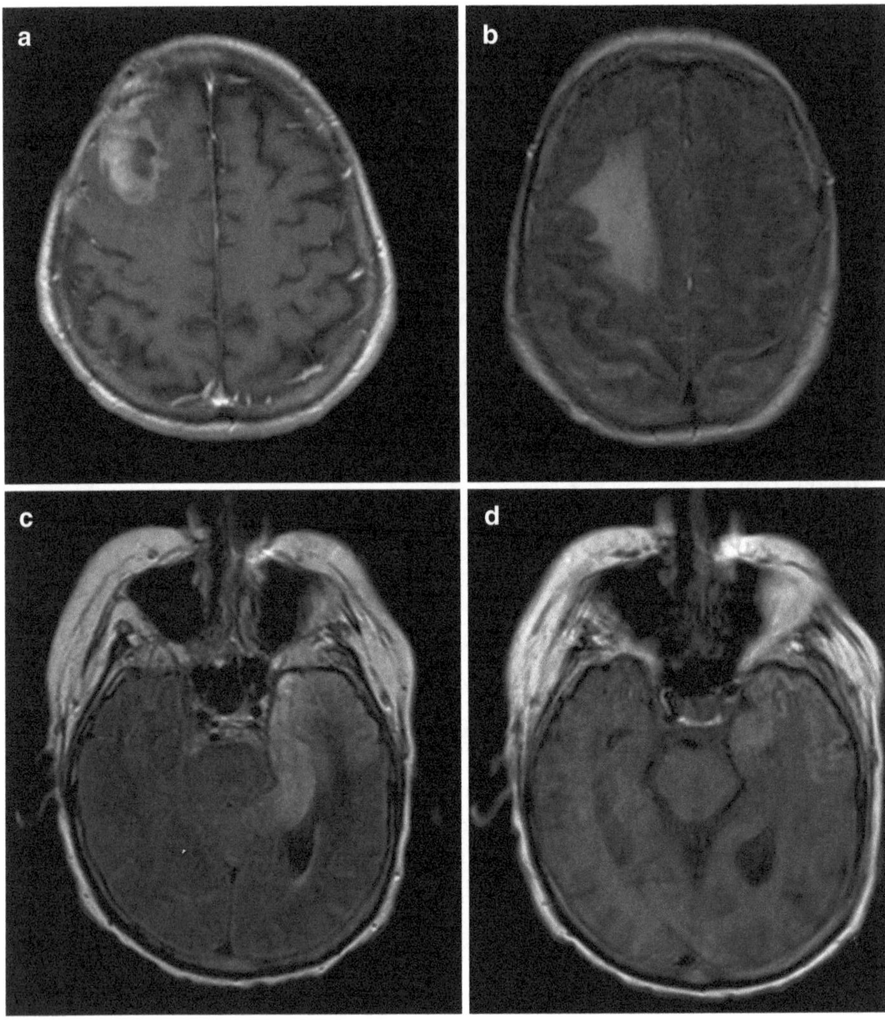

Fig. 14.1 Herpes simplex encephalitis concurrent with DRESS. A 57-year-old woman presented with seizures and was found to have a right frontal mass that proved to be a primary CNS lymphoma on biopsy of the gadolinium-enhancing area. (**a**) She was given phenytoin for seizures. During chemotherapy with methotrexate, temozolomide, and rituximab, her FLAIR signal remained about the same (**b**) but clinically she deteriorated, developing short-term memory problems and a diffuse maculopapular rash along with transaminase elevations. Scans showed expansion of the left temporal cortex (contralateral to the tumor) (**c**) with bright signal in the left temporal cortex on unenhanced T1 images consistent with cortical necrosis. (**d**) CSF had 56 WBC and PCR was positive for HSV. This case illustrates HSV infection concurrent with the DRESS syndrome (drug rash, eosinophilia, and systemic symptoms) due to antiepileptic drug hypersensitivity reaction. Radiation therapy also has been reported to provoke HSV or CMV encephalitis

appear after a several-day delay [11]. HHV6 (as well as cytomegalovirus (CMV)) lack thymidine kinase and are not sensitive to acyclovir, so ganciclovir, cidofovir, and foscarnet have been used individually or in combination, though there is no FDA-approved antiviral drug for this infection [12].

Middle Period (1–6 Months)

Varicella-Zoster Virus (VZV)

In the immunocompromised population, risk of VZV begins right after the procedure and extends for years. The most common syndromes are dermatomal VZV with a high risk of postherpetic neuralgia in patients with cancer and disseminated VZV [13]. Major complications of VZV include infratentorial and supratentorial stroke, retinal necrosis, pontine myelitis, cerebellar ataxia, cranial and spinal neuropathies, and spinal cord infarction. Multifocal VZV vasculopathy with temporal artery infection mimicking giant cell arteritis has been described recently [14, 15]. More than 35 % of patients have no rash and many have no pleocytosis. Any cancer patient with multifocal vasculopathy or unexplained radiculopathy should have CSF VZV PCR, which, however, may be positive in only slightly more than half of patients [16]. Diagnosis is more accurately confirmed by measuring anti-VZV IgG antibody in the CSF and documenting a reduced serum to CSF ratio.

Immunocompromised patients may not receive live attenuated VZV vaccine, and HCT recipients should receive prolonged valacyclovir prophylaxis. Active VZV infection is treated with IV acyclovir with addition of ganciclovir or foscarnet for treatment resistance and for retinal involvement [17].

Invasive Fungal Infections: *Candida* and *Cryptococcus* are likely to produce nonfocal meningeal syndromes, whereas *Aspergillus* and Mucoraceae invade sinuses and blood vessels producing cranial nerve palsies and stroke.

Cryptococcus neoformans

Cryptococcus neoformans is the most frequent cause of lymphocyte-predominant meningitis in patients with HIV. Other patients with T-lymphocyte defects, including all transplant recipients, are at risk for this fungus. The lungs are the most common extra-CNS site. Meningitis onset may be surprisingly indolent in patients who do not mount an effective inflammatory response. Markedly elevated intracranial pressure is frequent, and cell counts may be misleading in pancytopenic patients. Cryptococcal antigen in the CSF is a sensitive and specific diagnostic tool. A recent clinical trial demonstrated superiority of combined therapy with 5-flucytosine and amphotericin B over either drug alone [18]. IRIS has been observed with successful cryptococcal treatment in the non-HIV population.

Aspergillus

Patients at risk for *Aspergillus* infections often have AML or myelodysplastic syndromes. HCT recipients with active GVHD are also at risk as are those with long-term indwelling IV lines and long-term steroid use and use of fludarabine and alemtuzumab [19]. The disease has a high propensity to form aneurysms in vessels of the CNS, with a posterior fossa predilection, and may present with devastating intracerebral hemorrhage. Clues to this fungus' often-difficult presentation are sinusitis and headache, persistent fever with negative cultures, and persistent neutrophilic meningitis. Galactomannan detection in the CSF and sinus biopsy are two early diagnostically helpful tools. A similar clinical presentation can be seen with mucormycosis, a fungus that also can spread from the sinuses to the frontal lobes with frontal infarction.

Late Complications (>6 Months)

Posttransplantation Lymphoproliferative Disorders (PTLDs)

PTLDs are a diverse group of lymphoid proliferations occurring after HCT or SOT. They range from hyperplasia to aggressive, usually B cell lymphomas with CNS involvement in 10–15 %. Up to 70 % are Epstein-Barr virus (EBV) positive. EBV-negative PTLDs occur later after organ transplant. The pathogenesis involves defective T cell regulation of EBV-specific B cell proliferation. Median time from organ transplant to PTLDs is about 6 months but can occur many years later [20]. Multiple ring-enhancing lesions are often seen, but there is a wide spectrum of potential MRI characteristics.

Progressive Multifocal Leukoencephalopathy (PML)

Progressive multifocal leukoencephalopathy (PML) is a demyelinating disease caused by lytic infection of oligodendrocytes by a ubiquitous polyomavirus, the JC virus (John Cunningham virus). Primary infection, present in more than 50 % of the adult population, is asymptomatic, and the virus remains latent in the lymph nodes, bone marrow, kidney, and other host cells. Latency may also occur in the CNS, although this is less well established [21]. PML was originally recognized in 1958 as a rare condition in patients with hematologic malignancies. However, in the last three decades, there has been a 50-fold increase in PML incidence with the advent first of AIDS and then of intensive immunosuppressive regimens for organ transplantation and for a range of connective tissue and autoimmune conditions [22]. Table 14.3 summarizes the drugs that have been associated with increased risk of PML. In many instances, it is difficult to ascertain the relative risks posed by the underlying condition and by concurrently administered medicines. Table 14.3 derives from case reports, small series, and data from a disproportionality analysis

Table 14.3 Drug-related risk of progressive multifocal leukoencephalopathy

Generic drug	Molecular target	Neurological	Non-neurological	References
Natalizumab	A4 integrin CD49d	MS	Crohn's disease	NMSS [89]
Rituximab	CD20	MS, NMO, MMN, myasthenia gravis, inflammatory myositis	Lymphoma, autoimmune diseases (LE)	Clifford et al. [37, 72] Carson et al. [62] Tuccori et al. [68]
Alemtuzumab	CD52	MS	Hematologic malignancies	Piccinni et al. [60]
Efalizumab[a]	CD11a	None	Psoriasis	Tyler [70] Korman et al. [71]
Brentuximab	CD30	None	T cell lymphoma	Von Geldern et al. [75] Jalan et al. [76]
Ibritumomab	CD20	None	B cell NHL	Keene et al. [59]
Mycophenolate	Inhibitor inosine-5′-monophosphate dehydrogenase	Myasthenia gravis SLE Autoimmune glomerular disease	HCT and SOT NMO	Neff et al. [79] Mateen et al. [31] Berger [78]
Infliximab	Anti-TNF-α	Neurosarcoidosis	Sarcoidosis, RA	Keene et al. [59]
Adalimumab	Anti-TNF-α	None	RA	Keene et al. [59]
Fludarabine	Antimetabolite purine analogue	None	CLL HSCT	D'Souza et al. [69]
Azathioprine	Antimetabolite purine analogue	Myasthenia gravis NMO	SLE Sjogren's, vasculitis	Mateen et al. [31]
Tacrolimus, cyclosporine	Calcineurin inhibitors		HCT, SOT	Mateen et al. [31]

Data from Bosch et al. [24], Schmedt et al. [23], Berger [78], and other references noted in table
CLL, chronic lymphocytic leukemia; *HCT*, hematopoietic cell transplantation; *NMSS*, National Multiple Sclerosis Society; *NMO*, neuromyelitis optica; *RA*, rheumatoid arthritis; *SLE*, systemic lupus erythematosus; *SOT*, solid organ transplantation

[a]Withdrawn from market

of spontaneous reports within the US Adverse Event Reporting System [23]. Additional drugs were culled from the review by Bosch et al. using the BIOGEAS (Biological Agents in Autoimmune Diseases) registry [24]. The condition rarely has been described in patients with no prior known immunodeficiency state or with isolated CD8+ T-lymphocyte deficiency [25, 26].

While oligodendrocytes are the primary target of PML infection, other infected cells include granule cells leading to a pure cerebellar syndrome and fulminant JC virus encephalopathy of cortical pyramidal neurons [27, 28]. Definitive diagnosis requires the demonstration of enlarged oligodendroglial nuclei, bizarre astrocytes, and demyelination along with techniques confirming the presence of JCV. JCV by

PCR in the CSF in the absence of a better explanation for patient's symptoms is also used as a criterion [29]. Regardless of underlying immune deficiency, radiographic abnormality is usually an enlarging supratentorial white matter lesion or lesions with mass effect. Variable contrast enhancement can be seen with immune reconstitution. The posterior fossa is a favored site, but an increasingly broad spectrum of imaging features is recognized (Fig. 14.2) [30]. As illustrated by the examples in the figure, the differential diagnosis of PML varies with the underlying reason for immune compromise. For example, in a transplant recipient, PRES, EBV-associated PTLD, and de novo demyelinating disease are concerns. With rituximab, ADEM, PRES, mycobacterial disease, enteroviral meningitis, CMV, and WNV all could cause diagnostic confusion with PML. With TNF-alpha inhibitors, unmasking of demyelination may resemble PML as discussed later in this chapter. In the MS population on natalizumab, the disease may be difficult to sort out from MS exacerbation. Further, after withdrawal of the drug, IRIS may develop or IRIS and PML may coexist (Fig. 14.3 and discussion below).

PML in the transplant population occurs at a median time of 27 months in solid organ recipients versus 11 months among HCT recipients. Case fatality rate was 84 % in a recent series, a rate considerably higher than that of HIV patients on HAART or multiple sclerosis patients treated with natalizumab (see below) [31]. There is no effective therapy save for reduction in immunosuppression, if possible. A study of mefloquine in a group of largely HIV-positive patients showed no benefit [32].

PML provides an appropriate transition to consideration of the next section covering growing populations of at-risk patients immunocompromised not by cancer but by immunosuppressive therapies that alter B and T cell function. When PML is suspected, immunosuppressant or immunodulatory therapy should be suspended. If PML is associated with a therapy that has a long half-life, the use of plasma exchange (PLEX) is recommended. Immune restoration may lead to transient worsening of the disease [33] (Fig. 14.4).

Nonneoplastic Conditions

Multiple Sclerosis

Increasingly, patients with multiple sclerosis are treated with intensive immunosuppressive regimens that alter both B and T cell functions. Not surprisingly, some of these regimens have led to infectious complications not previously seen in this population group. The infection that has occasioned the greatest concern is PML in patients on natalizumab (Tysabri®), a humanized monoclonal antibody against the very late activating antigen-4 that prevents lymphocyte trafficking into the CSF. Three initial reports of PML led to the discontinuation of FDA's 2004 approval by early 2005 [34, 35]. One of the original three cases of PML associated with natalizumab received this drug for Crohn's disease [36]. As the risk of PML is related to

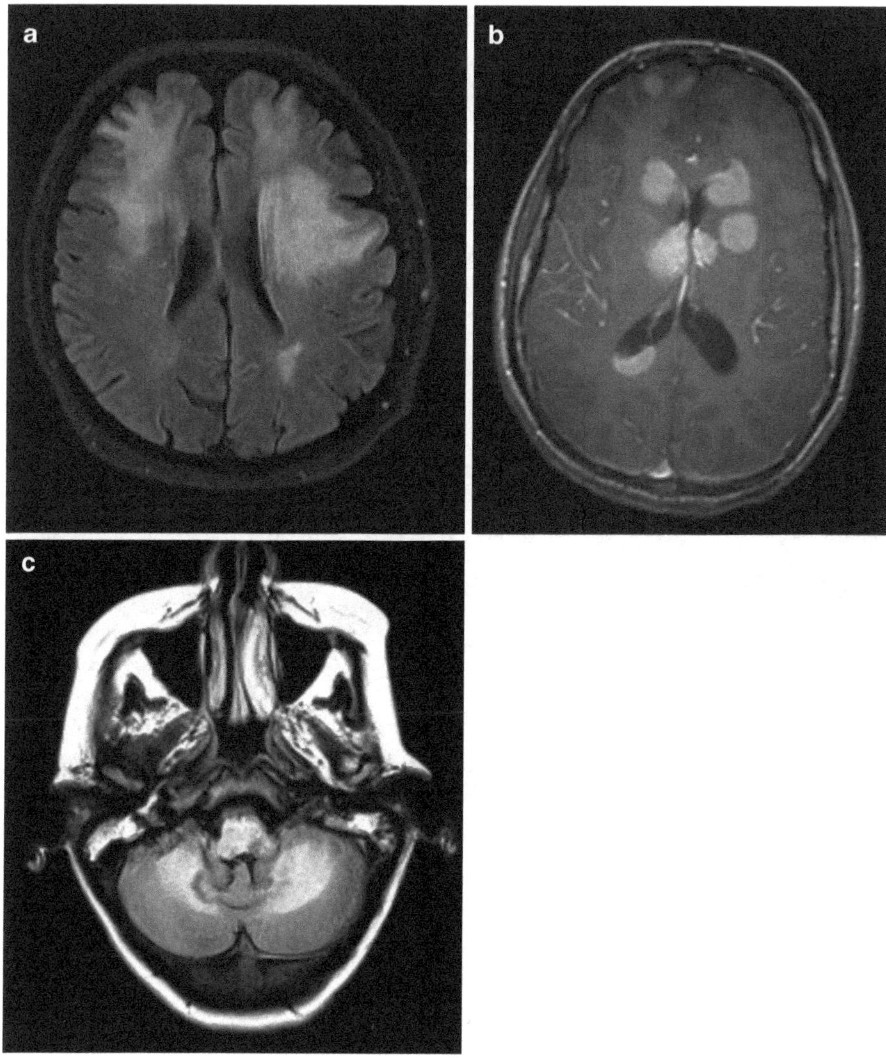

Fig. 14.2 Varied presentations of progressive multifocal leukoencephalopathy. (**a**) A patient with multiple myeloma received multiple chemotherapy regimens over a 2-year period and was on prednisone for much of this time as well as tacrolimus after an HST transplant. He presented with altered personality, abulia, and a nonenhancing multicentric process in the white matter shown on axial FLAIR images (**a**). The differential diagnosis included PRES, PML, or drug toxicity. JC virus was found in the CSF. (**b**) Hematopoietic cell transplant recipient presented 6 months after transplant with rapid onset of confusion and obtundation. Multifocal white matter lesions were found on FLAIR images (not shown), which enhanced vividly after gadolinium. EBV was found in the CSF. T1-weighted gadolinium-enhanced scan shows EBV-associated lymphoma. (**c**) Patient with untreated CLL developed facial numbness followed over 6 weeks by progressive ataxia and somnolence. JC virus was found in her acellular CSF. As she was untreated, the risk factor for opportunistic infection in this case appeared to be the hematologic malignancy itself rather than immunosuppressive therapy

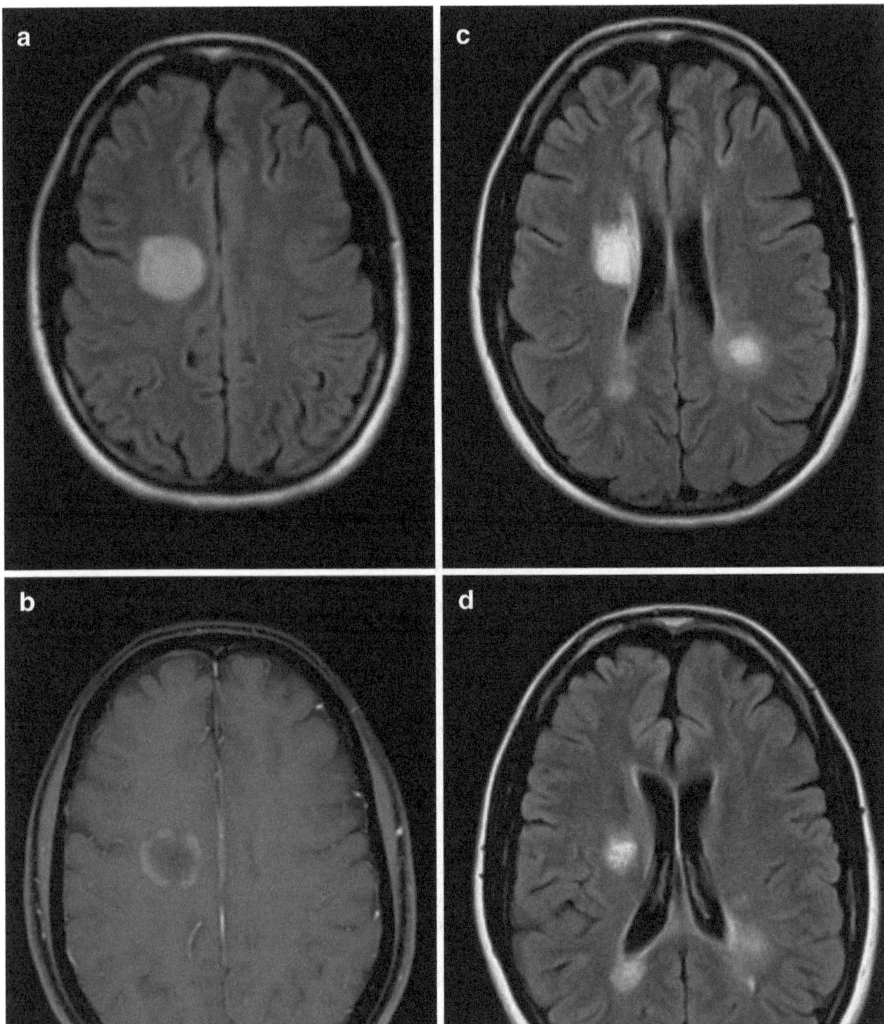

Fig. 14.3 Natalizumab-associated IRIS versus PML. A 28-year-old with multiple sclerosis had been on natalizumab for 2 years. Drug was discontinued in anticipation of conception, but after 4 months without established pregnancy, a follow-up scan at a time when the patient was asymptomatic showed a large FLAIR abnormality with partial ring enhancement (**a**, **b**). Seventeen days later the patient developed Gerstmann syndrome. The right hemisphere lesion no longer enhanced, but new lesions had developed in the left hemisphere and corpus callosum (**c**, **d**). In panel (**c**), the left hemisphere lesion shows concentric circles of hyperintensity consistent with demyelination. The differential diagnosis was PML versus natalizumab withdrawal-associated IRIS. JCV was negative in the CSF and patient recovered completely after high-dose corticosteroid treatment. Natalizumab treatment has been resumed for more than 1 year without complication usually hypointense on T1 and hyperintense on T2-weighted imaging compared to the normal white matter. Signal intensity and CT attenuation changes are subject to temporal changes. The subcortical arcuate (U) fibers are typically involved at first, creating sharp, scalloped margins (Fig. 14.1b, c). Rarely, faint marginal contrast enhancement may be encountered, particularly in the acute phase of demyelination. In HIV patients receiving antiretroviral therapy (HAART), marked enhancement can be observed, particularly during the immune reconstitution syndrome [8]

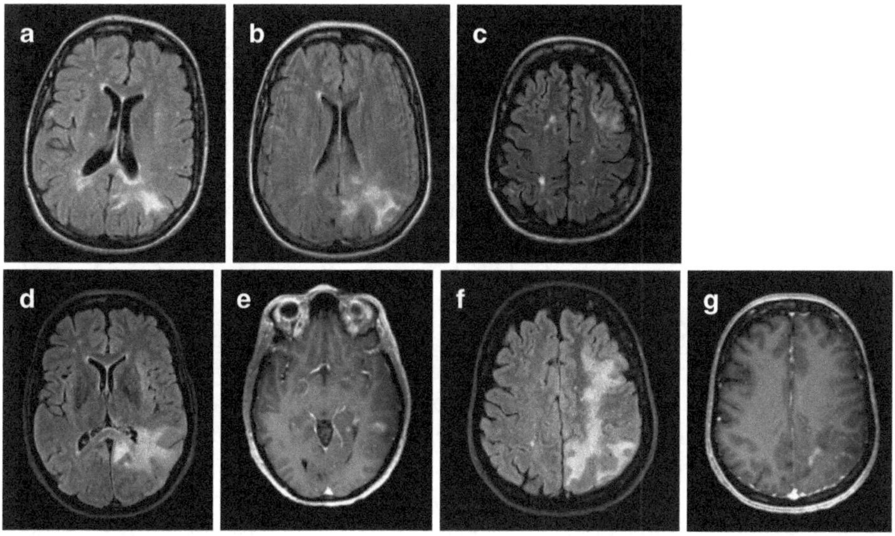

Fig. 14.4 Natalizumab-associated PML. After 25 courses of natalizumab, a 57-year-old patient complained of memory problems. New white matter lesion without enhancement was identified in the left parietal region (**a**). Lumbar puncture revealed JC virus and natalizumab was withdrawn. Seventeen days after the first scan, there is progression of the original area and new nonenhancing signal abnormality in the left frontal white matter (**b**, **c**). Eighteen days later, after 7 courses of plasmapheresis to remove natalizumab, clinical condition was worse with more extensive FLAIR abnormality in the original area (**d**) that now exhibits gadolinium contrast enhancement (**e**) as do parts of the now very extensive confluent left hemisphere affected areas (**f**, **g**) consistent with immune reconstitution (IRIS)

duration of immunosuppression, cases have continued to be reported. An early series comes from Clifford and colleagues who described 28 cases of natalizumab-associated PML. Eight of these were fatal. Median treatment duration prior to onset of symptoms was 25 months with impaired cognitive and motor performance being the major issues. Several patients had seizures. In all but one case, JCV was detected in the CSF. Plasma exchange (PLEX) led to exacerbation of symptoms and enlargement of MRI lesions within a few days to weeks after PLEX, indicating immune reconstitution inflammatory syndrome (IRIS), a phenomenon defined as worsening of symptoms during immune system recovery and not explained by recurrent infection or other process. IRIS appears to be more severe and frequent in these patients than in HIV patients [37]. In a subsequent series encompassing MedWatch reports from Biogen Idec, 42 cases of natalizumab-related PML were described. All except 2 were managed by PLEX and discontinuation of natalizumab. Twenty-three patients developed contrast enhancement after removal of natalizumab, while 17 had contrast enhancement on MRI before drug withdrawal. IRIS occurred in all patients. Early PML/IRIS was associated with worse survival and neurological outcome [38].

As of May 2013, 347 cases of PML had been reported to the FDA and the European Medicines Agency (EMA) teams (Biogen Idec, 2013). Data are available to physicians online to assist with explanation of risk to patients (medinfo.biogen-idec.com/medinfo). Twenty percent of these PML-infected MS patients have died and the survivors have varying degrees of disability. The lowest number of months on therapy before PML developed is 12. There are approximately 90,000 patients worldwide on the drug of which over 40,000 are in the USA. Prior immunosuppressive use (azathioprine, mycophenolate, mitoxantrone, methotrexate, or cyclophosphamide) raises risk of PML by fourfold [39]. Since 2011, a JCV serologic test (JCV Stratify) has been available. Gorelik and colleagues detected JCV seropositive in 54 % of MS patients [40]. In the non-MS population seropositivity increases steadily in each decade from 50 % at age 20–29 to 68 % in those 50–59 years old. Seropositivity for JC virus in the blood increases the incidence of natalizumab-associated PML to as much as 1 per 100 patients after 2 years of treatment [41]. However, seronegativity does not completely eliminate the possibility of PML. Recently patients receiving natalizumab for more than 2 years were analyzed for viremia. Viremia occurred in 35 % of 49 patients. Four of these were seronegative for JCV antibody. In some of these seronegative patients, the blood showed T cell responses to JC virus proteins. Chen showed that subclinical JCV reactivation is common in patients with MS on natalizumab and is related to transient reduction in the JCV-specific cellular immune response [42]. Stem cells and pre-B cells may migrate from the bone marrow as MS patients on natalizumab have increased circulating CD34+ cells. PML risk-stratification algorithms therefore remain imperfect, and a single measurement of JC virus antibody is insufficient as a complete risk-mitigation strategy [43]. Clinical vigilance and critical review of serial MRI scans remain essential.

Natalizumab appears rather specifically to increase risk for PML as other opportunistic infections are less common. A fatal case of HSV encephalitis has been reported and numerous cases of dermatomal VZV reactivation are recorded. PML risk may be related to the sustained reduction in lymphocyte counts in the CSF more than 6 months after cessation of therapy. With the latest figures, the PML risk can be quoted to patients as 1/100,000 in the first year, 127/100,000 in the second year, and 171/100,000 in the third year with an average risk of 1/1,000 in exposed individuals [44]. Because of the PML risk, natalizumab is available only through a restricted distribution program called the TOUCH® Prescribing Program.

A study looking at discontinuation of the drug for a holiday described relapse in 28 % with median time to relapse of 3 months. About a third of these were particularly severe relapses reminiscent of an IRIS phenomenon [45]. Very similar figures in a smaller number of patients are reported from the Netherlands [46]. Up to 40 % of patients in other series, again at median interval of 3 months from the end of therapy, experience significant relapses [47]. These observations have led to concern about discontinuation of therapy. In one recent series 38 % of patients experienced unusually widespread inflammatory activity on MRI exceeding that of their pre-natalizumab therapy and CSF findings were suggestive of IRIS [48]. Other infections may occur with possibly increased frequency in natalizumab-treated patients including herpes infections, *Pneumocystis jiroveci*, and *Mycobacterium avium intracellulare*.

For the clinician wary of MS relapse but concerned about opportunistic infection, the question becomes one of how to predict who is at risk. Clinically the differential diagnosis is difficult: symptoms and radiographic findings may be hard to sort out from new MS lesions except for a predominance of neurobehavioral, motor, language, and visual symptoms with PML. Unlike MS-related relapsing lesions, optic nerve and spinal cord lesions are not present. Blood testing for JCV has been of some value. Rudick and colleagues analyzed almost 13,000 blood and urine samples from almost 1,400 patients. JCV was found in plasma in four patients using a commercial test and two more using an ultrasensitive assay (detecting 10 copies per mL compared to 50 copies per mL). Thus, about 0.5 % of the entire study group was JCV positive. None of the patients went on to develop PML and none of the five patients in the studies who developed PML had detectable virus in the blood before developing disease [44]. Urine alone also is unhelpful, but a newer ELISA antibody test may be helpful [40]. These investigators used urine antibody test as a screen and then tested blood. Of these patients, 53.6 % were serum antibody positive and many urine-negative patients had positive serum antibody tests. One hundred percent (17/17) of the patients who went on to develop PML tested positive 16–180 months before symptoms. Thus, patients without detectable levels of anti-JCV antibodies are at low risk, but more patients are needed to confirm these findings. A particular note of caution is necessary here since after discontinuation of the drug, virus may persist [49]. In this study 11 of 13 MS patients had plasma exchange to remove natalizumab. Even though all 13 developed IRIS, 7 of the patients had persistent JC virus DNA in the CSF.

There are no known interventions that can adequately treat PML. Three to five sessions of plasma exchange (PLEX) over 5–12 days accelerate natalizumab clearance and are favored by many specialists. Steroids can help suppress the inflammation of IRIS. However, corticosteroids also have significant impact on the virus-specific T cell response to JCV, and a recent study suggests that methylprednisolone treatment decreased JCV-specific CD8+ T cells impairing control of JCV [50]. Thus, steroids likely should be used to treat but not to prevent PML-IRIS. Neurologists need to follow patients longitudinally because some of ongoing deficits after PML may be due to smoldering PML and not to MS.

Fingolimod

FDA approval of the first oral disease-modifying drug for multiple sclerosis fingolimod (Gilenya®) occurred in September 2010. Fingolimod is a sphingosine 1-phosphate receptor modulator. It inhibits egress of naïve and central memory lymphocytes from lymph nodes, but does not impede effector memory T cells. Numbers of lymphocytes in peripheral blood are reduced to approximately 30 % of baseline values. In the premarketing studies, an increased risk of dermatomal VZV was noted [51]. Serum VZV titers are obtained prior to the first drug dose, and antibody-negative patients are vaccinated before fingolimod treatment as recommended by the manufacturer Novartis' advisory, 2013. Following vaccination, fingolimod treatment should be postponed for 1 month. The use of live attenuated vaccines should be avoided during and for 2 months following treatment with fingolimod. While the manufacturer's guidelines emphasize cardiac precautions, there are no specific guidelines for dose reduction or discontinuation in patients with markedly lowered lymphocyte counts. Postmarketing experience includes case reports of VZV and multiple cranial neuropathies as well as VZV encephalitis and vasculopathy [52, 53]. In the past 3 years, IRIS after withdrawal of fingolimod has been reported as well.

Dimethyl Fumarate

Approved in April 2013 is dimethyl fumarate (Tecfidera®), a drug that has been available in Europe for the treatment of psoriasis for several years. PML has been described in four patients, two of whom had psoriasis and were on the drug for at least 3 years [54, 55]. Other immunosuppressives had been used in some of the patients as well. IRIS developed in at least one of these patients. Unlike other immune-based therapies associated with PML, this is not a monoclonal antibody, and prior exposure in other patients to treatment for sarcoidosis and cancer as well as efalizumab use, all known risk factors for PML, confounds interpretation. In total, there have been four reports of PML in patients treated with fumarates [56]. An immune deficiency panel with T-lymphocyte subsets is suggested before institution of therapy, and at the author's institution we also ascertain JCV status before using the drug.

Infections in Patients with Rheumatologic/Autoimmune Disorders

The diseases grouped here include rheumatologic conditions such as rheumatoid arthritis (RA) and systemic lupus erythematosus (SLE) and immune thrombocytopenia as well as diseases of immediate relevance to neurologists including myasthenia gravis and neurosarcoidosis. They share immunosuppressive and biological therapies that produce predictable risks for specific infections as well as a wide array of autoimmune diseases induced by the drugs themselves. More than 1,500 cases of nearly 50 different systemic autoimmune disease have been reported though one European registry of patients treated with biological therapies [57]. The long-term uses of corticosteroids and the more recent introduction of rituximab account for much of this risk. Two recent studies analyzed cases of PML with the FDA Adverse Event Reporting System in the setting of rheumatic diseases, mostly SLE and RA. The most frequently used drug was rituximab and, while the authors acknowledge limitations that preclude definite causality, a specific signal is emerging with regard to rituximab and PML [58]. Similar data came from an analysis of Health Canada Drug Product Database [59]. As more oral agents are approved, clinicians will need to be alert to similar infectious risks that perhaps may be specific to the individual agents. For example, alemtuzumab appears to be a potent immune modulator in multiple sclerosis patients and already has been reported to be associated with PML when given for hematologic malignancies [60].

In 2009, of a national estimate of hospitalized patients with PML, 82 % were HIV associated, 8.4 % had hematologic cancers and solid cancers (2.8 %), and rheumatic diseases including SLE, RA, and other connective tissue diseases accounted for fewer than 1 % [61]. Carson and colleagues reported 57 cases of PML occurring after rituximab use for rheumatologic disorders and noted that these cases, gleaned from a number of cancer and academic centers, from the manufacturer and from FDA reports probably represent an underestimate. Ninety percent of the cases were fatal [62]. The major clinically relevant demographic point is that the populations at risk are expanding [63].

Rituximab

After 13 years of clinical use, rituximab has found indications in various neoplastic and autoimmune disorders such as lupus, rheumatoid arthritis, non-Hodgkin lymphoma, and multiple sclerosis. It was approved by the US Food and Drug Administration in 1997 and by the European Medicines Agency in 1998. Directed against CD20, it has been associated with prolonged B cell depletion for many months though immunoglobulin levels are largely unchanged. Infectious complications with CNS implications either through direct involvement of the CNS or through organ dysfunction-related encephalopathy include reactivation of hepatitis B, PML, CMV, and enteroviral meningoencephalitis and increased severity of WNV, babesiosis, and *Pneumocystis jiroveci* [64–67]. Case series of PML in patients receiving rituximab in polychemotherapy regimens led to the black box warning. Retrospective study suggested that the inclusion of rituximab into standard chemotherapy for NHL cause was associated with a higher incidence of PML [68]. Another study of chronic lymphocytic leukemia associated PML with both fludarabine and rituximab at some point during their course [69].

The FDA, European Medicines Agency, and WHO have all issued warnings of PML following rituximab administration. Informed decision making and patient's informed consent for these therapies, ways to detect virus, and attempts to minimize immunosuppression must be investigated and emphasized in physician education [70]. Analyzing the role of specific drug toxicity is difficult in diseases that themselves produce some immunosuppression and that are often treated with multiple types of immune-altering drugs. For example, PML has been observed in RA and SLE without rituximab and in psoriasis patients treated with efalizumab alone or in combination with other immune suppressive regimens [71]. Sarcoidosis presenting as PML has been reported and the authors note that it may be responsive to cidofovir, a drug that has not proved helpful in the AIDS population raising the question of whether less heavily immunosuppressed patients may respond to therapies ineffective in AIDS patients [62]. Consistent subsequent series suggest an increased PML risk on the order of about 1 case per 25,000 RA patients. In these patients, inflammatory PML may occur even with low CD20 counts [72].

Other monoclonal antibodies such as adalimumab also have been associated with PML and other viral infections. Similarly, the fusion protein efalizumab as well as abatacept and anakinra confers increased PML risk when used for RA [22, 73, 74]. Brentuximab, an antibody-drug conjugate linking the antimicrotubule agent monomethyl auristatin E to a CD30 monoclonal antibody, has also been reported to produce PML with PML-IRIS in several patients [75, 76].

Mycophenolate mofetil (MMF) also has been associated with diffuse large B cell EBV-associated lymphoma in a patient with SLE [77, 78]. Increased risk in renal transplant recipients seems to occur with incorporation of MMF in the antirejection regimen [79]. PML can occur in patients with minimal immunosuppression, and the MRI appearance may differ considerably when host response produces an exuberant inflammatory response [25, 26].

Tumor Necrosis Factor Inhibitors

Inhibition of tumor necrosis factor (TNF-α) is an effective rheumatoid arthritis treatment for patients resistant to conventional diseases-modifying drugs, and this class of drugs is used also for ankylosing spondylitis, psoriatic arthritis, inflammatory bowel disease, and uveitis and as an alternative in steroid refractory neurosarcoidosis. Strangfeld and colleagues explored associations between anti-TNF-α therapy and viral disease from the German biologics registry. One-half of the cases of VZV they found were linked with adalimumab or infliximab and another 15 % had had etanercept. The VZV rate in this study was 11.1 per 1,000, a risk comparable to patients over age 80. The risk increased when patients were switched to adalimumab or infliximab but not to etanercept. One-fifth of the infections were severe enough to require hospitalization. The increased risk for this population therefore was considerably less than that of the transplant patients [80, 81]. However, the differential diagnosis may be complicated by concurrent infectious processes; for example, during *Listeria* sepsis while receiving infliximab, a patient also developed lesions that could be drug-related demyelination, and the future use of TNF-α inhibitors depends on the interpretation of this neurological complication (Fig. 14.5). Other drugs associated with an increased incidence of VZV when used in the RA population include cyclophosphamide, azathioprine, and prednisone, but not, at least in one survey, methotrexate [82]. Live virus VZV is contraindicated in patients receiving TNF-α inhibitor drugs. Therefore, administration of the vaccine before anti-TNF-α therapy appears reasonable [83].

As potent immunomodulators, TNF-α inhibitors and other biological therapies have been reported to cause the appearance of systemic autoimmune diseases (SLE, vasculitis, sarcoidosis) and organ-specific illnesses such as optic neuritis, multiple sclerosis, and forms of peripheral demyelinating neuropathy (CIDP, multifocal motor neuropathy with conduction block, and Lewis-Sumner syndrome) [24]. In anti-TNF-α-associated neurological syndromes, discontinuation of treatment does not always resolve the disorder and long-term immunotherapy may be required to control the condition.

The unmasking of clinically latent MS by this class of drugs is complicated by an often-ambiguous MRI appearance that generates a complicated differential

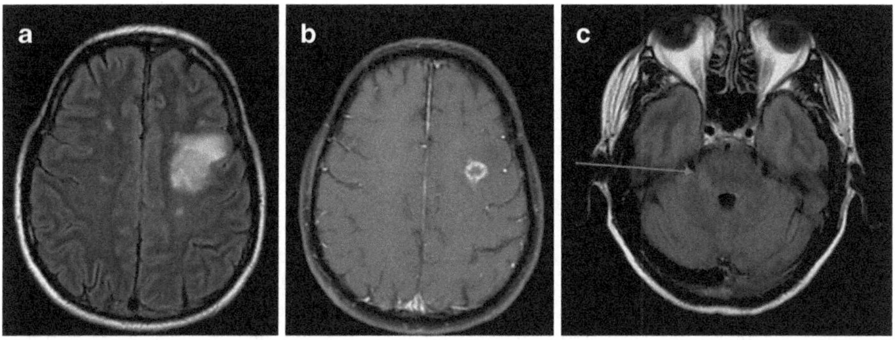

Fig. 14.5 Simultaneous drug toxicity and infection? A 58-year-old patient with steroid-refractory ulcerative colitis was started on infliximab therapy. After two courses of infliximab, abdominal pain, fever, and confusion led to diagnosis of *Listeria* bacteremia. CSF culture was negative and there was no pleocytosis. Seen on FLAIR and T1 gadolinium-enhanced scans is a ring-enhancing lesion that was assumed to be *Listeria* abscess (**a**, **b**). However, simultaneously multiple new areas of nonenhancing white matter abnormalities developed supratentorially and infratentorially (*arrow*) consistent with demyelination evoked by his recent TNF-α therapy (**a**, **c**). CSF was negative for both *Listeria* and oligoclonal bands and follow-up MRI showed resolution of all areas

diagnostic list of rapidly evolving sometimes enhancing multifocal lesions raising concern about PML, PTLD, and other infections. De novo appearance of demyelinating disease and both remission and exacerbation of preexisting MS have been reported in patients receiving this class of drugs. Etanercept is the most frequently implicated medicine [84]. Diagnosis can be difficult as is evident in the 21 reported cases of optic neuritis associated with TNF-α inhibition with adalimumab many of whom were receiving the drug for uveitis, iridocyclitis, and other primarily ocular conditions [85]. In this group of rheumatologic diseases, MS emerging in the context of immune dysregulation is reminiscent of cases described during immune reconstitution following HCT [86]. The MRI differential diagnosis is further complicated by the substantial proportion of patients with PRES who have underlying autoimmune conditions and whose multifocal abnormalities on MRI may cause diagnostic confusion [87]. While clinical evidence concerning the management of CNS or PNS neurological events arising while patients are receiving TNF-α antagonists remains inconclusive, this class of drugs should be avoided in patients with MS or other CNS demyelinating diseases [88].

References

1. Tan IL, McArthur JC, Ventaesan A, Nath A. Atypical manifestations and poor outcome of herpes simplex encephalitis in the immunocompromised. Neurology. 2012;79:2125–32.
2. Safdieh JE, Mead PA, Sepkowitz KA, Kiehn TE, Abrey LE. Bacterial and fungal meningitis in patients with cancer. Neurology. 2008;70(12):943–7.
3. Pruitt AA. CNS infections in patients with cancer. Continuum Lifelong Learning Neurol. 2012;18(2):384–405.

4. Kranick SM, Vinnard C, Kolson DL. Propionibacterium acnes brain abscess appearing 10 years after neurosurgery. Arch Neurol. 2009;66(6):793–5.
5. Pruitt AA. Central nervous system infections in cancer patients. Semin Neurol. 2010;30(3):296–310.
6. Clark AJ, Butowski NA, Chang SM, et al. Impact of bevacizumab chemotherapy on craniotomy wound healing. J Neurosurg. 2011;114(6):1609–16.
7. Suzuki HI, Hangaishi A, Hosoya N, et al. Herpes simplex encephalitis and subsequent cytomegalovirus encephalitis after chemoradiotherapy for central nervous system lymphoma: a case report and literature review. Int J Hematol. 2008;87(5):538–41.
8. Kocher M, Kunze S, Eich HT, et al. Efficacy and toxicity of postoperative temozolomide radiochemotherapy in malignant glioma. Strahlenter Onkol. 2005;181(3):157–63.
9. Pruitt AA, Graus F, Rosenfeld MR. Neurological complications of transplantation. Part I: hematopoietic cell transplantation. Neurohospitalist. 2013;3:24–38. Part II: solid organ transplantation. Neurohospitalist. 2013;3:152–66.
10. Siegal D, Keller A, Xu W, et al. Central nervous system complications after allogeneic hematopoietic stem cell transplantation: incidence, manifestations and clinical significance. Biol Blood Marrow Transplant. 2007;13(11):1369–79.
11. Bhanushali MJ, Kranick SM, Freeman AF, Cuellar-Rodriguez JM, Battiwalla M, Gea-Banacloche JC, et al. Human herpes 6 virus encephalitis complicating allogeneic hematopoietic stem cell transplantation. Neurology. 2013;80:1494–500.
12. Nath A, Berger JR. Complications of immunomodulatory therapy in neurological diseases. Curr Treat Options Neurol. 2012;14:241–55.
13. Nagel MA, Gilden DH. The protean neurologic manifestations of varicella-zoster virus infection. Cleve Clin J Med. 2007;74(7):489–94.
14. Salazar R, Russman AN, Nagel MA, et al. VZV temporal arteritis and subclinical temporal artery involvement. Arch Neurol. 2011;68:517–20.
15. Nagel MA, Russman AN, Feit DO, Schmid DS, Gilden D. VZV ischemic optic neuropathy and subclinical temporal artery infection without rash. Neurology. 2013;80:220–2.
16. Gilden D, Cohrs RJ, Mahalingam R, et al. Varicella zoster vasculopathies: diverse clinical manifestations, laboratory features, pathogenesis and treatment. Lancet Neurol. 2009;8(8):731–40.
17. Styczynski J, Reusser P, Einsele H, et al. Management of HSV, VZV and EBV infections in patients with hematological malignancies and after stem cell transplantation: guidelines from the Second European Conference on Infections in Leukemia. Bone Marrow Transplant. 2009;43(10):757–70.
18. Day JN, Chau TTH, Wolbers M, Mai PP, Dung NT, Mai NH, et al. Combination antifungal therapy for cryptococcal meningitis. N Engl J Med. 2013;268(14):1291–302.
19. Labbe AC, Su SH, Laverdiere M, et al. High incidence of invasive aspergillosis associated with intestinal graft-versus-host disease following nonmyeloablative transplantation. Biol Blood Marrow Transplant. 2007;13(10):1192–200.
20. Evens AM, Roy R, Sterrenberg D, et al. Post-transplantation lymphoproliferative disorders: diagnosis, prognosis and current approaches to therapy. Curr Oncol Rep. 2010;12(6):383–94.
21. Tan CS, Ellis LC, Wuthrich C, et al. JC virus latency in the brain and extraneural organs of patients with and without progressive multifocal leukoencephalopathy. J Virol. 2010;84:9200–9.
22. Tan CS, Koralnik IJ. Progressive multifocal leukoencephalopathy and other disorders caused by JC virus: clinical features and pathogenesis. Lancet Neurol. 2010;9:425–37.
23. Schmedt N, Andersohn F, Garbe E. Signals of progressive multifocal leukoencephalopathy for immunosuppressants: a disproportionality analysis of spontaneous reports within the US Adverse Event Reporting System (AERS). Pharmacoepidemiol Drug Saf. 2012;21:1216–20.
24. Bosch X, Saiz A, Ramos-Casals M, and the BIOGEAS Study Group. Monoclonal antibody therapy-associated neurological disorders. Nat Rev Neurol. 2011;7:165–72.
25. Gheuens S, Pierone G, Peeters P, et al. Progressive multifocal leukoencephalopathy in individuals with minimal or occult immunosuppression. J Neurol Neurosurg Psychiatry. 2010;81:247–54.

26. McGuire JL, Fridman V, Wuthrich C, Koralnik IJ, Jacobs D. Progressive multifocal leukoencephalopathy associated with isolated CD8+ T-lymphocyte deficiency mimicking tumefactive MS. J Neurovirol. 2011;17(5):500–3.
27. Koralnik IM, Wuthrich C, Dang X, et al. JC virus granule cell neuronopathy: a novel clinical syndrome distinct from progressive multifocal leukoencephalopathy. Ann Neurol. 2005;57:576–80.
28. Wuthrich C, Dang X, Westmoreland S, et al. Fulminant JC virus encephalopathy with productive infection of cortical pyramidal neurons. Ann Neurol. 2009;65:742–8.
29. Berger JR, Aksamit AJ, Clifford DB, Davis L, Koralnik IJ, Sejvar JJ, et al. PML diagnostic criteria: consensus statement from the AAN Neuroinfectious Disease Section. Neurology. 2013;80:1430–8.
30. Horger M, Beschorner R, Beck R, Nagele T, Schulze M, Ernemann U, Heckl S. Common and uncommon imaging findings in progressive multifocal leukoencephalopathy (PML) with differential diagnostic considerations. Clin Neurol Neruosurg. 2012;114:1123–30.
31. Mateen FJ, Muralidharan RN, Carone M, van de Beek D, Harrison DM, Aksamit AJ, et al. Progressive multifocal leukoencephalopathy in transplant recipients. Ann Neurol. 2011;70:305–22.
32. Clifford DB, Nath A, Cinque P, Brew BJ, Zivadinov R, Gorelik L, et al. A study of mefloquine treatment for progressive multifocal leukoencephalopathy: results and exploration of predictors of PML outcomes. J Neurovirol. 2013;19(4):351–8.
33. Brew BJ, Davies NWS, Cinque P, Cliffor DB, Nath A. Progressive multifocal leukoencephalopathy and other forms of JC virus disease. Nat Rev Neurol. 2010;6:667–79.
34. Kleinschmidt-DeMasters BK, Tyler KL. Progressive multifocal leukoencephalopathy complicating treatment with natalizumab and interferon beta-1a for multiple sclerosis. N Engl J Med. 2005;353:369–74.
35. Langer-Gould A, Atlas SW, Green AJ, et al. Progressive multifocal leukoencephalopathy in a patient treated with natalizumab. N Engl J Med. 2005;353:375–81.
36. Van Assche G, Van Ranst M, Sciot R, et al. Progressive multifocal leukoencephalopathy after natalizumab therapy for Crohn's disease. N Engl J Med. 2005;353:362–8.
37. Clifford DB, DeLuca A, Simpson DM, Arendt G, Giovannoni G, Nath A. Natalizumab-associated progressive multifocal leukoencephalopathy in patients with multiple sclerosis: lessons from 28 cases. Lancet Neurol. 2010;9:438–46.
38. Tan IL, McArthur JC, Clifford DB, Major E, Nath A. Immune reconstitution inflammatory syndrome in natalizumab – associated PML. Neurology. 2011;77:1061–7.
39. Linda H, von Heijne A, Major EO, et al. Progressive multifocal leukoencephalopathy after natalizumab monotherapy. N Engl J Med. 2009;361:1081–7.
40. Gorelik L, Lerner M, Bixler S, et al. Anti-JCV antibodies: implications for PML risk stratification. Ann Neurol. 2010;68:392–5.
41. Aksamit AJ. Progressive multifocal leukoencephalopathy. Continuum Lifelong Learning Neurol. 2012;18(6):1374–91.
42. Chen Y. Asymptomatic reactivation of JC virus in patients treated with natalizumab. N Engl J Med. 2009;361:1067–74.
43. Major EO, Frohman E, Douek D. JC viremia in natalizumab-treated patients with multiple sclerosis. N Engl J Med. 2013;368(23):2240–1.
44. Rudick RA, O'Connor PW, Goelz SE, et al. Assessment of JC virus DNA in blood and urine from natalizumab-treated patients. Ann Neurol. 2010;68:304–10.
45. West T, Cree B. Natalizumab dosage suspension: are we helping or hurting? Ann Neurol. 2010;68:395–9.
46. Killestein J, Vennegoor A, Striijbis EM, et al. Natalizumab drug holiday in multiple sclerosis: poorly tolerated. Ann Neurol. 2010;68:392–3935.
47. Lenhard T, Biller A, Mueller W, et al. Immune reconstitution inflammatory syndrome after withdrawal of natalizumab? Neurology. 2010;75:831–3.
48. Miravalle A, Jense R, Kinkel RP. Immune reconstitution inflammatory syndrome in patients with multiple sclerosis following cessation of natalizumab therapy. Arch Neurol. 2011;68:186–91.

49. Ryschkewitsch CF, Jensen PN, Major EO, et al. JC virus persistence following PML in MS patients treated with natalizumab. Ann Neurol. 2010;68:384–91.
50. Antoniol C, Jilek S, Schluep M, Mercier N, Canales M, Le Goff G, et al. Impairment of JCV-specific T-cell response by corticotherapy. Effect on PML-IRIS management. Neurology. 2012;79:2258–64.
51. Aktos O, Kury P, Kieseier B, et al. Fingolimod is a potential novel therapy for multiple sclerosis. Nat Rev Neurol. 2010;6:373–82.
52. Gross CM, Baumgartner A, Rauer S, Stich O. Multiple sclerosis rebound following herpes zoster infection and suspension of fingolimod. Neurology. 2012;79:2006–7.
53. Ratchford JN, Costell K, Riech DS, Calabresisi PA. Varicella zoster virus encephalitis and vasculopathy in a patient treated with fingolimod. Neurology. 2012;79:20020–2004.
54. Van Oosten BW, Killestien J, Barkhof F, Polman CH, Wattjes MP. PML in a patient treated with dimethyl fumarate from a compounding pharmacy. N Engl J Med. 2013;368(17):1658–9.
55. Ermis U, Weis J, Schulz JB. PML in a patient treated with fumaric acid. N Engl J Med. 2013;268(17):1657–8.
56. Sweetser MT, Dawson KT, Bozic C. Manufacturer's response to case reports of PML. N Engl J Med. 2013;368(17):1659–60.
57. Perez-Alvarez R, Perez-de-Lis M, Ramos-Casals M, on behalf of the BIOGEAS Study Group. Curr Opin Rheumatol. 2013;25(1):56–64.
58. Molloy ES, Calabrese LH. Progressive multifocal leukoencephalopathy associated with immunosuppressive therapy in rheumatoid diseases. Arthritis Rheum. 2012;64(9):3043–51.
59. Keene DL, Legare C, Taylor E, Gallivan J, Cawthorn GM, Vu D. Monoclonal antibodies and progressive multifocal leukoencephalopathy. Can J Neurol Sci. 2011;38:565–71.
60. Piccinni C, Sacripanti C, Poluzzi E, Motola D, Magro L, Moretti U, et al. Stronger association of drug-induced progressive multifocal leukoencephalopathy (PML) with biological immunomodulating agents. Eur J Clin Pharmacol. 2010;66:199–206.
61. Molloy ES, Calabrese LH. Progressive multifocal leukoencephalopathy: a national estimate of frequency in SLE and other rheumatic diseases. Arthritis Rheum. 2009;60:3761–5.
62. Carson KR, Focosi D, Major EO, Petrini M, Richey EA, West DP, Bennett CI. Monoclonal antibody-associated progressive multifocal leukoencephalopathy in patients treated with rituximab, natalizumab and efalizumab: a review from the Research on Adverse Drug Events and Reports (RADAR) project. Lancet Oncol. 2009;10:816–24.
63. Major EO. Progressive multifocal leukoencephalopathy in patients on immunomodulatory therapies. Annu Rev Med. 2010;61:35–47.
64. Gea-Banacloche JC. Rituximab-associated infections. Semin Hematol. 2010;47(2):187–98.
65. Ganjoo KN, Raman R, Sobel RA, et al. Opportunistic enteroviral meningoencephalitis: an unusual treatable complication of rituximab therapy. Leuk Lymphoma. 2009;50(4):673–5.
66. Levi ME, Quan D, Ho JT, et al. Impact of rituximab-associated B-cell defects on West Nile virus meningoencephalitis in solid organ transplant recipients. Clin Transplant. 2009;24(2):223–8.
67. Lee MY, Chiou TJ, Hsaiao LT, et al. Rituximab therapy increased post-transplant cytomegalovirus complications in non-Hodgkin lymphoma patients receiving autologous hematopoietic stem cell transplantation. Ann Hematol. 2008;87(4):285–9.
68. Tuccori M, Focosi D, Blandizzi C, Pelosini M, Montangni S, Maggi F, et al. Inclusion of rituximab in treatment protocols for non-Hodgkin's lymphomas and risk for progressive multifocal leukoencephalopathy. Oncologist. 2010;15:1214–9.
69. D'Souza A, Wilson J, Mukherjee S, Jaiyesimi I. Progressive multifocal leukoencephalopathy in chronic lymphocytic leukemia. A report of 3 cases and review of the literature. Clin Lymphoma Myeloma Leuk. 2010;10(1):E1–9.
70. Tyler KL. Progressive multifocal leukoencephalopathy: can we reduce risk in patients receiving biological immunomodulatory therapies? Ann Neurol. 2010;68(3):271–4.
71. Korman BD, Tyler KL, Korman NJ. Progressive multifocal leukoencephalopathy, efalizumab, and immunosuppression. A cautionary tale for dermatologists. Arch Dermatol. 2009;145(8):937–40.

72. Clifford DB, Ances B, Costello C, Rosen-Schmidt S, Andersson M, Parks D, et al. Rituximab-associated progressive multifocal leukoencephalopathy in rheumatoid arthritis. Arch Neurol. 2011;68(9):1156–64.
73. Salliot C, Dougados M, Gossec L. Risk of serious infections during rituximab, abatacept and anakinra treatments for rheumatoid arthritis: meta-analyses of randomised placebo-controlled trials. Ann Rheum Dis. 2009;68:25–32.
74. Schwab N, Ulzheimer JC, Fox RJ, et al. Fatal progressive multifocal leukoencephalopathy associated with efalizumab therapy: insights into the role of leukointegrin aLb2in JC virus control. Mult Scler. 2009;15:S271–7.
75. Von Geldern G, Pardo CA, Calabresi PA, Newsome SD. PML-IRIS in a patient treated with brentuximab. Neurology. 2012;79:2075–7.
76. Jalan P, Mahajan A, Pandav V, Bekker S, Koirala J. Brentuximab associated progressive multifocal leukoencephalopathy. Clin Neurol Neurosurg. 2012;114:1335–7.
77. Tsang HH, Trendell-Smith NJ, Wu AK, et al. Diffuse large B-cell lymphoma of the CNS in mycophenolate mofetil-treated patients with systemic lupus erythematosus. Lupus. 2010;19:330–3.
78. Berger JR. Progressive multifocal leukoencephalopathy and newer biological agents. Drug Saf. 2010;33(11):969–83.
79. Neff RT, Hurst GP, Falta EM, Bohen EM, Lentine KL, Dharnidharka VR, et al. Progressive multifocal leukoencephalopathy and use of mycophenolate mofetil after kidney transplantation. Transplantation. 2008;86:1474–8.
80. Strangfeld A, Lising J, Herzer P, et al. Risk of herpes zoster in patients with rheumatoid arthritis treated with anti-TNF-alpha agents. JAMA. 2009;301:737–44.
81. Whitfield RJ, Gnann JW. Herpes zoster in the age of focused immunosuppressive therapy. JAMA. 2009;301:774–5.
82. Wolfe F, Michaud K, Chakravarty EF. Rates and predictors of herpes zoster in patients with rheumatoid arthritis and non-inflammatory musculoskeletal disorders. Rheumatology. 2006;45:1370–5.
83. Harpaz R, Ortega-Sanchez IR, Seward JF. Advisory Committee on Immunization Practices (ACIP), Centers for Disease Control and Prevention. Prevention of herpes zoster: recommendations of the ACIP (published correction appears in MMWR Recomm Rep 2008;57:779). MMWR Recomm Rep. 2008;57(RR-5):1–30.
84. Lysandropoulos AP, Du Pasquier RA. Demyelination as a complication of new immunomodulatory treatments. Curr Opin Neurol. 2010;23:226–33.
85. Li S, Birnbaum AD, Goldstein DA. Optic neuritis associated with adalimumab in the treatment of uveitis. Ocul Immunol Inflamm. 2010;18:L475–81.
86. Armstrong RJE, Elston JS, Hatton CS, et al. De novo relapsing-remitting multiple sclerosis following autologous stem cell transplantation. Neurology. 2010;75:89–90.
87. Fugate JE, Claassen DO, Cloft HJ. Posterior reversible encephalopathy syndrome: associated clinical and radiologic findings. Mayo Clin Proc. 2010;85:427–32.
88. Nozaki K, Silver RM, Stickler DE, Abou-Fayssal NG, Giglio P, Kamen DL, et al. Neurological deficits during treatment with tumor necrosis factor-alpha antagonists. Am J Med Sci. 2011;342(5):352–5.
89. National Multiple Sclerosis Society (NMSS). 2013. Available from http://www.nationalmssociety.org.

Chapter 15
The Neurological Spectrum of HIV Infection

Iñigo Corral and Carmen Quereda

Abstract Neurological manifestations are frequent in human immunodeficiency virus (HIV)-infected patients and represent a great diagnostic and therapeutic challenge. They may be caused by many different mechanisms: the HIV, opportunistic infections or tumors, autoimmunity, and complications of systemic diseases or drugs, including the antiretrovirals. Patients may suffer several simultaneous neurological diseases, and the HIV and some opportunistic infections may affect simultaneously various levels in the nervous system. Highly active antiretroviral therapy (HAART) has produced a decline in opportunistic diseases and neurological disorders associated with severe immune depression. However, the prolonged survival of patients has increased morbidity due to chronic disorders, such as cerebrovascular disease and HIV-associated neurocognitive disorders. The central nervous system constitutes a reservoir for HIV replication in patients with controlled systemic disease. HAART itself is related to new emerging neurological problems: the specific neurotoxicity of the drugs and the appearance of neurological immune reconstitution inflammatory syndromes.

Keywords Human immunodeficiency virus • HIV-associated dementia • HIV-associated neurocognitive disorders • Immune reconstitution inflammatory syndromes • Toxoplasma encephalitis • Primary central nervous system lymphoma • Progressive multifocal leukoencephalopathy • Antiretroviral therapy • Cryptococcus

I. Corral, MD, PhD (✉)
Department of Neurology, Ramón y Cajal Hospital,
Carretera de Colmenar km 9,1, Madrid, 28034, Spain
e-mail: icorral.hrc@salud.madrid.org

C. Quereda, MD, PhD
Department of Infectious Diseases, Ramón y Cajal Hospital, Madrid, Spain

J.C. García-Moncó (ed.), *CNS Infections*,
DOI 10.1007/978-1-4471-6401-2_15, © Springer-Verlag London 2014

Introduction

The human immunodeficiency virus (HIV) infects both macrophages and CD4+ lymphocytes. Infected macrophages invade the central nervous system (CNS) and may cause direct CNS damage. CD4 lymphocyte depletion causes cellular immune depression, which may condition CNS opportunistic infections. In consequence, neurological manifestations are frequent in HIV-infected patients and tend to occur in advanced stages of HIV infection. Approximately 50 % of acquired immune deficiency syndrome (AIDS) patients will suffer neurological manifestations along the course of the disease [1] even a higher frequency of HIV-associated disorders (more than 75 % of cases) demonstrated in neuropathology studies [2].

After the introduction of HAART in 1996, a drastic decline in the incidence of opportunistic diseases and neurological disorders associated with severe immune depression was noted in developed countries [3, 4]. The prognosis and survival of patients with previously considered fatal diseases, such as progressive multifocal leukoencephalopathy (PML) and primary central nervous system lymphoma (PCNSL), have also substantially improved. Other concerns, however, emerged in the care of HIV-infected patients in the HAART era. The prolonged patient survival results in an increased morbidity due to chronic disorders, with particular relevance for those involving the CNS, including cerebrovascular disease and HIV-associated neurocognitive disorders (HAND). HAART itself is related to new emerging neurological problems that result from the specific neurotoxicity of these drugs and the appearance of neurological immune reconstitution inflammatory syndromes (IRIS). Nowadays, opportunistic CNS lesions present only as the first manifestation of disease, or in patients who do not adhere to treatment or with treatment failure due to drug resistance, or as IRIS.

Classification and Approach to the Patient

The approach to the patient with suspected neurological complications of HIV should consider three different yet complementary ways of classifying these disorders: (*a*) a pathogenic and etiological classification; (*b*) a chronologic classification, attending to the different stages of HIV infection regarding immune depression and antiretroviral treatment received; and (*c*) a neuroanatomical classification of the lesion. From a pathogenic point of view, the neurological disorders presenting in HIV-infected patients may be associated with (*1*) the infection of the nervous system by the HIV; (*2*) the disorder of cellular immunity, which facilitates opportunistic infections or tumors and may occasionally favor autoimmune neurological disorders; (*3*) the immune restoration induced by HAART; and (*4*) the neurological complications of other systemic diseases associated with the HIV and of the different drugs used in these patients, including the antiretrovirals. The wide spectrum of opportunistic CNS infections reported in AIDS patients may be classified according

Table 15.1 Pathogenic and chronologic classification of neurological complications of HIV infection

	Primary infection	Early stages (A, CD4 > 200/mm^3)	Late stages (B, C, CD4 < 200/mm^3)
HIV-associated	Acute encephalitis Aseptic meningitis Transverse myelitis	Mononeuritis multiplex HIV-associated myopathy	HIV-associated dementia Vacuolar myelopathy Distal symmetric polyneuropathy HIV-associated myopathy
Autoimmune	Guillain–Barré syndrome Acute disseminated encephalomyelitis Multiple sclerosis-like disease	Guillain–Barré syndrome Acute disseminated encephalomyelitis Multiple sclerosis-like disease Chronic inflammatory demyelinating polyneuropathy	-
Immune depression	–	–	Toxoplasma encephalitis Primary central nervous system lymphoma Progressive multifocal leukoencephalopathy Cryptococcal meningitis Tuberculosis Herpesvirus diseases Other opportunistic infections
Antiretroviral treatment	–	–	Zidovudine myopathy Antiretroviral neuropathy Immune reconstitution inflammatory syndrome Syndrome of neuromuscular weakness
Secondary disorders	–	–	Toxic–metabolic disorders

to the causing microorganism in bacterial (conventional bacteria, mycobacteria, nocardia), fungal, viral, and parasitic infections.

As the specific neurological disorders depend on the immunological status of the patient, they correlate with the stage of systemic HIV infection (Table 15.1). In primary HIV infection, neurological disease may be similar to that of other acute viral infections, presenting as acute encephalitis, aseptic meningitis, or transverse myelitis. In the early stages of HIV infection, including primary infection, autoimmune neurological disorders may occasionally occur. Cases of Guillain–Barré syndrome, chronic inflammatory demyelinating polyneuropathy, myasthenia gravis, acute disseminated encephalomyelitis, and multiple sclerosis-like disease have been reported. Opportunistic infections and HIV-associated disorders present almost exclusively in advanced stages of the disease, usually with a CD4+ lymphocyte count under 200/mm^3. In these stages, metabolic and toxic disorders are also common because of the frequency of systemic disease and the complexity of treatments received. Patients under HAART may suffer neurological IRISs in addition to the toxic effects of the drugs.

The neuroanatomical localization of the neurological syndrome presented by the patient will limit the differential diagnosis to the possible etiologies of the syndrome. A further limitation would be facilitated taking into account the stage of HIV infection, other clinical data, and the results of specific complementary studies (Table 15.2). However, the neurological diagnosis in patients with HIV infection is hampered by a number of difficulties. A major problem is that these patients may suffer several simultaneous neurological diseases. Autopsy studies frequently demonstrate more than one concomitant opportunistic disease, together with HIV-associated diseases [2]. In addition, the HIV and some opportunistic infections, such as cytomegalovirus (CMV) or varicella-zoster virus (VZV), may affect simultaneously various levels in the nervous system. Drug toxicity or withdrawal may complicate the picture in patients with illicit drug or alcohol abuse.

Encephalic Complications

The encephalic complications of HIV infection may be classified into focal lesions and diffuse encephalopathies (Table 15.2). Among the latter, a key point is whether the patient presents with attention deficit or alteration of the level of consciousness, in which case the patient probably suffers from diffuse infections or toxic–metabolic disorders. Attention and consciousness are preserved in HIV-associated neurocognitive disorders.

Focal lesions include opportunistic infections, primary or metastatic neoplasm, demyelinating lesions, and cerebrovascular diseases. The frequency of opportunistic infections of the CNS and PCNSL has dramatically decreased since the introduction of HAART, and CMV encephalitis is now rarely diagnosed [4, 5].

HIV-Associated Dementia

The HIV invades the SNC soon after primary infection, and inflammatory markers and evidence of neural damage are found in early HIV infection [6, 7]. Patients, however, remain asymptomatic until advanced stages of disease because a significant HIV infection of the CNS occurs only in the setting of severe immune depression [8], and thus the frequency of HIV-associated dementia (HAD) increases with the advance of systemic disease. The mean CD4 cell count in patients with HAD is approximately 100/mm^3. In patients with AIDS, the prevalence of dementia is close to 50 % [9], but the characteristic pathological features have been found in 11–90 % of autopsy cases [2, 10]. Risk factors associated with dementia are high plasma HIV

Table 15.2 Neuroanatomical and etiological classification of neurological complications of HIV infection

	Diffuse encephalopathies	Focal brain lesions	Myelopathies	Meningitis	Neuropathies
HIV	HIV-associated dementia Acute HIV encephalitis	–	Vacuolar myelopathy Transverse myelitis	Aseptic meningitis	Distal symmetric polyneuropathy Mononeuritis multiplex
Viral	CMV encephalitis	PML CMV encephalitis VZV encephalitis HSV encephalitis	Spastic tropical paraparesis CMV VZV HSV 1 and 2	VZV HSV 1 and 2 CMV	CMV polyradiculitis CMV neuropathy VZV polyradiculitis HSV 1 and 2 polyradiculitis
Bacterial	–	M. tuberculosis abscess or granuloma Bacterial abscess Nocardia abscess Syphilitic gumma	Epidural abscess Tuberculous granuloma Syphilis	M tuberculosis S. pneumoniae Listeria monocytogenes S. aureus Syphilis	M tuberculosis polyradiculitis Syphilis polyradiculitis
Fungal	–	Cryptococcal granuloma Aspergillus Mucor Candida	–	Cryptococcus Candida sp.	Cryptococcus
Parasitary	–	Toxoplasma encephalitis Cysticercosis	Toxoplasma	–	–
Tumor	–	Primary CNS lymphoma Gliomas Other primary neoplasms Metastatic neoplasms	Epidural metastasis Epidural lymphoma	Lymphomatous meningitis Meningeal carcinomatosis	Lymphomatous polyradiculopathy

(continued)

Table 15.2 (continued)

	Diffuse encephalopathies	Focal brain lesions	Myelopathies	Meningitis	Neuropathies
Autoimmune	–	ADEM Multiple sclerosis-like disease	–	–	Guillain–Barré syndrome CIDP
Other causes	Toxic–metabolic encephalopathy	Ischemic or hemorrhagic stroke	Vasculitis Disseminated intravascular coagulation		Antiretroviral neuropathy Other toxic neuropathies Cryoglobulinemia Diffuse infiltrative lymphocytosis syndrome Nutritional neuropathy Diabetic neuropathy Alcoholic neuropathy Uremic neuropathy

RNA level, low CD4 cell count, advanced age, female sex, the use of recreational drugs, and the presence of anemia and constitutional syndrome.

HAD can compromise cognitive, motor, and behavioral disorders. Any of these disorders may be the presenting symptom, and a psychiatric presentation with depression, acute psychosis, or mania is not uncommon. HAD usually begins insidiously, with difficulties in concentration, memory deficits, and psychomotor slowing progressing along weeks or months. The patient shows lack of motivation, apathy, irritability, emotional liability, and abnormal social behavior. These symptoms are frequently attributed to depression. Motor disorders include bradykinesia, incoordination, hypertonia, pyramidalism, and frontal regression signs. In the presence of vacuolar myelopathy, frequently associated with HAD, motor deficits in the legs may be present. HAD has been considered classically as a subcortical dementia. Cortical deficits, such as aphasia, apraxia, and agnosia are rare, but a frontal syndrome is common.

The diagnosis of HAD is clinical. Neuroimaging and CSF studies may support the diagnosis, but are oriented to exclude other neurological disorders. Information from the family or friends of the patient is essential to confirm cognitive or behavioral symptoms. A diagnosis of HAD should be postponed in the case of existing confounding factors, as active drug or alcohol abuse and systemic or neurological opportunistic diseases. Neuropsychological deficits must be confirmed with appropriate tests. To detect minor deficits, tests should explore memory, executive function, and complex attention [11]. The best screening tests are those exploring psychomotor speed (i.e., trail making test). The International HIV Dementia Scale is a rapid test useful for screening and follow-up [12].

Cranial tomography (CT) and magnetic resonance imaging (MRI) may show cerebral atrophy and leukoencephalopathy, which consists in symmetric and confluent areas of hyperintensity in T2 and fluid-attenuated inversion recovery (FLAIR)-weighted MRI sequences (Fig. 15.1). MRI spectroscopy may detect an early reduction in N-acetyl aspartate due neuronal loss, as well as an increase in choline, a marker of gliosis. CSF may show normal findings or nonspecific mild increase in protein concentration or lymphocytes. The presence of markers of immune activation in CSF (increased β_2-microglobulin or neopterin) supports the diagnosis. High levels of HIV RNA in CSF correlate with the presence of HIV encephalitis at autopsy [13], but there have been contradictory results regarding its value as a diagnostic test for dementia, especially in patients under HAART. The presence of HIV DNA in monocytes correlates with cognitive impairment, both before and after HAART, and increased levels differentiate patients with and without dementia [14].

A more inclusive classification now considered the HIV-associated neurocognitive disorders (HAND) has been recently divided into three categories: (1) HAD; (2) mild neurocognitive impairment (MNI), when cognitive deficits produce mild disability without dementia; and (3) asymptomatic neurocognitive impairment (ANI), when performance in neuropsychological test falls below that of controls, but there are no symptoms or functional impairment noted by the patient or informers [15]. The inclusion of ANI might overestimate the prevalence of HAND, as a percentage of the normal population would enter this category [16].

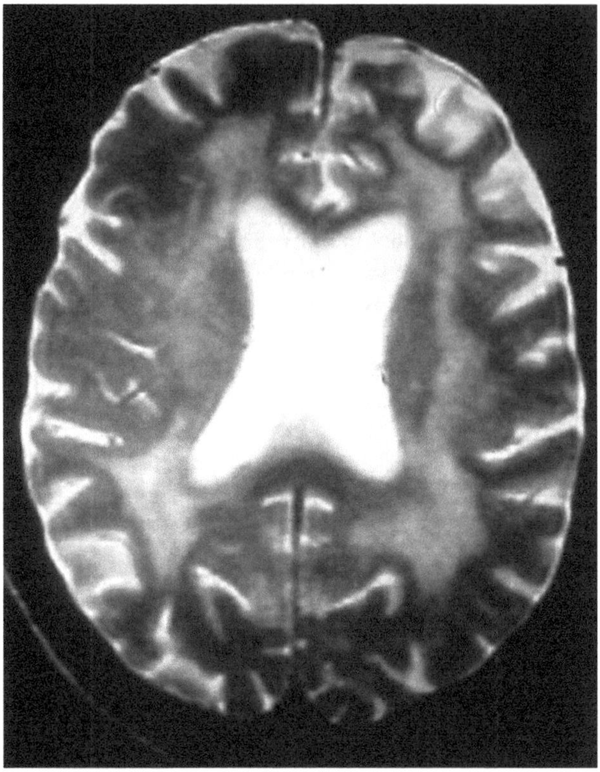

Fig. 15.1 Leukoencephalopathy of HIV-associated dementia. T2-weighted magnetic resonance imaging

Survival of HAD patients without treatment is less than 1 year. HAART is the standard therapy for HAD. The neuropsychological performance of HAD patients improves after months under HAART [17]. Maximal improvement occurs between weeks 24 and 36 of therapy, but may continue for more than 1 year [18]. In correlation with clinical improvement, HAART reduces CSF glutamate and other metabolites concentration, which are increased in HAD, lowers CSF HIV viral load, improves leukoencephalopathy in MRI, and reduces metabolic abnormalities of MR spectroscopy. However, many HAD patients improve incompletely or do not improve at all. Controlled trials of coadjutant treatment options for HAD have been disappointing [19].

HIV-Associated Neurocognitive Disorders in the HAART Era

In recent cohorts of patients receiving HAART, HAND was diagnosed in more than 50 % of patients, although fortunately many of them remained asymptomatic [19–23]. Many factors may condition this high prevalence. On the one hand, comorbidities may influence the diagnosis of HAND [21]. Cognitive performance can be influenced by the presence of vascular risk factors (hypertension, dyslipidemia, diabetes, obesity), hepatitis C virus (HCV) coinfection, drug abuse, or patient's age and educational level [20, 23–25]. On the other hand, the CNS damage caused by the HIV before treatment initiation or before HIV replication is controlled determines the persistence of cognitive deficits. HAND is associated with a lower pretreatment performance [20], a lower CD4 nadir [21, 26], a more advanced CDC stage, and a lower duration of controlled HIV replication [22]. Cerebral atrophy in MRI correlates with data of previous HIV infection, as are nadir CD4 count and duration of the infection [27]. These results highlight the need for early antiviral treatment to prevent HAND, before irreversible neuronal damage is established.

Persistent systemic HIV replication associates with higher frequency of HAND [21, 25, 26], but HAND prevalence is high even in patients with a successful control of HIV replication for years [22]. Markers of inflammation persist in CSF [19] and MRI spectroscopy [29] despite a controlled systemic replication. The presence of intramonocytic HIV DNA in treated patients has been associated with persistent HAND, suggesting a role of infected monocytes in the maintenance of neural injury through immune activation [28]. The possibility of escape replication of HIV within de CNS in patients with controlled systemic replication offers another hypothesis to explain the high prevalence of HAND. Recent reports of patients developing HAD after successful HAART due to CSF viral escape support this concept [30, 31]. In some patients with HAND, a compartmentalization of HIV in the CNS has been demonstrated by genetic differences between plasmatic and CSF viruses, especially in cases with controlled systemic replication and with drugs with low CNS penetration [32]. This may condition a different susceptibility pattern for antiretrovirals and a different macrophage tropism between plasma and CSF viruses. Antiretroviral combinations with a lower global CNS penetration might favor persistent CNS replication and HAND [33]. Indeed, HAART regimes with a higher penetration index give a better control of CNS replication, but contradictory results have been found regarding their effect on neuropsychological performance [18, 21, 29, 34–38]. On the contrary, antiretrovirals with high CNS penetration might have a negative effect on neuropsychological performance [34].

The pattern of cognitive impairment and cerebral atrophy in patients with HIV infection seems to have changed with HAART. In the pre-HAART era, there was a predominant involvement of motor skills, psychomotor speed, and verbal fluency, while in the HAART era, a greater impairment of memory and executive functions have been found [39], which correlates with greater temporal and frontal atrophy and less involvement of basal ganglia in MRI and pathological studies [21, 27]. Persistent inflammation associated with HIV infection might facilitate neurodegenerative disorders in patients with an increasing age [19]. There are some parallels between HAND and Alzheimer disease. In patients with HIV infection, an abnormal metabolism of β-amyloid protein is suggested [40], and APOE e4 allele is associated with HAND and cerebral atrophy [41]. The APOE e4 allele and older age are associated with the presence of amyloid plaques in the brain of HIV-infected patients and the probability of developing HAND [42]. In addition, familial history of dementia predicts HAND [43]. The present criteria for the diagnosis of HAND are not specific for the neural damage caused by the HIV and might not differentiate

HAND from other neurodegenerative disorders. CSF analysis can help in the differential diagnosis between HAND and mild Alzheimer disease, because, while both show a decrease in β-amyloid 1-42, tau and phosphorylated tau levels are decreased in the later [40].

In patients with HAART failure, a severe form of diffuse leukoencephalopathy has been reported. Pathological findings are similar to those of HIV encephalitis, with areas of demyelination and axonal damage, and intense perivascular infiltrates of lymphocytes and HIV-infected macrophages [44]. Patients with inadequate control of HIV infection and active cocaine abuse may suffer fulminant HIV encephalitis with predominant basal ganglia involvement in MRI [45].

Focal Brain Lesions

For the evaluation of focal brain lesions, clinical presentation, temporal evolution, and CSF and radiographic features should be considered. Opportunistic infections and tumors are usually present at advanced stages of disease (CD4 under $200/\text{mm}^3$) [3]. The spectrum of diseases that may cause focal lesions is wide. Three diseases constitute the great majority of diseases that contribute to focal lesions: toxoplasma encephalitis (TE), PCNLS, and PML. In patients under HAART PML seems the most frequent cause [3]. The evolution of the diseases is typically in hours or days in TE, days or weeks in PCNSL, and weeks or months in PML. A diagnostic algorithm is proposed in Fig. 15.2. In some patients, the presence of systemic infection might suggest the possible etiology. Ring enhancing lesions on CT or MRI are identical in abscesses caused by different microorganisms and may be difficult to distinguish from tumors. A definite diagnosis will frequently be established only by biopsy. If lumbar puncture is not contraindicated because of mass effect, it is helpful to perform specific CSF studies, such as cultures; polymerase chain reaction (PCR) for toxoplasma, mycobacteria, bacteria, JC virus (JCV), and Epstein–Barr virus (EBV); cytology; or immunophenotyping.

TE is the most frequent cause of focal brain lesions in AIDS. It usually results from reactivation of latent infection and, therefore, IgG antibodies against toxoplasma are detected in more than 90 % of cases. Clinical presentation consists in focal neurological deficits or seizures. Lesions most frequently locate at the cortico-subcortical union, but may affect the basal ganglia and, rarely, the brainstem or cerebellum. Multiple lesions are found in more than 50 % of patients. The characteristic lesions on CT are hypodense with perilesional edema and mass effect, with ring or nodular contrast enhancement. However, this pattern is unspecific and may not be present. A target sign highly suggests TE. The high frequency of TE justifies empiric treatment when it is suspected by radiology, even if serology is negative, which allows an *ex juvantibus* diagnosis. In a patient with negative serology under prophylaxis with cotrimoxazole, the probability of TE is very low, and empiric treatment is not indicated: a prompt brain biopsy should be scheduled [46]. CSF PCR for toxoplasma has high specificity but only 50 % sensitivity. Treatment consists in an induction phase with 2 drugs (pyrimethamine and sulfadiazine, or

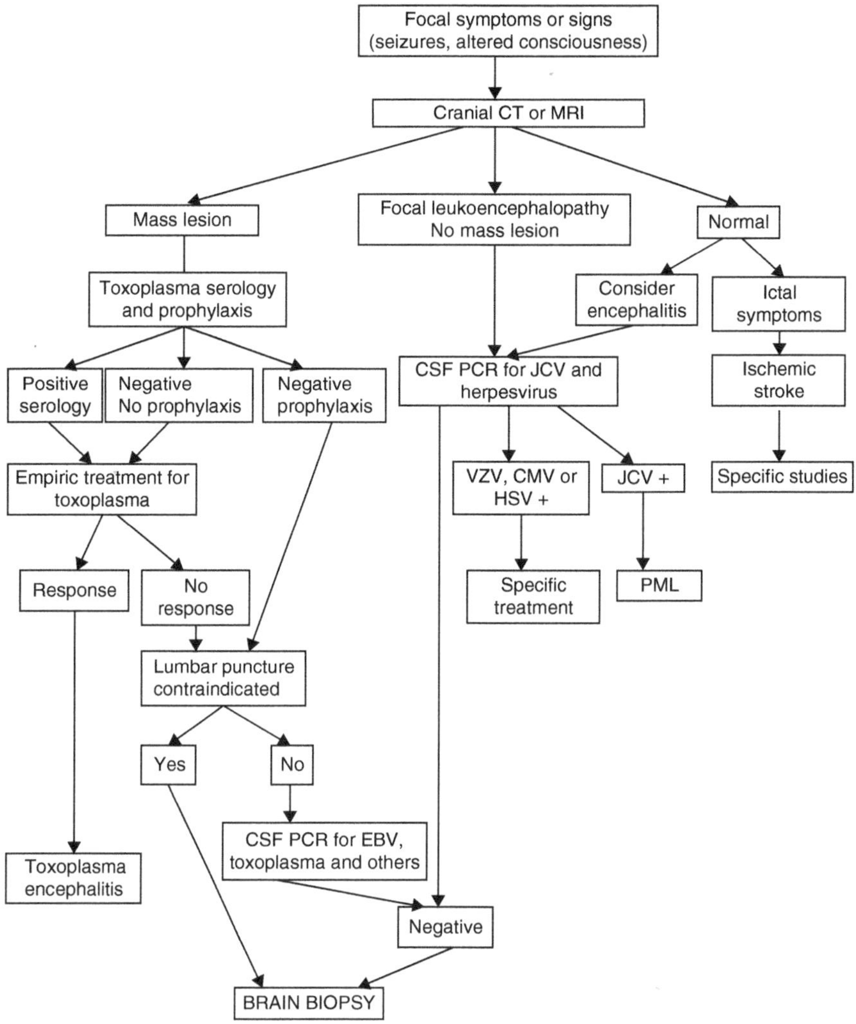

Fig. 15.2 Algorithm for the management of HIV-infected patients with focal brain lesions. Cranial tomography (CT) or magnetic resonance imaging (MRI) should be performed in every HIV-infected patient presenting with focal symptoms or signs, seizures, or altered state of consciousness. MRI is more sensitive to detect leukoencephalopathies, encephalitis, or posterior fossa lesions. If CT is normal and symptoms had ictal presentation, an ischemic stroke should be considered and the possible cause specifically investigated. In the presence of a mass lesion, empiric antitoxoplasma therapy is indicated in the case of a positive serology, but also if serology is negative if the patient has not received prophylaxis with cotrimoxazole. Biopsy is indicated if no clinical or radiological improvement is noted after 2 weeks of treatment or the patient has negative serology and received prophylaxis because in this case the probability of toxoplasma encephalitis is negligible. Before brain biopsy, if there is no contraindication for lumbar puncture because of the mass effect, an attempt for specific diagnosis by means of polymerase chain reaction (*PCR*) and other studies in cerebrospinal fluid (*CSF*) should be considered. If neuroimaging studies are normal, viral encephalitis must be considered, and CSF PCR for cytomegalovirus (*CMV*), herpes simplex virus (*HSV*), and varicella-zoster virus (*VZV*) should be performed. In the case of focal lesions suggesting focal leukoencephalopathy, CSF PCR for VZV or JC virus (*JCV*) may aid the diagnosis of VZV leukoencephalitis or progressive multifocal leukoencephalopathy (*PML*). If both are negative, brain biopsy is necessary

clindamycin, with folinic acid) for at least 6 weeks. Steroids may be added in the presence of significant mass effect. An indefinite maintenance therapy should be given to avoid relapses. In fact, relapses may occur in 20 % of cases and are related with inadequate maintenance therapy. In patients under HAART with more than 200 CD4/mm^3, maintenance therapy can be confidently suspended because the risk of relapse is very low in this setting [47].

PCNSL are diffuse B-cell or immunoblastic lymphomas, associated with the Epstein–Barr virus (EBV) [48]. PCNSL are multicentric in 40 % of patients (up to 72 % in autopsy series). They are most commonly supratentorial and frequently periventricular, and only 10 % locate infratentorial. Spinal and meningeal forms are rare. Most patients present focal neurological deficits. Intracranial hypertension, changes in mental status, and, occasionally, seizures may also occur. CT shows a hypodense, or sometimes hyperdense, lesion, with perilesional edema and mass effect, with ring enhancement after contrast, which can be indistinguishable from TE or other abscesses. Dissemination through the ependimary surface is a very characteristic radiological sign of PCNSL. Single photon emission computed tomography with thallium-201 and positron emission tomography with fluorodeoxyglucose may aid in the diagnosis and are useful for the differentiation between neoplastic and infectious lesions with high sensitivity and specificity. Detection of EBV in CSF by PCR has also shown a high diagnostic value for PCNSL. Radiotherapy is the most frequently employed treatment, along with steroids. Prognosis is fatal in patients without antiretroviral therapy, with a mean survival of 1 month, which can be prolonged to 3 months with radiotherapy or steroids. In patients receiving HAART survival is significantly prolonged, for years, and some complete remissions have been reported [49, 50]. Chemotherapy or combined treatments, as in patients without HIV infection, are options to consider in the era of HAART [50].

PML is a CNS demyelinating disease caused by oligodendrocyte infection by the JCV, a DNA virus of the polyomavirus family [51]. It affects 4 % of AIDS patients. JCV infection is practically universal in adults, and nonpathogenic strains may remain latent in the kidney and other organs [52]. Immune depression may favor replication of pathogenic strains (with rearrangements in the regulatory region of DNA), their hematogenous spread, and CNS infection. Alternatively, brain JCV latent infection may reactivate when immune surveillance fails. JCV binds serotoninergic 5-HT_{2A} and sialic acid receptors for integration in infected cells. Productive infection of neurons by a variant JCV has recently been demonstrated: infection of the granular cells of the cerebellum causes cerebellar syndrome without demyelination, and infection of pyramidal cells causes an acute encephalopathy [53].

PML manifests clinically as a slowly progressive focal deficit along weeks or months. It is often (47 % of cases) the first manifestation of AIDS. The most frequent initial symptoms are limb paresis, cognitive impairment, or visual symptoms. Seizures occur in 18 % of patients, are associated with juxtacortical lesions, and have a good response to antiepileptic drugs [54]. Neuroimaging studies are, in the clinical context, the main clue to suspect the diagnosis [55]. CT shows characteristic

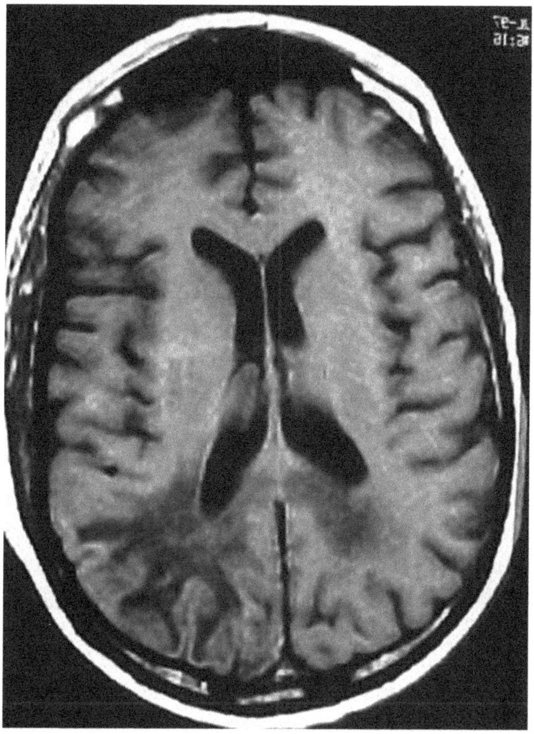

Fig. 15.3 Progressive multifocal leukoencephalopathy. T1-weighted magnetic resonance imaging

hypodense lesions, without mass effect or contrast enhancement, in the periventricular or subcortical white matter. Subcortical lesions display a geographic pattern as a consequence of U fibers involvement. MRI is more sensitive than CT for PML lesions. Lesions are hyperintense in T2- and FLAIR-weighted sequences and hypointense in T1-weighted images (Fig. 15.3). Gadolinium enhancement is exceptional (5–10 % of cases) and, when present, it is mild and peripheral. In diffusion sequences, there is restriction in the active borders of the lesions. A characteristic pattern in MRI spectroscopy may help in the diagnosis of PML: there is reduction of N-acetyl-aspartate and increase in choline, lipids, and myoinositol.

CSF is normal or can show mild protein elevation. The demonstration of JCV DNA in CSF has positive and negative predictive value of 88–100 % and 88.5–95 %, respectively, for the diagnosis of PML, although sensitivity is always below 75 % [56]. A negative result, however, does not exclude the diagnosis in 20–30 % of cases, but sensitivity can be increased with repeated CSF studies. In clinical practice, a diagnosis of PML can be established confidently with this technique, which avoids the need for brain biopsy. With clinical–radiological criteria and a positive CSF PCR, the probability of a correct diagnosis reaches 99 % [46]. The confirmation of LMP diagnosis requires demonstration of the characteristic pathological changes and of JCV in biopsy specimens or autopsy.

The differential diagnosis of PML includes other possible causes of leukoencephalopathy in patients with HIV infection. The leukoencephalopathy present in HAD may be confounded with PML. Aside from the clinical differences, the former is isodense in T1-weighted sequences, do not reach juxtacortical regions, and do not involve posterior fossa. VVZ vasculopathy and multiple sclerosis-like disease may have radiological similarities with PML [57]. Other diagnoses to consider are CMV encephalitis, posterior reversible leukoencephalopathy, leukoencephalopathy caused by heroin inhalation, ischemic stroke, and low-grade astrocytomas.

The natural course of PML is fatal within a mean of 4 months [51]. Factors associated with shorter survival are lower CD4 count, brainstem or cerebellar involvement, and high JCV viral load in CSF in quantitative PCR [58, 59]. A short percentage of patients may stabilize or improve spontaneously, with survival for more than 30 months or even complete remission. They have a higher CD4 count, some of them over 300/mm^3, and show frequently contrast enhancement due to inflammatory infiltrates [60].

Since the introduction of HAART, the prognosis of PML has improved drastically. More than 50 % improve or stabilize clinically, and the disease remains inactive after 1-year follow-up. MRI lesions also improve or stabilize in the majority of PML patients with HAART. Prolonged survival associates with restoration of the specific T-cell response against JCV [61, 62] and reduction or negativization of JCV load [58, 63]. However, efficacy of HAART is limited, since one-third of treated patients die due to progression of the lesions and half of survivors do not show significant neurological improvement [63]. A 3-year survival of only 27 % has been reported despite HAART [64]. PML is the AIDS-defining disease with higher mortality in the HAART era, after non-Hodgkin lymphoma [65]. No specific treatment for PML has shown efficacy in randomized studies [66]. Cidofovir, mefloquine, and mirtazapine have been reported to improve LMP in some patients, but their efficacy has not been proven.

Multiple infections can cause brain abscess in AIDS patients. Tuberculous granuloma or abscess and nocardia abscess should be considered (Fig. 15.4). Fungal granulomas or abscesses are uncommon and include those caused by aspergillus, mucor, histoplasma, cryptococcus, and candida. Cases of syphilitic gumma and cysticercosis have been reported in patients with HIV infection. Brain tumors may be secondary to Kaposi's sarcoma, systemic lymphoma, or other solid tumors, whose incidence are increased in HIV infection. Primary brain tumors, such as gliomas, seem also increased in these patients. Demyelinating diseases, either a multiple sclerosis-like disease or acute disseminated encephalomyelitis, have been reported in primary infection and early stages of HIV infection, but may occur also in advanced stages.

Encephalitis Caused by Herpesviruses

CMV is the most common herpesvirus causing neurological disease in AIDS patients. Risk for CMV diseases parallels the immune suppression and is maximal with CD4 counts below 50/mm^3. Median CD4 count in patients with CMV

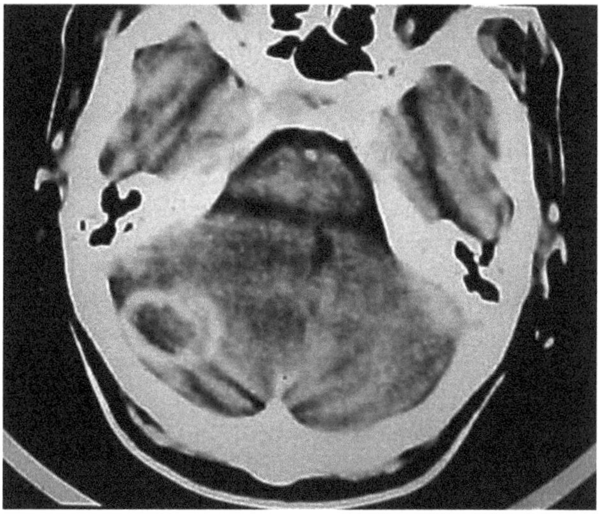

Fig. 15.4 Posterior fossa tuberculous abscess. Cranial computed tomography after intravenous contrast, showing a hypodense lesion, with ring enhancement and mass effect

encephalitis is 20/mm^3 (range 2–94) [67]. CNS involvement by CMV usually takes place in the context of systemic CMV infection, particularly retinitis, and encephalitis frequently develops despite maintenance therapy against CMV. An impressive reduction in the frequency of CMV disease, including CNS disease, followed the introduction of HAART, and, nowadays, it has practically disappeared in developed countries.

Two clinicopathologic forms of CMV encephalitis can be distinguished, as extremes of a spectrum where mixed forms are common: ventriculoencephalitis and diffuse micronodular encephalitis [67, 68]. In ventriculoencephalitis, there is destruction of the ependymal layer and necrosis of periventricular parenchyma. The most frequent clinical presentations are acute or subacute confusional state or depressed consciousness. Half of the patients present focal symptoms or signs, frequently revealing brainstem involvement (nystagmus, vertigo, ataxia, or cranial nerve palsy). Paraparesis may reflect associated polyradiculitis. In diffuse micronodular encephalitis, widespread microglial nodes and cytomegalic cells in gray matter suggest hematogenous dissemination. This condition presents as a subacute dementia difficult to differentiate from HAD. Confusion, hyponatremia, or focal brainstem symptoms may help in the diagnosis. This diagnosis should be considered in patients with systemic CMV disease presenting with cognitive impairment.

MRI has low sensitivity for CMV encephalitis and frequently has no specific findings. The most characteristic finding is periventricular contrast enhancement, with or without hydrocephalus. Cases of encephalitis presenting with progressive focal enhancing mass lesion have been reported [69]. CSF may show normal findings or pleocytosis. Detection of CMV DNA in CSF by PCR is the diagnostic test of choice for neurological CMV disease, with a reported sensitivity of 82–92 % and specificity of 94–99 % [56, 70].

CMV CNS disease is usually fatal in a few weeks. Mean survival of ventriculoencephalitis from the first symptom is 42 days [67]. Antiviral drugs against CMV are not effective in most cases, but a combined regimen with foscarnet and ganciclovir may produce clinical improvement or stabilization in a high proportion of cases [71], until immune reconstitution with HAART.

Herpes simplex virus (HSV) encephalitis in AIDS patients can show identical presentation as that of immunocompetent patients [72] or can present with atypical clinical or pathological presentations due to immune suppression. While HSV-2 encephalitis is rare in immunocompetent patients, it has been reported frequently in HIV-infected patients [73]. Concomitant HSV-1 or HSV-2 and CMV encephalitis may also occur [73]. The demonstration of HSV DNA in CSF by PCR has high diagnostic value for HSV encephalitis [73]. Acyclovir is the treatment of choice, although resistant strains may cause disease in AIDS. A bad response is the rule in cases with severe immune depression, usually associated with CMV encephalitis [73].

A wide spectrum of neurological complications of VZV has been described in patients with HIV infection, including encephalitis (or leukoencephalitis), ventriculoencephalitis, myelitis, aseptic meningitis, polyradiculitis, optic neuritis, and other cranial neuritis [74, 75]. The risk of herpes zoster complications increases with immune depression. They can present months after cutaneous lesions or even without them. VZV encephalitis or leukoencephalitis is considered to represent actually a vasculopathy caused by the virus [76]. Small artery vasculopathy produces demyelination or necrotizing leukoencephalitis with a multifocal distribution and sometimes with hemorrhages; large artery vasculopathy causes cerebral infarction. This condition manifests clinically with a progressive encephalopathy with variable impairment of consciousness and focal signs, which may take a chronic course. Sometimes the encephalitis is limited to the brainstem. Demyelinating lesions, mimicking those of PML, can be seen in CT or MRI. The association of multiple ischemic and hemorrhagic lesions is highly suggestive of VZV vasculopathy. Cerebral angiography may show arterial narrowing indicative of vasculitis. CSF usually contains high proteins without pleocytosis. Demonstration of VZV DNA in CSF may be useful for the diagnosis of VZV neurological complications. Intrathecal synthesis of IgG antibodies against VZV is more sensitive than PCR for the diagnosis [76]. Treatment with acyclovir may improve VZV encephalitis. Steroids are indicated as coadjutant therapy for vasculitis.

Stroke in Patients with HIV Infection

The frequency of stroke is highly increased in AIDS patients compared to an age-matched population. Patients with HIV infection may suffer a stroke due to a wide spectrum of mechanisms and etiologies [77–79]. Ischemic stroke may be caused by infections, most of them associated with immune depression, such as vasculitis associated with opportunistic meningitis (bacterial, including tuberculous, cryptococcal, or candidal), VZV, or CMV infection. Meningovascular syphilis should also be considered. Cardioembolic stroke may be related to AIDS-related cardiomyopathy, nonbacterial thrombotic endocarditis, and, particularly, infectious endocarditis in intravenous drug users. Between hematological causes, the high frequency of antiphospholipid antibodies and protein S deficit should be borne in mind, although it is sometimes difficult to establish a causal relationship. Acute stroke may occur also in the context of disseminated intravascular coagulation. Atherothrombotic stroke is also common, especially in older patients [78]. HIV per se may cause large vessel vasculopathy, sometimes with formation or large aneurysms, which may be the cause of up to 20 % of strokes in these patients [79]. In many cases stroke cause cannot be finally demonstrated.

In recent years, there has been concern about a possible risk of accelerated atherosclerosis associated with HAART, particularly with protease inhibitors, which may cause metabolic syndrome, with dyslipidemia and insulin resistance. The risk increases with the time of HAART exposure, but also with the presence of vascular risk factors [80]. The incidence of ischemic stroke in HAART-treated patients is also increased with respect the general population [81], and a substantial rise in patients hospitalized for stroke with coexisting HIV infection has been noticed in the United States [82]. However, the causes of the stroke in these patients are also multiple, and as yet it is not been shown that HAART increases the frequency of atherothrombotic strokes [78, 81].

Meningitis

Causes of meningitis among HIV-infected patients are multiple, including viral, bacterial, and fungal infections, together with carcinomatous meningitis. Clinical and CSF findings may be similar in all types of meningitis in HIV-infected patients. In some patients, CSF analysis can be entirely normal. Therefore, an exhaustive processing of CSF samples covering all the possible etiologies is warranted in cases with suspected meningitis. However, the low diagnostic yield of CSF microbiological studies forces empirical treatment in many patients. *Cryptococcus* and *Mycobacterium tuberculosis* meningitis are the most frequent etiological agents of meningitis in these patients. Aseptic lymphocytic meningitis may be caused by the HIV and herpesviruses, particularly VZV. The incidence of conventional bacterial meningitis is highly increased in comparison with the general population, even in the HAART era, and carries out a worse prognosis [83]. *Streptococcus pneumoniae* is the most frequent agent. *Listeria* meningitis may be increased in HIV-infected patients. *Staphylococcus aureus* causes meningitis in intravenous drug users, sometimes associated with endocarditis. Meningitis due to *Candida* spp. has been reported in HIV-infected patients usually in the presence of other predisposing factors, such as intravenous drug use and previous antibiotics [84].

The clinical manifestations of tuberculous meningitis are similar in patients with and without HIV infection [85]. Presentation is with subacute or chronic (occasionally acute) meningeal syndrome with fever, headache, and frequently altered mental status.

Cranial nerve involvement is common, and focal neurological symptoms may be the consequence of vasculitic infarctions or granulomas. Most patients have extraneurological tuberculosis and 50 % have lung infiltrates. CT and MRI may reveal hydrocephalus, meningeal enhancement, and, occasionally, granulomas. CSF contains a variable pleocytosis, which is usually lymphocytic, but sometimes polymorphonuclear, elevated proteins and low levels of glucose. Sensitivity of the Ziehl-auramine stain is low (20 %), as is the yield of CSF cultures for mycobacteria. Adenosine deaminase activity in CSF has been considered useful in the early diagnosis of tuberculous meningitis, but in HIV-infected patients has low sensitivity and specificity [86]. CSF PCR for *M. tuberculosis* in CSF may aid in the diagnosis because of its high sensitivity and specificity. Meningitis caused by opportunistic mycobacteria is rare.

Cryptococcal meningitis may be indistinguishable from tuberculous meningitis on clinical grounds or in CSF findings [87]. A characteristic finding in MRI is the presence of hyperintensities in T2-weighted sequences in the basal ganglia caused by dilatation of the Virchow–Robin spaces. CSF India ink can demonstrate the fungal capsule in 75 % of cases. Cryptococcal antigen is positive in 90–100 % of patients in CSF and in 75–99 % in serum, always with high specificity. Treatment of choice is amphotericin B associated with 5-fluocytosine. A maintenance therapy with fluconazole is mandatory because of the high risk of relapse. In patients under HAART, maintenance therapy can be suppressed after 3 months with CD4 over $100/mm^3$ and undetectable HIV viral load [47].

Myelopathies

Myelopathies affecting patients with HIV infection are best classified in segmentary myelopathies, which tend to present with an acute or subacute course, and diffuse myelopathies, usually with a progressive chronic or subacute presentation, as is the case with vacuolar myelopathy.

Vacuolar myelopathy is the most common cause of myelopathy in these patients [88]. It has been found in 50 % of autopsies of AIDS patients, although only one-fourth of them were evident clinically. Pathological anomalies predominantly involve the lateral and dorsal columns of dorsal region, resembling subacute combined degeneration. It presents clinically as slowly progressive (along weeks or months) and symmetric spastic paraparesis. Gait ataxia or sensory symptoms are also common presentations. Sphincter symptoms are late. HAD is present in 60 % of the patients. Neurological exam reveals that vibration and position senses are more severely affected than pain or light touch. There are symmetric pyramidal signs, but hyperreflexia might be absent in the case of associated peripheral neuropathy. Vacuolar myelopathy progresses slowly to spastic paraplegia. Diagnosis is mainly clinical, after other possible causes of myelopathy are excluded by means of spinal MRI and CSF studies. MRI shows atrophy of the spine and, occasionally, hyperintensities in the lateral or dorsal columns. There is no specific treatment. There have been reports of patients who improved after HAART. The other chronic diffuse myelopathy to consider in patients with HIV infection is tropical spastic paraparesis caused by HTLV-I, particularly in patients from countries were this infection is prevalent. Contrary to what happens with vacuolar myelopathy, this disease does not occur necessarily in patients with significant immune depression [89].

Among the segmentary myelopathies, viruses are the most frequent causes. HIV may cause transverse myelitis during primary infection. VZV myelitis develops more frequently in immunocompromised patients [90]. Weakness progresses in weeks, but may show a chronic course over several months. MRI may be normal or show spinal hyperintensities in T2-weighted sequences, which may enhance after gadolinium. CSF may also be normal or demonstrate a variable inflammatory response. CMV can cause necrotizing myelopathy, which may be associated with encephalitis or polyradiculitis. The HSV-1 and more frequently the HSV-2 in association with genital herpes are other possible causes of myelopathy. Concomitant HSV-2 and CMV myelopathy has also been reported. Other causes of segmentary myelopathies are toxoplasmosis, tuberculous granuloma, epidural tumor or abscess, and vascular lesions due to syphilis or disseminated intravascular coagulation. Primary intramedullary tumors, as gliomas or lymphomas, are rare.

Neuropathies

Peripheral neuropathy is very common in HIV infection. In the pre-HAART era, the prevalence of symptomatic neuropathy was 35 %, while 20 % had asymptomatic neuropathy [91]. A similar prevalence has been found in HAART-treated patients, despite controlled HIV infection [92]. For the clinical management of patients with suspected neuropathy, it is useful to classify neuropathies according to the clinical and electrophysiological pattern [93]. We will consider four groups: demyelinating neuropathies, axonal polyradiculopathies, mononeuritis multiplex, and distal symmetric polyneuropathy.

Distal symmetric polyneuropathy is the most frequent pattern. It is an axonal predominantly sensory polyneuropathy, caused most commonly by the HIV itself and by antiretroviral toxicity [93]. These two etiologies are practically indistinguishable from the clinical or electrophysiological point of view. Other causes of predominantly sensory distal neuropathy in these patients are alcoholism, malnutrition and vitamin deficits, diabetes, and uremia. A clinical picture similar to distal sensory polyneuropathy may occur with CMV nerve infection. HIV-associated distal sensory polyneuropathy characteristically presents with symmetric distal painful paresthesias and affects mainly the legs. Only occasionally a motor deficit exists. Examination may disclose hypesthesia with a stocking and glove distribution and distal hyporeflexia. Treatment is only symptomatic. Tricyclic antidepressants and antiepileptic drugs as gabapentin and lamotrigine are widely used, but unfortunately only topic capsaicin and cannabis have demonstrated efficacy in controlled studies [93]. Antiretroviral toxic neuropathy is caused by the nucleoside reverse transcriptase inhibitors didanosine, zalcitabine, and stavudine. Combined therapy has a synergistic toxic effect. It affects between 15 and 30 % of treated patients. They cause a sensitive, dose-dependent, distal axonal neuropathy. Treatment consists in drug suppression and symptomatic treatment as used for VIH-associated neuropathy. Other drugs used in HIV-infected patients may cause toxic neuropathy: vincristine, isoniazid, dapsone, metronidazole, and thalidomide. Autonomic nervous system dysfunction can be demonstrated in a high percentage of HIV-infected patients in advanced stages, frequently in association with distal neuropathy, but it is rarely symptomatic.

Demyelinating inflammatory neuropathies are an uncommon cause of neuropathy in HIV-infected patients. Guillain–Barré syndrome and chronic inflammatory demyelinating polyneuropathy in HIV-infected patients have the same clinical, electrophysiological, and pathological characteristics as in uninfected patients [94]. CSF may contain mild pleocytosis, but not in all cases. Both present in patients without significative immune depression or in primary HIV infection.

Acute lumbosacral polyradiculitis, or cauda equina syndrome, is a well-defined clinical syndrome in AIDS patients with multiple causes [95, 96]. Most cases are caused by CMV infection. Tuberculosis is the second most frequent cause. Other reported etiologies are VZV and HSV, often associated with myelitis, cryptococcal or bacterial meningitis, syphilis, and meningeal lymphomatosis. All these causes have similar clinical presentation and CSF findings. CMV polyradiculitis presents with acute or subacute progressive leg weakness, often accompanied with paresthesias and radicular pain and urinary retention. Encephalopathic symptoms are frequent in final stages due to associated encephalitis. CSF contains variable pleocytosis, which may be polymorphonuclear in the most typical cases, increased proteins, and normal or low glucose. CSF viral cultures have low yield, but CSF PCR for CMV is useful for diagnosis. Lumbar MRI is needed to exclude other causes of cauda equina syndrome. It may show normal results or demonstrate contrast enhancement in the roots and conus medullaris. This disease is fatal in most untreated cases. Treatment with ganciclovir or foscarnet has been successful in many patients. The most important factor for treatment response is early institution of therapy [97]. Therefore, rapid initiation of empirical antiviral treatment is mandatory when the disease is suspected.

Mononeuritis multiplex in HIV-infected patients is due mainly to two causes: the HIV itself and CMV infection. Less common causes are cryoglobulinemia associated with HCV, peripheral nerve infiltration by lymphoma, and diffuse infiltrative lymphocytosis syndrome. Mononeuritis multiplex associated with HIV is caused by peripheral nerve vasculitis and presents in early stages, whereas CMV neuropathy presents in severely immunocompromised patients [98]. The latter is a multifocal sensory and motor neuropathy with a subacute or chronic course, which often presents with patchy areas of dysesthesia and paresthesia. CSF is usually normal. It may improve with ganciclovir or foscarnet.

Myopathies

Two myopathies, difficult to differentiate form each other, may present in HIV-infected patients. One is HIV-associated myopathy and the other is AZT myopathy. HIV-associated myopathy may present at any moment in the course of HIV infection [99]. Clinical and pathological findings are similar to those of polymyositis. The patient experiences symmetric limb weakness, with a predominantly proximal distribution, progressing in months. Patients improve with steroids. AZT myopathy has a similar clinical presentation, but has a distinctive pathological pattern [100]. It improves after suppression of AZT. The probable cause of this myopathy is mitochondrial dysfunction caused by the drug, although mitochondrial anomalies have been found also in untreated HIV-infected patients. Cases of severe rhabdomyolysis caused by other antiretroviral drugs, such as didanosine and raltegravir, have been reported. Other causes of myopathy in HIV-infected patients include focal myositis caused by toxoplasma and pyomyositis of diverse etiologies, frequently associated with venous puncture in drug addicts.

Neurosyphilis and HIV

Neurosyphilis may occur in any stage of HIV infection. However, the prevalence is higher than in patients without HIV infection and greater in patients with CD4 counts under 350/mm^3 [101]. In HIV-infected patients, neurosyphilis appears mainly in early stages of the syphilitic infection. For this reason, some authors have recommended CSF analysis in every patient with syphilis and HIV infection. However, CSF analysis is not considered necessary in cases of primary, secondary, or early latent syphilis, if neurological, visual, or auditory symptoms are not present. In HIV-infected patients, neurosyphilis may be asymptomatic or present the usual range of presentations in the general population that include lymphocytic meningitis, cranial neuropathies (VIII nerve), optic neuropathy, meningovascular syphilis, meningomyelitis, meningoradiculitis, cerebral gummas, general paresis, or tabes dorsalis. Some difficulties for the diagnosis of neurosyphilis may be present in these patients. CSF pleocytosis is one of the clues for the diagnosis of neurosyphilis, but it is common in HIV infection. Occasionally non-treponemal tests for syphilis, VDRL (Venereal Disease Research Laboratory) and RPR (rapid plasma reagin), are negative in CSF. Treatment is the same as for patients without HIV infection. Reports of HIV-infected patients correctly treated for primary syphilis who had meningovascular relapse have induced some authors to recommend treating with doses for neurosyphilis every HIV-infected patient with syphilis.

Neurological Complications Associated with HAART

Neurological Immune Reconstitution Inflammatory Syndromes

Following the initiation of HAART, there is a rapid fall in plasma levels of HIV RNA and an increase in T lymphocytes, accompanied by significant functional improvement. Due to the restoration of the capability to develop an inflammatory response against infectious and noninfectious antigens, some patients may suffer clinical deterioration. This phenomenon is designated as immune reconstitution inflammatory syndrome (IRIS) [102]. Some autoimmune diseases presenting after initiation of HAART may be considered part of this entity. IRIS may represent the debut of a previously unknown disease (unmasking IRIS) or a paradoxical clinical deterioration of a known disease (paradoxical IRIS) after the beginning of HAART. IRIS affects between 15 and 35 % of patients receiving HAART, and 1 % suffer neurological IRIS [102, 103]. Risk factors for IRIS are a higher immune depression before HAART and a more rapid immunological response. IRIS usually presents in the first weeks or months of therapy, but may be retarded for more than 1 year. Recognizing this clinical entity is essential for the appropriate management of the patient, without compromising antiretroviral or anti-infective treatment.

IRIS presents in 30 % of all patients with a diagnosis of tuberculosis who initiate HAART, and 12 % of them may be neurological syndromes [104]. Intracranial tuberculomas, meningitis, or myeloradiculitis may appear or deteriorate, after a mean of 14–43 days. Steroids improve the inflammation and clinical course. In patients with a diagnosis of tuberculosis, HAART initiation must be retarded until several weeks of antituberculous drugs have been completed. IRIS may present in 17 % of cryptococcal meningitis [105]. Early initiation of HAART after the diagnosis of cryptococcal meningitis has a high risk of IRIS, and therefore, it is recommended retarding several weeks the beginning of HAART [106]. Latent meningitis may be unmasked. In addition to the clinical deterioration of the patient, there is increased inflammatory reaction in CSF and meningeal enhancement in neuroimaging studies, and granulomas may appear. Patients may improve with steroids or spontaneously.

PML may also present as IRIS or suffer paradoxical deterioration after HAART [107–109]. PML presenting as IRIS constitute up to 20 % of all recent PML cases. After the clinical deterioration produced by IRIS, the patient may improve spontaneously, but occasionally the course is fatal. Thus, while effective HAART initiated early is essential for the improvement of PML patients, this treatment may result in death for some patients. A case of fatal inflammatory PML has presented after more than 2 years of HAART [110]. Global mortality of PML patients with or without IRIS is similar, but patients with paradoxical IRIS have higher mortality than those with unmasking IRIS. In neuroimaging studies the inflammatory component can be demonstrated as contrast enhancement of the lesions in 60 % of cases (Fig. 15.5). CSF may also show inflammatory signs, something unusual in PML. CSF PCR for JCV is frequently negative because the host immune response can control JCV replication. PML IRIS may improve after HAART suppression or with steroids [109].

The incidence of herpes zoster increases up to five times in patients with HAART. Most cases (86 %) present between the second and fourth months of treatment [111]. Zoster may be a manifestation of IRIS related to an increase in CD8 T cells, which may be involved in VZV reactivation [111]. VZV myelitis and encephalitis has also been reported as IRIS [102]. Other neurological IRIS reported are associated with TE, *Candida* meningitis, CMV ventriculoencephalitis, and primary cerebral lymphomatoid granulomatosis [102, 112]. The HIV itself might be the triggering

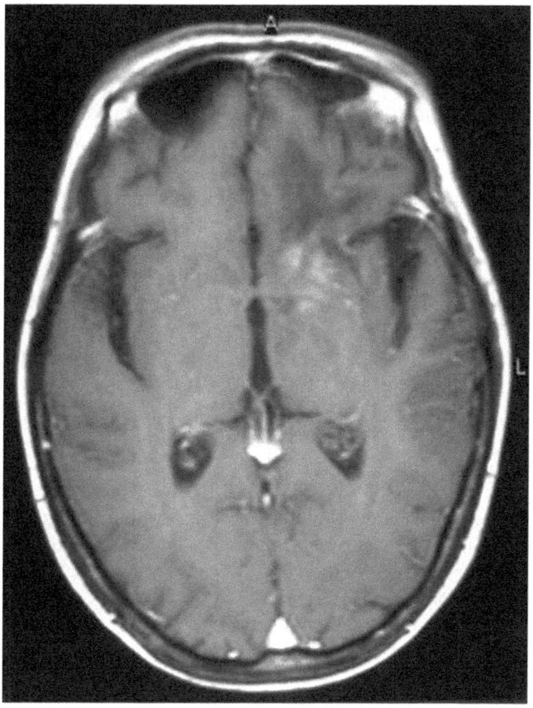

Fig. 15.5 Contrast enhancement in a patient with progressive multifocal leukoencephalopathy-associated immune reconstitution inflammatory syndrome

antigen of a neurological IRIS, causing encephalitis with multiple enhancing lesions and CD8 lymphocyte infiltration in pathological studies [113, 114]. Chronic form of CNS-IRIS might be an important component of HAND [102].

After the initiation of HAART, the possible appearance of autoreactive T cells might trigger autoimmune diseases, such as Guillain–Barré syndrome and demyelinating leukoencephalopathies [102].

Neuromuscular Weakness Associated with HIV

Patients undergoing HAART may present a syndrome of acute or subacute neuromuscular weakness associated with lactic acidosis [115]. In most cases, an axonal neuropathy is demonstrated in electrophysiological and pathological studies, but some patients have a myopathy (15 %) or both. This picture resembles axonal Guillain–Barré syndrome. One-third of patients have sensory symptoms, and some have cranial nerve involvement. Hyperlactacidemia causes systemic symptoms, vomiting, and abdominal pain. Mortality of this syndrome is 13 %. It has been related to nucleoside reverse transcriptase inhibitors, particularly stavudine, the antiretrovirals most frequently associated with lactic acidosis. The pathogenesis is not known, but it is considered to be probably caused by mitochondrial dysfunction.

References

1. Brew BJ. Medical management of AIDS patients. Central and peripheral nervous system abnormalities. Med Clin North Am. 1992;76:63–81.
2. Gray F, Gherardi R, Scaravilli F. The neuropathology of the acquired immune deficiency syndrome (AIDS). A review. Brain. 1988;111(Pt 2):245–66.
3. Tan IK, Smith BR, von Geldern G, Mateen FJ, McArthur JC. HIV-associated opportunistic infections of the CNS. Lancet Neurol. 2012;11:605–17.
4. Maschke M, Kastrup O, Esser S, Ross B, Hengge U, Hufnagel A. Incidence and prevalence of neurological disorders associated with HIV since the introduction of highly active antiretroviral therapy (HAART). J Neurol Neurosurg Psychiatry. 2000;69:376–80.
5. Sacktor N, Lyles RH, Skolasky MA, Kleeberger MAS, Selnes OA, Miller EN, et al. HIV-associated neurologic disease incidence changes: Multicenter AIDS Cohort Study, 1990-1998. Neurology. 2001;56:257–60.
6. Valcour V, Chalermchai T, Sailasuta N, Marovich M, Lerdlum S, Suttichom D, et al. Central nervous system viral invasion and inflammation during acute HIV infection. J Infect Dis. 2012;206:275–82.
7. Peluso MJ, Meyerhoff DJ, Price RW, Peterson J, Lee E, Young AC, et al. Cerebrospinal fluid and neuroimaging biomarker abnormalities suggest early neurological injury in a subset of individuals during primary HIV infection. J Infect Dis. 2013;207:1703–12.
8. Wiley CA, Achim C. Human immunodeficiency virus encephalitis and dementia. Ann Neurol. 1995;38:559–60.
9. Navia BA, Jordan BD, Price RW. The AIDS-dementia complex: I. Clinical features. Ann Neurol. 1986;19:517–24.
10. Janssen RS. Epidemiology and neuroepidemiology of human immunodeficiency virus infection. In: Berger JR, Levy RM, editors. AIDS and the nervous system. Philadelphia: Lippincott-Raven; 1997. p. 13–37.
11. Maruff P, Currie J, Malone V, McArthur-Jacson C, Mulhall B, Benson E. Neuropsychological characterization of the AIDS dementia complex and rationalization of a test battery. Arch Neurol. 1994;51:689–95.
12. Sacktor NC, Wong M, Nakasujja N, Skolasky RL, Selnes OA, Musisi S, et al. The International HIV Dementia Scale: a new rapid screening test for HIV dementia. AIDS. 2005;19:1367–74.
13. Cinque P, Vago L, Ceresa D, Mainini F, Terreni MR, Vagani A, et al. Cerebrospinal fluid HIV-1 RNA levels: correlation with HIV encephalitis. AIDS. 1998;12:389–94.
14. Valcour VG, Shiramizu BT, Sithinamsuwan P, Nidhinandana S, Ratto-Kim S, Ananworanich J, et al. HIV DNA and cognition in a Thai longitudinal HAART initiation cohort The SEARCH 001 Cohort Study. Neurology. 2009;72:992–8.
15. Antinori A, Arendt G, Becker JT, Brew BJ, Byrd DA, Cherner M, et al. Updated research nosology for HIV-associated neurocognitive disorders. Neurology. 2007;69:1789–99.
16. Gisslén M, Price RW, Nilsson S. The definition of HIV-associated neurocognitive disorders: are we overestimating the real prevalence? BMC Infect Dis. 2011;11:356.
17. Cohen RA, Boland R, Paul R, Tashima KT, Schoenbaum EE, Celentano DD, et al. Neurocognitive performance enhanced by highly active antiretroviral therapy in HIV-infected women. AIDS. 2001;15:341–5.
18. Cysique LA, Vaida F, Letendre S, Gibson S, Cherner M, Woods SP, et al. Dynamics of cognitive change in impaired HIV-positive patients initiating antiretroviral therapy. Neurology. 2009;73:342–8.
19. Fessel WJ. Impaired neurocognition in HIV-infected patients: antecedents and treatment. AIDS. 2009;23:1731–3.
20. Tozzi V, Balestra P, Bellagamba R, Corpolongo A, Salvatori MF, Visco-Comandini U, et al. Persistence of neuropsychologic deficits despite long-term highly active antiretroviral therapy in patients with HIV-related neurocognitive impairment: prevalence and risk factors. J Acquir Immune Defic Syndr. 2007;45:174–82.

21. Heaton RK, Clifford DB, Franklin D, Woods S, Ake C, Vaida F, et al. HIV associated neurocognitive disorders (HAND) persist in the era of potent antiretroviral therapy: The CHARTER Study. Neurology. 2010;75:2087–96.
22. Simioni S, Cavassini M, Annoni JM, Rimbault Abraham A, Bourquin I, Schiffer V, et al. Cognitive dysfunction in HIV patients despite long-standing suppression of viremia. AIDS. 2010;24:1243–50.
23. McCutchan JA, Marquie-Beck J, FitzSimons JA, Letendre SL, Ellis RJ, Heaton RK, et al. Role of obesity, metabolic variables, and diabetes in HIV-associated neurocognitive disorder. Neurology. 2012;78:485–92.
24. Wright EJ, Grund B, Robertson K, Brew BJ, Roediger M, Bain MP, et al. Cardiovascular risk factors associated with lower baseline cognitive performance in HIV-positive persons. Neurology. 2010;75:864–73.
25. Gannon P, Khan MZ, Kolson DL. Current understanding of HIV-associated neurocognitive disorders pathogenesis. Curr Opin Neurol. 2011;24:275–83.
26. Ellis RJ, Badiee J, Vaida F, Letendre S, Heaton RK, Clifford D, et al. CD4 nadir is a predictor of HIV neurocognitive impairment in the era of combination antiretroviral therapy. AIDS. 2011;25:1747–51.
27. Cohen RA, Harezlak J, Schifitto G, Hana G, Clark U, Gongvatana A, et al. Effects of nadir CD4 count and duration of human immunodeficiency virus infection on brain volumes in the highly active antiretroviral therapy era. J Neurovirol. 2010;16:25–32.
28. Shiramizu B, Ananworanich J, Chalermchai T, Siangphoe U, Troelstrup D, Shikuma C, et al. Failure to clear intra-monocyte HIV infection linked to persistent neuropsychological testing impairment after first-line combined antiretroviral therapy. J Neurovirol. 2012;18: 69–73.
29. Harezlak J, Buchthal S, Taylor M, Schifitto G, Zhong J, Daar E, et al. Persistence of HIV-associated cognitive impairment, inflammation, and neuronal injury in era of highly active antiretroviral treatment. AIDS. 2011;25:625–33.
30. Peluso MJ, Ferrett F, Peterson J, Lee E, Fuchs D, Boschini A, et al. Cerebrospinal fluid HIV escape associated with progressive neurologic dysfunction in patients on antiretroviral therapy with well controlled plasma viral load. AIDS. 2012;26:1765–74.
31. Del Palacio Tamarit M, Quereda C, González-Rozas M, Corral I, Casado JL. HIV type 1 viral encephalitis after development of viral resistance to plasma suppressive antiretroviral therapy. AIDS Res Hum Retroviruses. 2012;28:83–6.
32. Soulie C, Fourati S, Lambert-Niclot S, Tubiana R, Canestri A, Girard PM, et al. HIV genetic diversity between plasma and cerebrospinal fluid in patients with HIV encephalitis. AIDS. 2010;24:2412–4.
33. Letendre S, Marquie-Beck J, Capparelli E, Best B, Clifford D, Collier AC, et al. Validation of the CNS penetration effectiveness rank for quantifying antiretroviral penetration into the central nervous system. Arch Neurol. 2008;65:65–70.
34. Marra CM, Zhao Y, Clifford DB, Letendre S, Evans S, Henry K, et al. Impact of combination antiretroviral therapy on cerebrospinal fluid HIV RNA and neurocognitive performance. AIDS. 2009;23:1359–66.
35. Smurzynski M, Wu K, Letendre S, Robertson K, Bosch RJ, Clifford DB, et al. Effects of central nervous system antiretroviral penetration on cognitive functioning in the ALLRT cohort. AIDS. 2011;25:357–65.
36. Robertson K, Jiang H, Kumwenda J, Supparatpinyo K, Evans S, Campbell TB, et al. Improved neuropsychological and neurological functioning across three antiretroviral regimens in diverse resource-limited settings: AIDS Clinical Trials Group study a5199, the International Neurological Study. Clin Infect Dis. 2012;55:868–76.
37. Dahl V, Lee E, Peterson J, Spudich SS, Leppla I, Sinclair E. Fuchs, et al. Raltegravir treatment intensification does not alter cerebrospinal fluid VIH-1 infection or immunoactivation on suppressive therapy. J Infect Dis. 2011;204:1036–45.
38. Cysique LA, Waters EK, Brew BJ. Central nervous system antiretroviral efficacy in HIV infection: a qualitative and quantitative review and implications for future research. BMC Neurol. 2011;11:148.

39. Heaton RK, Franklin DR, Ellis RJ, McCutchan JA, Letendre SL, Leblanc S, et al. HIV-associated neurocognitive disorders before and during the era of combination antiretroviral therapy: differences in rates, nature, and predictors. J Neurovirol. 2011;17:3–16.
40. Clifford DB, Fagan AM, Holtzman DM, Morris JC, Teshome M, Shah AR, et al. CSF biomarkers of Alzheimer disease in HIV-associated neurologic disease. Neurology. 2009;73:1982–7.
41. Chang L, Andres M, Sadino J, Jiang CS, Nakama H, Miller E, et al. Impact of apolipoprotein E ε4 and HIV on cognition and brain atrophy: Antagonistic pleiotropy and premature brain aging. Neuroimage. 2011;58:1017–27.
42. Soontornniyomkij W, Moore M, Gouaux B, Soontornniyomkij B, Tatro ET, Umlauf A, et al. Cerebral β-amyloid deposition predicts HIV-associated neurocognitive disorders in APOE e4 carriers. AIDS. 2012;26:2327–35.
43. Moore DJ, Arce M, Moseley S, McCutchan JA, Marquie-Beck J, Franklin DR, et al. Family history of dementia predicts worse neuropsychological functioning among HIV infected persons. J Neuropsychiatry Clin Neurosci. 2011;23:316–23.
44. Langford TD, Letendre SL, Marcote TD, Ellis RJ, McCutchan JA, Grant I, et al. Severe, demyelinating leukoencephalopathy in AIDS patients on antiretroviral therapy. AIDS. 2002;16:1019–29.
45. Newsome SD, Johnson E, Pardo C, McArthur JC, Nath A. Fulminant encephalopathy with basal ganglia hyperintensities in HIV-infected drug users. Neurology. 2011;76:787–94.
46. Antinori A, Ammassari A, De Luca A, Cingolani A, Murri R, Scoppettuolo G, et al. Diagnosis of AIDS-related focal brain lesions: a decision-making analysis based on clinical and neuroradiologic characteristics combined with polymerase chain reaction assays in CSF. Neurology. 1997;48:687–94.
47. Kirk O, Reiss P, Uberti-Foppa C, Bickel M, Gerstoft J, Pradier C, et al. Safe interruption of maintenance therapy against previous infection with four common HIV-associated opportunistic pathogens during potent antiretroviral therapy. Ann Intern Med. 2002;137:239–50.
48. Flinn IW, Ambinder RF. AIDS primary central nervous system lymphoma. Curr Op Neurol. 1996;8:373–6.
49. Diamond C, Taylor TH, Im I, Miradi M, Wallace M, Anton-Culver H. Highly active antiretroviral therapy is associated with prolonged survival among patients with AIDS-related primary central nervous system non-Hodgkin's lymphoma. Curr HIV Res. 2006;4:375–8.
50. Newell ME, Hoy JF, Cooper SG, DeGraaff B, Grulich AE, Bryant M, et al. Human immunodeficiency virus-related primary central nervous system lymphoma: factors influencing survival in 111 patients. Cancer. 2004;100:2627–36.
51. Cinque P, Koralnik IJ, Gerevini S, Miro JM, Price RW. Progressive multifocal leukoencephalopathy in HIV-1 infection. Lancet Infect Dis. 2009;9:625–36.
52. Tan CS, Koralnik IJ. Progressive multifocal leukoencephalopathy and other disorders caused by JC virus: clinical features and pathogenesis. Lancet Neurol. 2010;9:425–37.
53. Wüthrich C, Cheng YM, Joseph JT, Kesari S, Beckwith C, Stopa E, et al. Frequent infection of cerebellar granule cell neurons by polyomavirus JC in progressive multifocal leukoencephalopathy. J Neuropathol Exp Neurol. 2009;68:15–25.
54. Lima MA, Drislane FW, Koralnik IJ. Seizures and their outcome in progressive multifocal leukoencephalopathy. Neurology. 2006;66:262–4.
55. Sahraian MA, Radue EW, Eshaghi A, Besliu S, Minagar A. Progressive multifocal leukoencephalopathy: a review of the neuroimaging features and differential diagnosis. Eur J Neurol. 2012;19:1060–9.
56. Cinque P, Scarpellini P, Vago L, Linde A, Lazzarin A. Diagnosis of central nervous system complications in HIV-infected patients: cerebrospinal fluid analysis by polymerase chain reaction. AIDS. 1997;11:1–17.
57. Corral I, Quereda C, García-Villanueva M, Casado JL, Perez-Elias MJ, Navas E, et al. Focal monophasic demyelinating leukoencephalopathy in advanced HIV infection. Eur Neurol. 2004;52:36–41.

58. De Luca A, Giancola ML, Ammassari A, Grisetti S, Paglia MG, Cingolani A, et al. The effect of potent antiretroviral therapy and JC virus load in cerebrospinal fluid on clinical outcome of patients with AIDS-associated progressive multifocal leukoencephalopathy. J Infect Dis. 2000;182:1077–83.
59. Garcia De Viedma D, Diaz Infantes M, Miralles P, Berenguer J, Marin M, Muñoz L, et al. JC virus load in progressive multifocal leukoencephalopathy: analysis of the correlation between the viral burden in cerebrospinal fluid, patient survival, and the volume of neurological lesions. Clin Infect Dis. 2002;34:1568–75.
60. Berger JR, Levy RM, Flomenhoft D, Dobbs M. Predictive factors for prolonged survival in acquired immunodeficiency syndrome-associated progressive multifocal leukoencephalopathy. Ann Neurol. 1998;44:341–9.
61. Khanna N, Wolbers M, Mueller NJ, Garzoni C, Du Pasquier RA, Fux CA, et al. JC virus-specific immune responses in human immunodeficiency virus type 1 patients with progressive multifocal leukoencephalopathy. J Virol. 2009;83:4404–11.
62. Marzocchetti A, Tompkins T, Clifford DB, Gandhi RT, Kesari S, Berger JR, et al. Determinants of survival in progressive multifocal leukoencephalopathy. Neurology. 2009;73:1551–8.
63. Miralles P, Berenguer J, Garcia de Viedma DV, Padilla B, Cosin J, Lopez-Bernaldo-de-Quiros JC, et al. Treatment of AIDS-associated progressive multifocal leukoencephalopathy with highly active antiretroviral therapy. AIDS. 1998;12:2467–72.
64. Falcó V, Olmo M, Villar del Saz S, Guelar A, Santos JR, Gutiérrez M, et al. Influence of HAART on the clinical course of HIV-1–infected patients with progressive multifocal leukoencephalopathy: results of an observational multicenter study. J Acquir Immune Defic Syndr. 2008;49:26–31.
65. Antiretroviral Therapy Cohort Collaboration. Variable impact on mortality of AIDS-defining events diagnosed during combination antiretroviral therapy: Not all AIDS-defining conditions are created equal. Clin Infect Dis. 2009;48:1138–51.
66. Hernández B, Dronda F, Moreno S. Treatment options for AIDS patients with progressive multifocal leukoencephalopathy. Expert Opin Pharmacother. 2009;10:403–16.
67. Arribas JR, Storch GA, Clifford DB, Tselis AC. Cytomegalovirus encephalitis. Ann Intern Med. 1996;125:577–87.
68. Grassi MP, Clerici F, Perin C, d'Arminio MA, Vago L, Borella M, et al. Microglial nodular encephalitis and ventriculoencephalitis due to cytomegalovirus infection in patients with AIDS: two distinct clinical patterns. Clin Infect Dis. 1998;27:504–8.
69. Huang PP, McMeeking AA, Stempien MJ, Zagzag D. Cytomegalovirus disease presenting as a focal brain mass: report of two cases. Neurosurgery. 1997;40:1074–8.
70. Quereda C, Corral I, Laguna F, Valencia ME, Tenorio A, Echeverría JM, et al. Diagnostic utility of a multiplex herpesvirus PCR assay performed with cerebrospinal fluid from human immunodeficiency virus-infected patients with neurological disorders. J Clin Microbiol. 2000;38:3061–7.
71. Anduze-Faris BM, Fillet AM, Gozlan J, Lancar R, Boukli N, Gasnault J, et al. Induction and maintenance therapy of cytomegalovirus central nervous system infection in HIV-infected patients. AIDS. 2000;14:517–24.
72. Tan SV, Guiloff RJ, Scaravilli F, Klapper PE, Cleator GM, Gazzard BG. Herpes simplex type 1 encephalitis in acquired immunodeficiency syndrome. Ann Neurol. 1993;34:619–22.
73. Cinque P, Vago L, Marenzi R, Guidici T, Weber R, Corradini D, et al. Herpes simplex virus infections of the central nervous system in human immunodeficiency virus-infected patients: clinical management by polymerase chain reaction assay of cerebrospinal fluid. Clin Infect Dis. 1998;27:303–9.
74. Glesby MJ, Moore RD, Chaisson RE. Clinical spectrum of herpes zoster in adults infected with human immunodeficiency virus. Clin Infect Dis. 1995;21:370–5.
75. Corral I, Quereda C, Antela A, Pintado V, Casado JL, Martín-Dávila P, et al. Neurological complications of varicella-zoster virus in human immunodeficiency virus-infected patients: changes in prevalence and diagnostic utility of polymerase chain reaction in cerebrospinal fluid. J Neurovirol. 2003;9:129–35.

76. Gilden D, Cohrs RJ, Mahalingam R, Nagel MA. Varicella zoster virus vasculopathies: diverse clinical manifestations, laboratory features, pathogenesis, and treatment. Lancet Neurol. 2009;8:731–40.
77. Pinto AN. AIDS and cerebrovascular disease. Stroke. 1996;27:538–43.
78. Ortiz G, Koch S, Gomano JG, Forteza AM, Rabinstein AA. Mechanisms of stroke in HIV-infected patients. Neurology. 2007;68:1257–61.
79. Tipping B, de Villiers L, Wainwright H, Candy S, Bryer A. Stroke in patients with human immunodeficiency virus infection. J Neurol Neurosurg Psychiatry. 2007;78:1320–4.
80. The Writing Committee of the D:A:D: Study Group. Cardio- and cerebrovascular events in HIV-infected persons. AIDS. 2004;18:1811–7.
81. Corral I, Quereda C, Moreno A, Pérez-Elías MJ, Dronda F, Casado JL, et al. Cerebrovascular ischemic events in HIV-1-infected patients receiving highly active antiretroviral therapy: incidence and risk factors. Cerebrovasc Dis. 2009;27:559–63.
82. Ovbiagele B, Nath A. Increasing incidence of ischemic stroke in patients with HIV infection. Neurology. 2011;76:444–50.
83. Domingo P, Suarez-Lozano I, Torres F, Pomar V, Ribera E, Galindo MJ, et al. Bacterial meningitis in HIV-1-infected patients in the era of highly active antiretroviral therapy. J Acquir Immune Defic Syndr. 2009;51:582–7.
84. Casado JL, Quereda C, Oliva J, Navas E, Moreno A, Pintado V, et al. Candidal meningitis in HIV-infected patients: Analysis of 14 cases. Clin Infect Dis. 1997;25:673–6.
85. Berenguer J, Moreno S, Laguna F, Vicente T, Adrados M, Ortega A, et al. Tuberculous meningitis in patients infected with the human immunodeficiency virus. N Engl J Med. 1992;326:668–72.
86. Corral I, Quereda C, Navas E, Martín-Dávila P, Pérez-Elías MJ, Casado JL, et al. Adenosine deaminase activity in cerebrospinal fluid of HIV-infected patients: limited value for diagnosis of tuberculous meningitis. Eur J Clin Microbiol Infect Dis. 2004;23:471–6.
87. Sánchez-Portocarrrero J, Pérez-Cecilia E, Jiménez-Escrig A, Martín-Rabadán P, Roca V, Ruíz-Yagüe M, et al. Tuberculous meningitis. Clinical characteristics and comparison with cryptococcal meningitis in patients with human immunodeficiency virus infection. Arch Neurol. 1996;53:671–6.
88. Del Pan GL, Glass JD, McArthur JC. Clinicopathologic correlations of HIV-1 associated vacuolar myelopathy. An autopsy-based case control study. Neurology. 1994;44:2159–64.
89. Beilke MA, Japa S, Moeller-Hadi C, Martin-Schild S. Tropical spastic paraparesis/human T leukemia virus type 1-associated myelopathy in HIV type 1-coinfected patients. Clin Infect Dis. 2005;41:57–63.
90. Gilden DH, Beinlich BR, Rubinstein EM, Stommel E, Swenson R, Rubinstein D, et al. Varicella-zoster virus myelitis: An expanding spectrum. Neurology. 1994;44:1818–23.
91. Schiffito G, McDermott M, McArthur J. Incidence and risk factors for HIV-associated distal sensory polyneuropathy. Neurology. 2002;58:1764–8.
92. Evans SR, Ellis RJ, Chen H, Yeh T, Lee AJ, Schifitto G, et al. Peripheral neuropathy in HIV: prevalence and risk factors. AIDS. 2011;25:919–28.
93. Centne CM, Bateman KJ, Heckmann JM. Manifestations of HIV Infection in the peripheral nervous system. Lancet Neurol. 2013;12:295–309.
94. Cornblath DR, McArthur JC, Kennedy PGE, Witte AS, Griffin JW. Inflammatory demyelinating peripheral neuropathies associated with human T-cell lymphotropic virus type III infection. Ann Neurol. 1987;21:32–40.
95. So YT, Olney RK. Acute lumbosacral polyradiculopathy in acquired immunodeficiency syndrome: experience in 23 patients. Ann Neurol. 1994;35:53–8.
96. Corral I, Quereda C, Casado JL, Cobo J, Navas E, Pérez-Elías MJ, et al. Acute polyradiculopathies in HIV-infected patients. J Neurol. 1997;244:499–504.
97. Cohen BA, McArthur JC, Grohman S, Patterson B, Glass JD. Neurologic prognosis of cytomegalovirus polyradiculomyelopathy in AIDS. Neurology. 1993;43:493–9.

98. Roullet E, Assuerus V, Gozlan J, Ropert A, Saïd G, Baudrimont M, et al. Cytomegalovirus multifocal neuropathy in AIDS: Analysis of 15 consecutive cases. Neurology. 1994;44:2174–82.
99. Simpson DM, Bender AN. HIV associated myopathy: Analysis of 11 patients. Ann Neurol. 1988;24:79–84.
100. Mhiri C, Baudrimont M, Bonne G, Geny C, Degoul F, Marsac C, et al. Zidovudine myopathy: a distinctive disorder associated with mitochondrial dysfunction. Ann Neurol. 1991;29:606–14.
101. Zetola NM, Klausner JD. Syphilis and HIV infection: An update. Clin Infect Dis. 2007;44:1222–8.
102. Johnson T, Nath A. Immune reconstitution inflammatory syndrome and the central nervous system. Curr Op Neurol. 2011;24:284–90.
103. McCombe JA, Auer RN, Maingat FG, Houston S, Gill MJ, Power C. Neurologic immune reconstitution inflammatory syndrome in HIV/AIDS: outcome and epidemiology. Neurology. 2009;72:835–41.
104. Pepper DJ, Marais S, Maartens G, Rebe K, Morroni C, Rangaka MX, et al. Neurologic manifestations of paradoxical tuberculosis-associated immune reconstitution inflammatory syndrome: a case series. Clin Infect Dis. 2009;48:e96–107.
105. Bicanic T, Meintjes G, Rebe K, Williams A, Loyse A, Wood R, et al. Immune reconstitution inflammatory syndrome in HIV-associated cryptococcal meningitis: a prospective study. J Acquir Immune Defic Syndr. 2009;51:130–4.
106. Bisson GP, Molefi M, Bellamy S, Thakur R, Steenhoff A, Tamuhla N, et al. Early versus delayed antiretroviral therapy and cerebrospinal fluid fungal clearance in adults with HIV and cryptococcal meningitis. Clin Infect Dis. 2013;56:1165–73.
107. Tan K, Roda R, Ostrow L, McArthur J, Nath A. PML-IRIS in patients with HIV infection. Clinical manifestations and treatment with steroids. Neurology. 2009;72:1458–64.
108. Safdar A, Rubocki RJ, Horvath JA, Narayan KK, Waldron RL. Fatal immune restoration disease in human immunodeficiency virus type 1-infected patients with progressive multifocal leukoencephalopathy: impact of antiretroviral therapy-associated immune reconstitution. Clin Infect Dis. 2002;35:1250–7.
109. Martinez JV, Mazziotti JV, Efron ED, Bonardo P, Jordan R, Sevlever G, et al. Immune reconstitution inflammatory syndrome associated with PML in AIDS: a treatable disorder. Neurology. 2006;67:1692–4.
110. Di Giambenedetto S, Vago G, Pompucci A, Scoppettuolo G, Cingolani A, Marzocchetti A, et al. Fatal inflammatory AIDS-associated PML with high CD4 counts on HAART: a new clinical entity? Neurology. 2004;63:2452–3.
111. Domingo P, Torres OH, Ris J, Vázquez G. Herpes zoster as an immune reconstitution disease after initiation of combination antiretroviral therapy in patients with human immunodeficiency virus type-1 infection. Am J Med. 2001;110:605–9.
112. González-Valcárcel J, Corral I, Quereda C, Alonso-Cánovas A, Aparicio Hernandez M, de Felipe Mimbrera A, et al. Primary cerebral lymphomatoid granulomatosis as an immune reconstitution inflammatory syndrome in AIDS. J Neurol. 2010;257:2106–8.
113. Lescure FX, Moulignier A, Savatovsky J, Amiel C, Carcelain G, Molina JM, et al. CD8 encephalitis in HIV-infected patients receiving cART: a treatable entity. Clin Infect Dis. 2013;57:101–8.
114. Gray F, Lescure FX, Adle-Biassette H, Polivka M, Gallien S, Pialoux G, et al. Encephalitis with infiltration by CD8+ lymphocytes in HIV patients receiving combination antiretroviral treatment. Brain Pathol. 2013;23:525–33.
115. Simpson D, Estanislao L, Evans S, McArthur J, Markus K, Truffa M, et al. HIV-associated neuromuscular weakness syndrome. AIDS. 2004;18:1403–12.

Index

J.C. García-Moncó (ed.), *CNS Infections*,
DOI 10.1007/978-1-4471-6401-2, © Springer-Verlag London 2014

D

H

V

FSC
www.fsc.org
MIX
Papier | Fördert
gute Waldnutzung
FSC® C083411

Kolibri 360 GmbH
Ferdinand-Jühlke-Straße 7
99095 Erfurt, Deutschland
produktsicherheit@kolibri360.de